WEIGHT LOSS HYPNOSIS:

This Book Includes:

Rapid Weight Loss Hypnosis for Women and Hypnotic Gastric Band. 247 Affirmations; Meditation; The 21-Day Technique. Burn Fat Today or Hate Yourself Tomorrow

---

Cleopatra Johnson

© **Copyright 2020 - All rights reserved.**

The content contained within this book may not be reproduced, duplicated or transmitted without direct written permission from the author or the publisher. Under no circumstances will any blame or legal responsibility be held against the publisher, or author, for any damages, reparation, or monetary loss due to the information contained within this book. Either directly or indirectly.

Legal Notice:

This book is copyright protected. This book is only for personal use. You cannot amend, distribute, sell, use, quote or paraphrase any part, or the content within this book, without the consent of the author or publisher.

Disclaimer Notice:

Please note the information contained within this document is for educational and entertainment purposes only. All effort has been executed to present accurate, up to date, and reliable, complete information. No warranties of any kind are declared or implied. Readers acknowledge that the author is not engaging in the rendering of legal, financial, medical or professional advice. The content within this book has been derived from various sources. Please consult a licensed professional before attempting any techniques outlined in this book.

By reading this document, the reader agrees that under no circumstances is the author responsible for any losses, direct or indirect, which are incurred as a result of the use of information contained within this document, including, but not limited to, — errors, omissions, or inaccuracies.

THIS BOOK INCLUDES

BOOK1: 10 (PAGE)

RAPID WEIGHT LOSS HYPNOSIS FOR WOMEN

Burn Fat, Blast Calories; Kill Obesity Through 189 Affirmations, Positive Meditation, Powerful Hypnotic Techniques and The Motivation Code. Change Your Body.

BOOK2: 264 (PAGE)

HYPNOTIC GASTRIC BAND

A Complete Guide to Achieve Weight Loss and Eat Healthy Through Gastric Band Hypnosis, Meditation, Affirmations and Motivation. Change Your Mind, Change Your Body.

RAPID WEIGHT LOSS HYPNOSIS FOR WOMEN

Burn Fat, Blast Calories; Kill Obesity Through 189 Affirmations, Positive Meditation, Powerful Hypnotic Techniques and The Motivation Code. Change Your Body.

Cleopatra Johnson

Table of Contents

Introduction 10

Chapter 1: What Is Self-Hypnosis? 14

Chapter 2: Techniques About Rapid Weight Loss Hypnosis 20

Chapter 3: Self-Hypnosis Session 24

Chapter 4: Re-Program Your Mind 32

Chapter 5: The Golden Protocol: The Hypnotic Method Of 21 Days With Daily Statements 38

Chapter 6: Healing The Body With Self-Hypnosis 46

Chapter 7: The Power Of Meditation For Rapid Weight Loss ... 52

Chapter 8: The Power Of Positive Affirmations 56

Chapter 9: Positive Affirmations For Rapid Weight Loss 62

Chapter 10: Repetition Of A Mantra 70

Chapter 11: How To Practice Every Day 76

Chapter 12: Using Positive Affirmations To Lose Weight 82

Chapter 13: Harnessing Positive Affirmation And Meditation For Rapid Weight Loss 88

Chapter 14: Rapid Weight Loss Through Affirmation 94

Chapter 15: Weight Loss Affirmations 100

Chapter 16: How Do I Pick And Use Affirmations For Rapid Weight Loss? 106

Chapter 17: What Are Beliefs, Patterns, And Blocks Of Hypnosis Therapy To Weight Loss? 114

Chapter 18: Sharp Your Mind To Shape Your Body 122

Chapter 19: Overcoming Negative Habits 130

Chapter 20: Stop Sugar Cravings Hypnotic Session 136

Chapter 21: Rapid Weight Loss Hypnosis Sessions 142

Chapter 22: Rapid Weight Loss Without Diet 146

Chapter 23: Create Reasonable Goals 152

Chapter 24: Change Bad Eating Habits Through Hypnosis 158

Chapter 25: Mistakes To Avoid 166

Chapter 26: Additional Tips To Help You Lose Weight 170
Chapter 27: Mindful Eating Habits 176
Chapter 28: Frequently Asked Questions 180
Chapter 29: From Fat To Thin Thinking 188
Chapter 30: Overcoming Emotional Eating 194
Chapter 31: The Mindfulness Diet 200
Chapter 32: Control Your Calories 206
Chapter 33: Emotional Eating Hypnosis 212
Chapter 34: Types Of Food To Avoid Losing Weight 220
Chapter 35: Hypnosis To Control Food Portion 224
Chapter 36: Your Path To Your Perfect Weight 232
Chapter 37: Why Do We Struggle With Weight? 240
Chapter 38: What Are Body Goals? 246
Chapter 39: How Do I Love My Body If There Is No Reason? 250
Conclusion 256

Introduction

I can comprehend how hard it can be to be overweight. As a matter of fact, I handled a problem with my weight some time ago. When I was getting a bit older, I felt as if there was nothing that could be done to overcome it.

After discovering the connection between Hypnosis and weight reduction, nevertheless, I realized the power in it, and I took advantage of it.

I'll have to admit, I was a bit skeptical about going through with Hypnosis when I initially considered it. Many of my buddies had attempted it and were somewhat successful with losing weight and keeping it off, which I discovered to be fairly excellent.

I had always heard that Hypnosis was mind control, but I didn't realize that it was a medical procedure that was frequently carried out by a qualified therapist. The possibilities of Hypnosis and weight reduction began to give me a bit of hope.

The one choice that I had to make was whether to go through a hypnosis and weight reduction program in the presence of a certified professional or do it in the house myself.

There were several different self-hypnosis courses that I was checking out; the majority looked rather promising. Instead of being something mystical, it turned out to be something that simply gave me the strength that I needed to overcome my ingrained mediocre meals and workout routines. I take every chance that I can, at this point to inform people about how effective hypnosis and weight loss programs can be.

If you're anything like I was, fighting with your weight, you feel like you'll be fighting this problem for the rest of your life. This doesn't have to be true. Hypnosis and weight-loss can lead you to find a long-term method of losing weight and keeping it off without the constant battle.

What is the link between Hypnosis and rapid weight-loss? Hypnosis is something we usually consider as a kind of entertainment but have you ever thought about Hypnosis for weight loss? It's trying to use Hypnosis to deal with an issue as serious as weight problems, but perhaps it's not as ludicrous as it sounds. Hypnosis for weight-loss is an appealing idea—it offers people a reasonably simple out of their weight problem, by stopping their yearnings for food at the source.

One problem with weight loss through Hypnosis is the same issue that afflicts other weight reduction solutions. There are a lot of scams out there, and the individuals behind them will not hesitate about trying to take your money for a product that does not do anything at all. Hypnosis has the very same problem. You might be able to trust some claims about hypnosis weight reduction treatment; however, there are just as lots of ones that have lots of lies.

If you find claims that state that Hypnosis can alter the way the mind works to prevent eating, they're probably deceptive. A session of Hypnosis will not make you into some sort of robot that's immune to yearnings and programmed not to overindulge. What it can do, however, is make a person most likely to follow a correct dietary strategy. The effects are entirely psychological. Hypnosis can't "persuade" your body to accelerate weight loss, it can only implant the concept in your brain that maybe you do not require to eat that 2nd piece of cake.

People looking for rapid weight loss hypnosis treatments should be especially careful of group hypnosis sessions. To work, Hypnosis needs to be customized specifically to the person getting it. Group sessions plainly will not work, as the therapist cannot connect with any single person on his or her own. You should also be warned against hypnosis cassettes or videos, as they share this same issue.

Hypnosis for weight reduction is a tempting thought. If you can train your mind to minimize your yearnings and increase your self-discipline, you'll be well on your way to dropping weight. The vital thing to have in mind is to be cautious and study all the alternatives before you buy an item or see a hypnotherapist, or else you may end with nothing at all.

The Ultimate Challenge to Weight Watchers

Not everybody goes on the journey to lose weight because of their health. You might choose to lose weight since you perceive weight loss as a means to appear appealing to others and to enhance your self-image. By attempting these steps, people around the world are spending thousands and even millions every year to lose weight.

Weight loss is a multi-million market. Do these procedures always assist you in reducing weight? Not, constantly I suppose might be your response. The real response may sound essential to you, but it is real. The magic answer is this little fundamental trick of weight loss. You should change the method you consider food and yourself. Take this scenario. Did you keep in mind those events when you were on that expensive wonder diet, which you have carefully watched your weight but yet had a hard time to keep your eyes off that velvety dessert after meals or did not even feel brave enough to shut down the craving for chocolate?

Hang on to this situation for a while, and I will also explain why you have a hard time keeping your weight down despite your vigorous exercise regime, diet classes, and the slimming pills.

You might discover it tough to think, but I can inform you that the reason you feel you are losing the fight is fundamental. The reason is that you have not altered your old idea patterns about how you used to think about the velvety desert and the bar of chocolate and more significantly about yourself. This example is to show you why your idea patterns can influence your weight reduction.

As people, our feelings or thoughts affect our behavior, which then leads us to react to a situation in a specific way. After having your meals, those little thoughts you used to have about the sweet dessert or the chocolate would have led you on to pick to overlook the desert or just to take a bite and, after that, complete all of it. Your recent action regrettably would be to the detriment of your attempt to lose some weight.

On the other hand, you can also manage your thoughts or make ideas in your mind to change how you feel about the chocolate and the desert. Fortunately, is you can manage your feelings or make suggestions to your account on how you respond to the desert or the pudding without jeopardizing your weight loss program. A rapid weight loss hypnosis treatment will teach you how to make these recommendations in your mind to manage your ideas.

CHAPTER 1:

What Is Self-Hypnosis?

Self-hypnosis is still considered a mystical phenomenon by many people, even though this technique can be seen as prayer. You are alone and you concentrate on your well-being. If you like, you ask God or a supreme being you believe in to help you. This practice also includes meditation (just like praying does), as well as chanting, mantras, inner confirmation or affirmation. When you have to perform at work or at college, you make such statements like "I don't fear; I'm fine"; "I can do it" or exactly the opposite, like "I can't do it. Everybody is better than me," etc. Even when we imagine ourselves in a different scenario from what is currently happening, we are programming ourselves. What you are doing is continuously hypnotizing yourself. Self-hypnosis helps us to come into contact with the unconscious through the use of a specific language, aimed at awakening some parts of ourselves by leveraging archetypal symbols.

However, we must learn to pray or let's say hypnotize ourselves accurately! Self-hypnosis is the ability to apply techniques and procedures alone to stimulate the unconscious to become our ally and involve it directly in the realization of our goals. By learning the essential elements of communication with the unconscious mind, it is possible to become able to reprogram activities of our unconscious. Self-hypnosis is a method that does not dismiss the support of a professional but has the advantage of being able to be performed independently. This is possible through the use of CDs and DIY courses made by hypnotists to make this practice accessible to a larger number of people with significant advantages, even from an economic point of view!

What Is Self-Hypnosis For?

It was Milton H. Erickson, founder of modern hypnotherapy, who gave an exhaustive illustration of the effects and purposes of hypnosis and self-hypnosis. The scholar stated that the aim of this practice is to communicate with the subconscious of the subjects through the use of metaphors and stories full of symbolic meanings (Tyrrell, 2014).

If incorrectly applied, self-hypnosis can certainly not harm, but it may not be useful in attaining the desired results, with the risk of not feeling motivated to continue a constructive relationship with the unconscious. However, to do it as efficiently as possible, we need to be in a relaxed state of mind. So, accordingly, we start with relaxation to gather the attention inside, while suspending conscious control. Then we insert suggestions and affirmations to the unconscious mind. At the end of the time allocated for the process, a gradual awakening procedure facilitates the return to the state of permanent consciousness. When you are calm, your subconscious is 20–25% more programmable than when you are agitated. Also, it effectively relieves stress (you can repair a lot of information and stimuli you understand), aids regeneration, energizes, triggers positive physiological changes, improves concentration, helps you find solutions, and helps you make the right decisions. If the state of conscious trance is reached, then if the patient manages to let himself go by concentrating on the words of the hypnotist, progressively forgetting the external stimuli, then the physiological parameters undergo considerable variations. The confirmation comes from science, and in fact, it was found that during hypnosis, the left hemisphere, the rational one, decreases its activity in favor of the more creative hemisphere, the right one (Harris, n. d.).

You can do self-hypnosis in faster and more immediate ways, even during the course of the various daily activities after you have experienced what state you need to reach during hypnosis.

A better understanding of communication with the unconscious mind highlights how indispensable our collaboration is to slip into the state outside the ordinary consciousness. In other words, we enter an altered state of consciousness because we want it, and every form of hypnosis, even if induced by someone else, is always self-hypnosis.

We wish to access the extraordinary power of unconscious creativity; for this, we understand that it is necessary to put aside for a while the control of the rational mind and let ourselves slip entirely into relaxation and into the magical world of the unconscious where everything is possible. Immense benefits can be obtained from a relationship that becomes natural and habitual with one's own unconscious. Self-hypnosis favors the emergence of constructive responses from our being, can allow us to know ourselves better, helps us to be more aware of our potential, and abler to express them and use them to foster our success in every field of possible application.

How Do You Do Self-Hypnosis?

There are several self-hypnosis techniques out there; however, they are all based on one concept: focusing on a single idea, object, image, or word. This is the key that opens the door to trance. You can achieve focus in many ways, which is the reason why there are so many different techniques that can be applied. After a period of initial learning, those who have learned a method, and have continued to practice it, realize that they can skip certain steps. In this part, we will take a look at the essential self-hypnosis techniques.

The Betty Erickson Method

Here I'll summarize the most practical points of this method of Betty Erickson, wife of Milton Erickson, the most famous hypnotist of 1900.

Choose something you don't like about yourself. Turn it into an image, and then turn this image into a positive one. If you don't like your body shape, take a picture of your body, then turn it into an image of your beautiful self with a body you would like to have. Before inducing self-hypnosis, give yourself a time limit before hypnotizing yourself by mentally or better yet, saying aloud the following sentence, "I induce self-hypnosis for X minutes." Your mind will take time like a Swiss watch.

How Do You Practice?

Take three objects around you, preferably small and bright, like a door handle, a light spot on a painting, etc. and fix your attention on each one of them. Take three sounds from your environment, traffic, fridge noise, etc., and fix your attention on each one. Take three sensations you are feeling, the itchy nose, tingling in the leg, the feeling of air passing through the nose, etc. It's better to use unusual sensations, to which attention is not usually drawn, such as the sensation of the right foot inside the shoe. Don't fix your attention for too long, just enough to make you aware of what you are seeing, feeling or trying. The mind is quick. Then, in the same way, switch to two objects, two sounds, two sensations. Always be calm, while switching to an object, a sound, a sensation. If you have done things correctly, you are in a trance, ready for the next step.

Now let your mind wander, as you did in class when the teacher spoke and you looked out of the window, and you were in another place, in another time, in another space, in a place where you would have liked to be, so completely forget about everything else. Now recall the initial image. Perhaps the mind wanders, from time to time it gets distracted, maybe it goes adrift, but it doesn't matter. As soon as you can, take the initial image, and start working on it. Do not make efforts to try to remind you of what it means or what it is. Your mind works according to mental associations, let it work at its best without unnecessarily disturbing it: it knows what it must do. Manipulate the image, play with it a little. See if it looks brighter, or if it is smaller, or it is more pleasant.

If it is a moving image, send it back and forth in slow motion or speed it up. When the initial image always gets worse, replace it instantly with the second image.

CHAPTER 2:

Techniques about Rapid Weight Loss Hypnosis

Meditation Exercise 1: Release of Bad Habits

Sit comfortably. Relax your muscles, close your eyes. Breathe in and breathe out. Do not cross your feet because this will lock you away from the desired experience. Hold your hands together to connect your logical brain hemisphere with your instinct.

Concentrate on your back now and notice how you feel in the bed or chair you are sitting in. Take a deep breath and let your stress leave your body. Now focus on your neck. Observe how your neck is joined to your shoulders. Lift your shoulders slowly. Breathe in slowly and release it. Feel how your shoulders loosen. Lift your shoulders again a little bit, then let them relax. Observe how your neck muscles are tensing and how much pressure it has. Breathe in and breathe out slowly. Release the pressure in your neck and notice how the stress is leaving your body. Repeat the whole exercise from the beginning. Observe your back. Notice all the stress and let it go with a profound breath. Focus on your shoulders and neck again. Lift up your shoulders and hold it for some moments, then release your shoulders again and let all the stress go away. Sense how the stress is going away. Now, focus your attention on your back. Feel how comfortable it is. Focus on your whole body. While breathing in, let relaxation come, and while you are breathing out, let frustration leave your body. Notice how much you are relaxed.

Concentrate on your inner self. Breathe slowly in and release it. Calm your mind. Observe your thoughts. Don't go with them because your aim is to observe them and not to be involved. It's time to let go of your overweight self that you are not feeling good about. It's like your body is wearing a bigger, heavier top at this point in your life. Imagine stepping out of it and laying it on an imaginary chair facing you. Now tell yourself to let go of these old, established eating and behavioral patterns. Imagine that all your old, fixed patterns and all the obstacles that prevent you from achieving your desired weight are exiting your body, soul, and spirit with each breath. Know that your soul is perfect as it is, and all you want is for everything that pulls away to leave. With every breath, let your old beliefs go, as you are creating more and more space for something new. After spending a few minutes with this, imagine that every time you breathe in, you are inhaling prana, the life energy of the universe, shining in gold. In this life force, you will find everything you need and desire: a healthy, muscular body, a self that loves itself in all circumstances, a hand that puts enough nutritious food on the table, a strong voice to say no to sabotaging your diet, a head that can say no to those who are trying to distract you from your ideas and goals. With each breath, you absorb these positive images and emotions.

See in front of you exactly what your life would be like if you got everything you wanted. Release your old self and start becoming your new self. Gradually restore your breathing to regular breathing. Feel the solid ground beneath you, open your eyes, and return to your everyday state of consciousness.

Meditation Exercise 2: Forgiving Yourself

Imagine a staircase in front of you! Descend it, counting down from ten to one.

You reached and found a door at the bottom of the stairs. Open the door. There is a meadow in front of us. Let's see if it has grass, if so, if it has flowers, what color, whether there is a bush or tree, and describe what you see in the distance.

Find the path covered with white stones and start walking on it.

Feel the power of the Earth flowing through your soles, the breeze stroking your skin, the warmth of the sun radiating toward you. Feel the harmony of the elements and your state of well-being.

From the left side, you hear the rattle of the stream. Walk down to the shore. This water of life comes from the throne of God. Take it with your palms and drink three sips and notice how it tastes. If you want, you can wash yourself in it. Keep walking. Feel the power of the Earth flowing through your soles, the breeze stroking your skin, the warmth of the sun radiating toward you. Feel the harmony of the elements and your state of well-being. In the distance, you see an ancient tree with many branches. This is the Tree of Life. Take a leaf from it, chew it, and note its taste. You have arrived at the Lake of Conscience, no one in this lake sinks. Rest on the water and think that all the emotions and thoughts you no longer need (anger, fear, horror, hopelessness, pain, sorrow, anxiety, annoyance, self-blame, superiority, self-pity, and guilt) pass through your skin and you purify them by the magical power of water. And you see that the water around you is full of gray and black globules that are slowly recovering the turquoise-green color of the water.

You feel the power of the water, the power of the Earth, the breeze of your skin, the radiance of the sun warming you, the harmony of the elements, the feeling of well-being.

You ask your magical horse to come for you. You love your horse; you pamper it, and let it caress you too. You bounce on its back and head to God's Grad. In the air, you fly together, become one being. You have arrived. Ask your horse to wait.

You grow wings, and you fly toward the Trinity. You bow your head and apologize for all the sins you have committed against your body. You apologize for all the sins you have committed against your soul. You apologize for all the sins you committed against your spirit. You wait for the angels to give you the gifts that help you. If you can't see yourself receive one, it means you don't need one yet. If you did, open it and look inside. Give thanks that you could be here. Get back on your horse and fly back to the meadow. Find the white gravel path and head back down to the door to your stairs. Look at the grass in the meadow. Notice if there are any flowers. If so, describe the colors, any bush or tree, and whatever you see in the distance. You arrive at the door, open it, and head up the stairs. Count from one to ten. You are back, move your fingers slowly, open your eyes.

Meditation Exercise 3: Rapid Weight Loss

See yourself in every detail. Describe your hair, the color of your clothes, your eyes. See your face, your nose, your mouth. Set aside this image for a moment. Now imagine yourself as you would like to be in the future. Imagine that your new self-approaches your present self and pampers it. See that your new self-hugs your present self. Feel the love that is spread in the air. Now see that your present self leaves the scene and your new self takes its place. See and feel how happy and satisfied you are. You believe that you can become this beautiful new self. You breathe in this image and place it in your soul. This image will always be with you and flow through your whole body. You want to be this new self. You can be this new self.

CHAPTER 3:

Self-Hypnosis Session

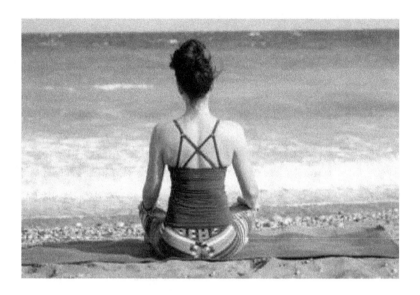

Simple Steps for Self-Hypnosis

Now we will go over 10 simple and succinct steps to perform a successful and fruitful and positively effective session of self-hypnosis. I will list the steps first and follow up with a step-by-step breakdown featuring a brief and easy to understand the description of what each step should entail for you in your journey.

- **Step 1:** Preparation of Self

- **Step 2:** Preparation of Time

- **Step 3:** Preparation of Space

- **Step 4:** Preparation of Goal and Motive

- **Step 5:** Relaxation of the Physical Body

- **Step 6:** Relaxation of the Soul and the Mind

- **Step 7:** Realization of Trance

- **Step 8:** Active Repetition of Mantra or Performance of Script

- **Step 9:** Preparation for Exiting the Trance State

- **Step 10:** Returning to Earth

As you read those steps, I'm sure they bring forth images in your mind. It may seem apparent already what you have to do, and ideas for how to guide yourself through this self-hypnosis you are preparing for are blossoming like wildfire in your mind. Let us go more in-depth to further prepare and become aware of all that you can do to make your self-hypnosis as easy and effective as your soul will wish to better yourself in the most transformative way possible.

Step 1: Preparation of Self

So, as you are aware, one of the first and foremost goals is to become as relaxed as possible—before, during, and after entering the trance-state. Relaxation is the key that helps us enter the trance-state, and the trance-state further facilitates relaxation of the entire being both during the active self-hypnosis and afterward, for positive benefits of your being. To achieve the most successful self-hypnosis possible, we must first prepare ourselves, our minds and our physical bodies, for what we desire to achieve, a state of heightened relaxation in which we can become hyper-aware of the inner machinations of the mind, to achieve a closer union with them, to bond with them, and to converse with them on the most intimate level possible. The popularity of this music exists because people desire for sounds that will lull them into a more peaceful state. Maybe you would like to try something like this. Some people prefer silence; some people prefer a peaceful noise, a sort of hypnotizing drone that guides them into a more relaxed state of being. White noise, be it from a fan, a laundry machine, running water, or a white noise machine made specifically for the purpose of filling the air with a light white noise, can also be effective for this purpose. Anything that has the desired effect on you will serve this purpose. Another thing you can do is to drink a nice herbal tea of your choosing; find a blend that is relaxing to you as an individual. Some common choices would be lavender-orange teas or chamomile teas. These will set a space internally for you to prepare yourself for entering your trance-state.

Step 2: Preparation of Time

It goes without saying that if an alarm clock goes on when you are in your trance-state, the effectiveness of your self-hypnosis session will be largely inhibited. It is necessary, if you wish for an effective and transformative session of self-hypnosis, that you make sure a certain amount of time is allotted where you will be safe, secure, at peace, and uninterrupted by your daily responsibilities. Many things can get in the way of this. Common inhibitors of time include children, chores, spouses, day-to-day noise, and work. If you have children, maybe you can have a relative or a reliable babysitter watch them for a certain amount of time. Maybe you could ask your spouse to take the children out for an hour or two and explain to them your intentions of performing a transformative inner-journey that requires the utmost relaxation possible. Situations in which you have a large burden of responsibility, ironically, are the types of situations that can make necessary long and fruitful journeys into self-hypnosis. It takes planning and care to make sure that, while all responsibilities are met, there is a designated and a specified time for you to go into your journey with the utmost confidence and care that you will be able to do what you need to do, and come out the other end as enlightened as possible.

Step 3: Preparation of Space

It also should go without saying that a crowded, busy subway station at peak times of the day is no place for you to go about your most effective journeys into self-hypnosis or the trance-like state. Place is of the essence. Just as your body temple must be totally clean and prepped and ready for the ascension, so must your surrounding area be prepared for you to feel as comfortable as possible to allow for the most successful transition into a strong and malleable trance-like state, allowing for the most successful self-hypnosis possible? As always, it is different for different people, depending on beliefs, religion, and personal comforts. Feel free to experiment and find what makes you most comfortable. No one knows how to make you as comfortable as possible, like yourself. Trusting yourself is both one of the biggest keys and one of the biggest goals of self-hypnosis in general, so you must trust yourself here.

Step 4: Preparation of Goal and Motive

One of the critical factors of self-hypnosis is having a plan for what specific change or changes you wish to enact once having entered the trance state, and how you plan to achieve them. This is where the narratives you wish to express, the prayers, or the mantra or mantras you wish to repeat to yourself, come into play. What do you hope to achieve in your self-hypnosis session? It is always different for different people and at different times. But there is always at least one goal, and preparation for achieving that goal is a must when it comes to performing a successful and fruitful and transformative self-hypnosis session. Imagine you are about to have a very important conversation with a very important person in your life. You are crossing a river one stepping stone at a time, putting one foot in front of the other, and you will make it across if you stay steady, attentive, and aware of your surroundings. Be calm, be collected, and be prepared for what you are about to do.

Step 5: Relaxation of the Physical Body

Now we begin. There are many schools of thought on the best ways to relax the body. One very common through-line in all of these is the act of deep, conscious breathing. Breathe in, breathe out, be aware of your breaths, and be in control of each one of them. The goal here is mainly to become aware of every single voluntary and involuntary action of the physical body and slow it down. Feel your heartbeat. Be aware of it. Envision it slowing down. Relax. Expand the space and the length of each breath. Focus on certain areas of the body and watch them become more and more still.

Step 6: Relaxation of the Soul and the Mind

So to relax the mind, we can perform a series of steps very similar to those shown when relaxing the body but carried over to another plane. Just as in relaxing the physical body our goal was to become totally aware of all voluntary and involuntary actions of the body, so as to slow them down to a point where they are more malleable and understandable, so too here, we must become aware of all the voluntary and involuntary actions of the mind, so as to slow them down to a point where they are more malleable and understandable. It is like slowly zooming in with a microscope, so things that were once small, almost imperceptible, become very large and monolithic. Our goal is to achieve a state of hyper-awareness.

Step 7: Realization of Trance

Now you are here, and you have willfully affected the realization of the trance-like state that is the initial aim of a good, effective session of proper self-hypnosis.

Don't be afraid to reach out and touch the light. Fully immerse yourself in this experience that you have prepared for. Know that you are achieving a very important and personal goal, be glad, grateful, ecstatic and proud of where you are. Feel the ball of light at your core, your solar plexus, emanating out like a shining star, like the sun, like the soil. It may be orgasmic. You may be taken aback by the power you have tapped into, the infinite potential. Focus on the awareness of the self and see who you are.

Step 8: Active Repetition of Mantra or Performance of Script

Now you have journeyed into space. Speak.

Speak the words you wish to speak to yourself. Each repetition of the mantra will completely change the landscape that you have found yourself in seismic waves. You will feel a growing energy completely under your control swarm over your entire being and beyond. You are in charge here. What you say goes. You are the ruler of this land, and you are going to take care of it well and make sure it is a prosperous paradise. Watch the negative thoughts, the images, the shadows, the memories you feared, the people you hate, the guilt, the pain, watch it shrivel into dust and evaporate before your very eyes, melted into oblivion by the sheer overwhelming power you have achieved.

Step 9: Preparation for Exiting the Trance State

Just as when you fully submersed, take a moment after you are done with your action to appreciate the beauty of what you are witnessing. Just be here now in this state. It is an eternal state. You will leave, and you will go back to the physical world, but this state will stay untouched, eternal, waiting for you to return. This is heaven. Know that you are about to return, and you are about to feel very different than you have ever felt before. Embrace these differences. It may be odd and imperfect at first, but it is a learning experience. The physical reality still awaits you as always—a different eternal experience. The rest of your life will be spent juxtaposing these two very different and very real planes and finding the perfect balance where you are in absolute control, yet in total surrender and synchronicity.

Step 10: Returning to Earth

Open your eyes. Where are you? Who are you? You may feel like this is something equally new as the realm you have just left. But there is a feeling of familiarity. You are awakened to the infinite possibilities of life. You see that your perspective can change in infinite ways, and with that change in perspective leads a portal to infinite different realties experienced through the multi-faceted crystal that exists. You may be stunned. You will be changed.

CHAPTER 4:

Re-Program Your Mind

Visualization

If you want to reshape the reality of your life, start by visualizing how you want your ideal life to be. Our subconscious mind's main language is emotions and images. Write a script of your ideal life and then play it like a movie in your imagination. The more detailed, vivid, and emotional you make it, the more your subconscious will think it is real because it cannot tell the difference. Remember, the subconscious is your captive audience. You can transfer your ideas from your conscious imagination to your subconscious to make success happen for you. Do your visualization for 10 to 15 minutes daily.

- For visualization you can also use a vision board, which is covered in.

Affirmations

The trick to saying affirmations that work and can program your subconscious mind is confidence and perceived truth. Simply put, although our subconscious does not know the difference between real or fantasy, our affirmations should not raise internal objections because it is too farfetched. For example, if you are currently broke and unemployed. In that case, it might be a stretch for your subconscious to believe the affirmation "I'm going to be a billionaire by this December" as compared to "The ideal job is already mine."

My finances are improving every day."

- Write affirmations that have corresponding feelings, focus on the positive, and have no opposing views.

- Face a mirror, take a deep breath and speak your affirmation a few times in the morning, noon, and evening. When saying your affirmation, focus on the meaning and feeling of your words.

- Another method is to write your affirmation several times on a piece of paper daily.

- Repetition and feelings are the key to reinforcing affirmations to your subconscious.

Listening to brainwaves audio program

Neuroscientists have discovered that different types of brainwaves can influence our creativity, habits, behavior, thoughts, and moods.

There are 5 types of brainwaves:

a) Beta brainwaves are associated with our waking consciousness and are important for our state of alertness, logic, and critical reasoning.

b) Alpha brainwaves are present in deep relaxation, meditation, or dreaming states. This is also the optimal brainwave when we need to program our subconscious mind for success as it is when our imagination and visualization are at their peak.

c) Theta brainwaves are present during light sleep, REM sleep, and meditation. These are also optimal waves for mind programming, vivid visualization, creativity, and insight.

d) Delta brainwaves are the slowest brainwaves that happen during deep, dreamless sleep and transcendental meditation. During these brainwaves, our body is healing and regenerating.

e) Gamma brainwaves are the fastest brainwaves, which are associated with high-level processing and insight.

For subconscious programming, you can use either alpha or theta brainwaves to help you while you are doing your visualization work. There are many apps and online audio programs that you can download, such as Brainwaves—Binaural Beats, Brainwave Tuner Lite, Binality, edenBeats for Android and iPhone users.

Hypnosis

Typically, in hypnosis, a qualified hypnotist will put you in a relaxed and suggestible state before programming positive and empowering messages into your subconscious mind.

Techniques for Health

We explained the emotions that harm our health and the mind-body connection where we feel an emotion and it activates certain neural pathways in our brain. Whether you're looking to improve a specific area of your health or your total well-being, the first step is to be aware of negative emotions that might be hampering your health. This step is like removing the weeds from your garden before you can start planting good seeds. The good news is once you have identified these negative emotions, you can work towards healthy subconscious programming.

- Be aware of your inner dialogue because every feeling, thought, and emotion carries energetic effects that can influence your body. For example, if you keep saying to yourself, "I feel sad," it will cause stress, damage, and increase cortisol and adrenaline in your body. Imagine the long-term damage this does to your body if you do this repeatedly.

- Many diseases are manifested by our consistent toxic emotions and thoughts.

- Are you stuck in toxic emotions, such as anger or sadness, which are sending a negative feedback loop to your mind and body? Manage and take charge of your negative emotions otherwise, they will control and deplete your mental strength.

- If you are currently undergoing treatment for any ailment, focus your mind on how the treatment or medication is going to help you get better. Let's say you are undergoing physical therapy for your bad knee. Instead of being passive and just going through the motions, you need to start seeing and believing that the therapy is indeed making your knee better. Use the power of your mind to expect your treatment to work.

- All sickness, be it the common flu or an incurable disease, can be reversed by releasing negative thoughts and replacing them with positive thoughts of health; healing through the mind works harmoniously with medicine.

- Our bodies respond to thoughts from our subconscious mind. Therefore, if you focus your thoughts on being healthy, you will create more health.

Steps:

1. Ask for what you desire e.g., "I am healthy, and my body is perfect in every way."

2. Every day, look at yourself in the mirror and say aloud your health affirmation "I am healthy, and my body is perfect in every way."

3. Visualize your body in perfect health. Imagine yourself doing all the things you thought you couldn't do e.g.; your bad knee prevents you from running.

4. To help you visualize better, cut out pictures of healthy-looking people that inspire you and paste it next to your mirror where you do your daily health affirmation.

5. Every day, try to do things that are relaxing and de-stressing to help you let go of toxic emotions and thoughts e.g., watching funny movies or playing with your children.

6. Be thankful and act like you already have a healthy body. If you want to accelerate your progress, keep a gratitude journal and write down three things you are grateful for before you sleep. The purpose is to let these positive thoughts sink into your subconscious and expand your awareness before you drift off to sleep.

7. To keep your state of health, avoid people who are negative or focus too much on your illness.

8. Read (or listen) to books on health and well-being.

9. Lastly, believe and have faith that once you ask, your body is already whole.

10. Suggested daily affirmations for health.

E.g.

1. "I am getting stronger and healthier every day in every way."
2. "I am perfectly healthy and full of energy."
3. "I take good care of my body by eating healthy and nutritious food."
4. "I am filled with energy and physical stamina."
5. "I want wholeness and healing for my body."
6. "Healing power flows through my body in all ways."
7. "I am kind, loving and gentle to my body."
8. "I love food and food loves me back."
9. "I am at my perfect weight with a beautiful and healthy body."

CHAPTER 5:

The Golden Protocol: The Hypnotic Method of 21 Days with Daily Statements

The 21-day entrancing technique with day by day certifications

Would you like to free your life of uneasiness, show your fantasy list, and praise energy surrounding you? In case you're not kidding about utilizing the Law of Attraction, one of the best approaches to supercharge your inspiration and center your essentialness is to follow a 21-day challenge plan! You can use this methodology with any objective, regardless of whether little or extraordinary. Its motivation is to give you honed center and upgrade your capacity to show anything you desire.

Keep perusing to find your free printable sheet and manual for the 21-day challenge just as point by point clarifications of the specific activities and strategies to utilize every day.

Day 1: Clear Your Mind

Go through this day discreetly, doing fundamental breathing activities, and purposely relinquishing any burdens that may have been keeping you down lately. You need a fresh start to draw in energizing new things. Here is a straightforward breathing activity to kick you off today.

- Take a deep breath in through the nose. Fill your lungs and feel your stomach grow. Hold this for 4 seconds.
- Discharge the breath through your mouth, similar to you is letting out a significant moan.
- You're completely done! Rehash as regularly as you have to.

Day 2: Make Space in your Life

Look at your living spaces and clean up things that help you to remember negative considerations or bind you also firmly to the past (for instance, protests that help you to recall past connections). Encircle yourself with things you partner with good faith, development, and enthusiasm. These aides may help you while doing a 'spring clean' of your home:

- Instructions to Declutter Your Home: 9 Questions to Ask Yourself When Tidying
- Instructions to Improve Your Bedroom for MAX Energy Level
- 150+ Things to Throw Away Today

Day 3: Explore Your Goal

Consider what you trust you need. Presently ask yourself these inquiries…

- For what reason do you need it?
- Do you need it?
- When thinking about your objective, envision it showing in various ways until you get a feeling of the particular purpose you're genuinely taking a stab at.

Day 4: Put Your Goal into the Words

Investigation with methods of stating what you need to show. Change the words around until you simply realize you've found the correct ones.

Record them and put them up someplace you can see. One helpful method is to put them by or on your restroom reflect!

Day 5: Make a Step-by-Step Plan

Note each progress you'll have to take to meet your definitive objective. This assists with guaranteeing you're progressing in the direction of something achievable and makes each stage concrete and genuine in your brain.

Day 6: Create a Dream Board

This engaging activity just expects you to pick magazine patterns, photos, and words that best speak to the thing you need to pull in and join them such that you find moving. Be as imaginative as you like!

For instance, if you are attempting to show your perfect partner, you may cover your fantasy board in pictures of sound connections, you know. You could likewise include statements of what you are searching for in an accomplice.

You can utilize physical arrangement for this, for example, using photos and patterns as portrayed above or utilize online assets. Numerous individuals like to utilize locales like Pinterest as a type of fantasy board. Get more motivation for your fantasy board today with your free dream board toolbox!

Day 7: Pick a Manifestation Song

Discover a tune that catches all the sentiments you partner with your fantasy. For instance, you may pick a triumphant song of praise in case you're moving in the direction of a vocation or wellness objective, and a fantastic melody in case you're searching for adoration. Play it, move to it, sing it, and associate with it.

Day 8: Basic Visualization

Put aside, in any event, ten minutes in a tranquil spot where you won't be upset, and focus on building a maximally striking picture of the thing you need. Here are the absolute most helpful hints for improving your perception procedures:

Envision not just the sight and sentiment of the thing you need to show yet, besides the various faculties. Picture the scents, sounds, and sensations as well.

The utilization of reflection or hypnotherapy can likewise help dig further into your representation by shutting out interruptions and expanding your core interest.

You can likewise utilize craftsmanship, composing, and music for perception! Draw, paint, or write your vision. Centerfold girl your work in a generally noticeable region, so you are helped to remember it regularly. Submerge yourself in this procedure, permitting yourself to feel it as if it's going on. It before long will be!

Day 9: Design Your Affirmations

Utilize the expression (or expressions) from day four to assemble attestations that fortify your conviction that you can draw in what you need. Let's assume them into the mirror, grin, and let them resound. You'll likely get the best outcomes on the off chance that you state them consistently. For instance, attempt a portion of the accompanying positive every day certifications:

- "I acknowledge my capacity."
- "All aspects of my life are copious and filling."
- "Each experience I have is ideal for my development."
- "I merit adoring. There is love surrounding me."

- Make sure to get a definitive assertion to manage in your one of a kind LOA toolbox!

Day 10: Write About Your Dream

Let your psyche meander unfiltered, and record as much as possible about your fantasy. For instance:

- What it resembles.
- Why you need it.
- How it'll be to live it.
- Try not to blue pencil yourself by any stretch of the imagination, regardless of whether you get negative musings or emotions sneaking in.

Day 11: Uncover Negative Thinking Patterns

Check whether you can spot regions where constraining convictions and suspicions may hold you down and gaze them in the face. It is astounding what the number of our contemplations is subliminally negative! Take a stab at asking yourself the accompanying inquiries…

- What are your uncertainty and tensions?
- How 'reasonable' are your presumptions?

What messages did you get when you were youthful that may lead you to figure you can't show your wants? At the point when you figure out how to respond to these inquiries, you can begin to reveal why you have explicit reasoning examples you do and how to recognize and battle whenever you get yourself on edge.

Day 12: Challenge Negative Thinking Patterns

For each constraining conviction, you found in the past exercise, record a clarification of why you hold it. At that point, compose another, positive reasoning that you need to use to supplant the negative old one. You can utilize these to structure new attestations or simply look at the definite rundown once every day.

Day 13: Take Stock of the Value You Have

Days 11 and 12 can be hard, so go through day 13 on self-care and consider things that support your confidence. On the off chance that it helps, take a stab at checking ten things you love and incentive about yourself. You have the right to have all that you need!

Day 14: Connect With an Object

Discover something that speaks to your objective, for example, a stone, a bit of gem, or an adornment. Practice a perception while holding the article; at that point, ensure that the thing remains with you for the rest of the 21 days. It will ground you and help you to remember your latent capacity. Additionally, consider examining the various advantages of gem recuperating. A scope of different gems and stones can help center the Law of Attraction work and lift your appearance power.

Day 15: Multi-Perspective Visualization

Add another layer to your perceptions by envisioning your fantasy from an outsider point of view. Notice new subtleties, develop a much increasingly amazing and energizing picture of what you'll accomplish.

Day 16: Start a Gratitude Journal

Record 3–5 things that cause you to feel appreciative every day or every week, contingent upon your way of life. The reason for this errand is to fill you with vigorous positive imperativeness that causes you to vibrate at a high recurrence and improves your capacity to draw in progressively positive things to you.

On the off chance that this is hard, make sure to consider what you underestimate every day. Things may not stand apart as something to be thankful for, yet envision your existence without specific things.

Day 17: Revisit Your Plan

Come back to the arrangement you made on day five and consider where you are. Does anything have to change? Alter as vital, and be satisfied with the means you've taken.

Day 18: Look for Signs

The Universe regularly conveys signs to direct you towards the things you need; however, to see those signs, you have to get to your instinct. Today, keep your eyes stripped for rehashing expressions, incidents, or shock solicitations. These sorts of things may help you on your way. (P.S. Make sure to likewise pay a one of a kind psyche to these seven great karma signs and otherworldly change manifestations!)

Day 19: Give Love

Commit the day to consideration, empathy, and liberality, causing companions and outsiders the same to feel great. This, similar to your appreciation diary, encourages you to vibrate on a recurrence of wealth as opposed to one of need, placing you in the perfect space to show what you need. Here are only several thoughts of interesting points doing today just as instructional exercises to assist you with accomplishing the immediate objective:

- 20 Actions of Kindness That You Can Do for Loved One's Today
- Step-by-step instructions to Be Kind to Yourself
- 10 Exercises You Should Try for Increased Happiness
- Step-by-step instructions to Help Someone with Depression and Anxiety

Day 20: Live "As though"

Make arrangements like you will have an accomplice, investigate excursions like you'll have the cash to pay for them, or buy garments like you'll fit into them how you need. This limits the vibrational hole among you and the thing you need.

Day 21: Release What You Desire

At last, you have to figure out how to consider them to be in life all things considered and acknowledge that the Universe will send what you need precisely when you need it. Put stock in your capacity to show, yet discharge your longing and have a sense of security in the information you can and will have the life of your dream.

CHAPTER 6:

Healing the Body with Self-Hypnosis

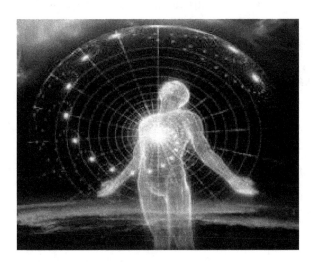

What does your body tell you in your own life of the need to heal the wound? Every day, the body sends out signals which let you know how safe it really is in general. Aches and pains are usually a warning inside that something is wrong. Some of the origins are a little more obvious than others. It is up to you to take the time to listen to the hints about your overall health that your body offers.

Positive Thought

Nearly every religion in the world states that positive thinking plays a significant role in healing. When it is a necessity for you to heal the body, it is a good idea to spend a little time thinking positively each day. You may just find that in this age-old philosophy, you have made a believer out of yourself in no time when you start to experience the power of positive thinking working inside your body to build a healthier you.

Exercise

It is an exercise that is one of the most neglected factors in healing the body. Over the years, it has been reduced to a fitness role and is equated with the need to keep in shape or assist in that goal rather than a balanced practice in and of itself. Exercise releases endorphins to provide relief from pain and a sense of happiness and well-being at large.

Good Diet

A balanced diet is a wonderful resource for healing your body as much as it can cause you to know it. To maintain maximum health, you need other nutrients. Unfortunately, we live in a world of fast food, and very few people get the nutrients required for optimum health. That's why it's important to bear in mind other choices like vitamin supplements—although they're not nearly as successful as getting the nutrients through your diet.

Adopt Healthy Habits

There are some behaviors that you can adopt that will promote improved health. Replace antibacterial soap with your regular hand soap. Often wash your hands and wash them well. Teach your family how to wash their faces, cover their mouths, and use sanitizing hand wipes or liquid cleaners in public to reduce the risk of taking home infections and diseases. Such practices can seem too simplistic but may result in prevention, which is often the best treatment, allowing the body to heal.

Protecting the body with hypnosis Self-hypnosis is just another means of protecting the body from illnesses of all kinds. There are many ways that mastering the art of self-hypnosis can help in your struggle, whether you are trying to reject cancer that is just as hard to take over or ward off the common cold. Hypnosis can help you relax, open your mind to positive thinking, help the nutrients get where they are best served, and help boost immunity, among other great things.

Take control of your healing process. It is time for you to take control of your body and its process of healing. Whether you are using one or all of the above techniques, if you listen to your body and react accordingly—for the best possible health outcome—you can find real help when it comes to healing the body.

Hypnosis is a powerful mode that literally can help your body stop unwanted habits and then start to heal and rejuvenate your body. It's all about the computer device situated within the brain.

After about 5 years, smoking stops being fun, and you realize how reliant you are becoming on that smelly habit. Does anyone really enjoy the desperation and mental obsession with a dried leaf filled with those little white papers that have become your best friend? It's true; it's that bad negative friend you have to take with you everywhere you go. Those "cigs" will be with you 24 hours a day and 7 days a week, and you'll want to press the panic button if by chance you run out. That's how it has been for me. For a period of 30 years, I smoke tons of cigarettes a day. Before the day I was hypnotized and quit smoking forever, I knew nothing about the strength of my subconscious. It's why I became a Hypnotherapist, too.

Stress creates the need to smoke, or does it cause stress? It is very difficult to go cold-turkey in this modern-day world where tension is a daily occurrence. Hypnotherapy is often the last option, and yet smoking cessation is the most successful strategy than any prescription medication designed to quit smoking.

Stress will manifest itself in all sorts of scenarios... Ranging from being depressed to violent. Contrary to common opinion, medications just exacerbate the condition while making huge bucks for the pharmaceuticals. Seek your nearest Hypnotherapist first before you go to get medication to be healthy again. You're going to be happier faster, and it's going to last a lot longer!

Will they hypnotize you? Hey! The condition you strive to achieve is one of absolute relaxation as though you're about to fall asleep. You are still very much in charge because we are enhancing your drive to do what you set out to do.

Hypnosis is essentially a form of deep relaxation that allows the client to take an imagined journey. The imagination is where you build a new, vibrant vision for what you want to be like in your future.

When your critical mind is in a very deep relaxed state, it calms down from that constant thinking that says: "I can't just leave," or "It's just too hard to quit." Side-stepping the critical mind lets you become motivated to accomplish what you felt was impossible before. Not only does it work well with smoking, but it also works well in sports, handling discomfort, and even taking exams.

Old habits of thinking can be replaced quickly and lovingly with fresh, wonderful optimistic thoughts that can make leaving such a positive force in your life. Only imagine if you can avoid obsessing about a question, you can actually do something, be, have anything. You broke the habit, and YOU CAN ACHIEVE ANYTHING SET OUT TO DO. Your level of confidence goes sky-high!

The most popular problem is that after stopping smoking, customers assume they'll gain weight. Luckily, when the body recovers from the smoking effects, the weight would inevitably result in a benefit or loss. It is a positive thing meaning that the body is in the healing process. You can also eradicate the habit with hypnosis, and stop replacing one oral obsession with another. The subconscious mind is already planting the new thought cycle, and when you listen to your private session's mp3, you can really reduce the weight tension.

I suggest that you choose a hypnotherapist who has your mind— rejuvenating your heart and lungs back to an age you feel tremendous strength and energy. A successful hypnotherapist can even get your liver to detoxify your body very gently so that the tar and nicotine or even heavy metals can be extracted very quickly and easily. The body is in the healing process until they leave the workplace and will remain there for a few months.

Hypnotherapy will help move the body into new wellness. Your cells can be ordered to heal through the science of Epigenetics. Hypnosis is the best way to help cancer patients help the body cure at faster speeds, particularly with surgeries. Studies that show hypnosis heals the body have been performed to minimize bleeding, swelling, and bruises, as well as speed up the recovery process 10 times faster. In addition to that, it has been established that 10 minutes of hypnosis actually reduce blood pressure and lower cholesterol.

If you want to quit smoking, eradicate a phobia, help heal cancer or pain, then just use your strong and focused mind to seek it out without medication. It is a lot easier than you could ever imagine. You become a champion, and you'll be shocked by how strong you are.

CHAPTER 7:

The Power of Meditation for Rapid Weight Loss

Meditation is one of the extraordinary eastern practices that have begun to grab hold in western culture. Individuals everywhere throughout the world are profiting by it, both in mind and body. Anyway, for what reason isn't everybody pondering? It may be the case that not every person is aware of all the astounding advantages like expanded unwinding and diminished degrees of uneasiness and melancholy. This article contains an overview of just a portion of the numerous advantages of meditation and a lot of guidelines for beginning your meditation practice.

This article is part of two principal segments. To start with, we talk about the advantages of meditation. From that point onward, we talk about how you can begin your meditation practice. If you don't know about the numerous advantages of meditation, we suggest you read through the following segment. It will assist with persuading you to stay with your training. If you know the advantages of meditation, don't hesitate to avoid forward.

Advantages of Meditation

There have been numerous examinations performed on meditation in the most recent decade attempting to comprehend its belongings, just as how it finds out how to help us with such a great amount of, both in mind and body.

An investigation into meditation has exhibited that thinking for a brief timeframe expands alpha waves, which causes us to feel progressively loose, while at the same time diminishing our sentiments of nervousness and misery. Alpha waves course through cells in the brain's cortex, where we process tactile data. These waves help stifle insignificant or diverting tangible data, permitting us to center. The more alpha waves we have, the better we center. There are a couple of particular meditation techniques that an individual can practice. The critical thing is to find a meditation technique that you approve of and endeavor to remain with that one. On the off chance that you will see by and large skip around starting with one meditation strategy, then onto the next, you won't get the full focal points of meditation. Meditation has various focal points, both truly, intellectually, and significantly. A segment of these consolidates lower circulatory strain, improved skin tone, peppy perspective, less weight, and just a general feeling of thriving. Today we are just going to give a short system of five of the critical meditation strategies. Mantra The accompanying meditation strategy is Mantra Meditation. Mantra Meditation is the spot you express a word, for instance, ohm over and over in your mind. In Mantra Meditation, the word exhibitions like a vehicle that takes you to a state of no thought. When repeating the mantra or word, it is incredibly standard for the mind to gliding off into various thoughts. Right, when this happens, the individual needs to fragile return their insights to the mantra and start repeating it before long. In Mantra Meditation, the word that is reiterated is unequivocal to change the person supernaturally. Regularly a mantra will be given to a meditator by an ace.

Chakra

The third meditation technique is Chakra Meditation. There are seven noteworthy chakras in the human body. When performing Chakra Meditation, the individual will focus on a specific chakra to wash the door empowering that chakra. Chakra Meditation can restore a person's body through the cleansing, resuscitating method. As the chakras are interrelated, it is urged in the first place the root chakra and work your way up when performing Chakra Meditation. While doing Chakra Meditation, you can moreover use the guide of valuable stones to help in the cleansing, restoration process. Chakra Meditation can be powerful for repairing and liberating from negative emotions.

Vipassana

The forward meditation technique is Vipassana Meditation. Vipassana Meditation is presumably the most settled kind of meditation and is used to get information into one's nature and the possibility of this present reality. The goal of Vipassana Meditation is to get done with moping over the individual. This is drilled by executing the three conditions, which are incidental quality, suffering, and not-self. In the wake of practicing Vipassana Meditation for a noteworthy stretch, the meditator ought to go to a point where they separate these three conditions from themselves and achieving nirvana. It is acknowledged that all physical and states of mind are not part of the authentic self or the "I" and should be cleared out with the demonstration of Vipassana Meditation.

CHAPTER 8:

The Power of Positive Affirmations

Affirmation has to be appreciated, and people should believe in them so that they can work well.

However, for this to work well, you must have a strong belief. Your belief will make you comprehend affirmation for a healthy diet.

You can genuinely achieve all affirmations if, at all, you put more effort and faith in managing. Nothing can't be grasped either conceived, and that's why for you to come up with the best affirmation, then a little effort and faith has to be employed. Before you move further with all these, it would be better for you to understand the real functions or rather the real purpose of affirmation. That's what they do in your daily life. It also appears as their primary function and purpose. The statement will highly motivate you and adds you with more power of urge to move ahead. In this, they not only keep you focused on your daily goals but also maintain that positive feeling in you. In that, they can affect your subconscious and conscious mind n. Affirmation always has that hidden ability to change your way of thinking and behaving. That's, they can control or have an effect on how you reason, especially about yourself. As a result of this, you are placing in a better position in which you will be able to transform every part of your world, that's both external and inner worlds. In short, affirmation is all about being extremely positive about yourself and having no space of negative thoughts in your life. You can also define it as having positive and straightforward thinking about yourself. You can also talk of it as an essential phrase that helps you in achieving some of your roles.

Affirmations are always honest words and phrases that you take your little time to speak to yourself. These phrases usually capture your physical health level. Everything that you want in life and how you will achieve them revolves around affirmation. Now that you have known this, you should understand all the affirmations for a healthy diet and body image in detail form. The following declarations have been approved as the most influential and have been grouped into different categories to help you transparently understand them.

Preparing Meals Affirmation

These affirmations are positive phrases you say to yourself while preparing food. They include the following:

Healthy meal planning is a kind of joy. You derive pleasure in making food that has got everything needed in terms of quality. You feel delighted having prepared all these plans, and this will reflect on how you feel about yourself. The right diet that you planned will boost your morale and gives you that anxious feeling about your body. It implies that planning healthy food or somewhat having a healthy diet plan will help you to have the right ingredients for a better meal.

Many studies have found that the proper meal has a positive effect on your body image in that it improves it to a certain level.

"Hi Kitchen, forever my center of nourishment." You look at your kitchen as a center of pleasure where you get all forms of nourishment. When you have positive affirmation thoughts like these, you understand that feeling of relaxed. Do this every day by reassuring yourself that, indeed, your kitchen is just a darling to you. That it is the only place where you can get that kind of nourishment your body needed. After that, spend as much as possible time in your darling kitchen. And make yourself a healthy diet that will help you improve not only to your inner world but also to the rest of the external world.

Appreciate your healthy diet. Your diet has helped you a lot in making sure that you can prepare those delicious meals. These meals are not only sumptuous but also highly nutritious. Without your healthy diet, then you couldn't have been in a position to prepare food with such qualities. It is better to note that preparing these kinds of food makes you even healthier. Also, this will make you feel even more joyous, relaxed, and at the end of the day, give you that kind of body shape you have always admired. Remember, healthy diet preparation is the cornerstone of your health. Without this, then you are doomed. Appreciate this affirmation and make it your daily phrase.

A healthy diet enables you to have a healthy meal plan. These meal plans have every ingredient required in making healthy food. You will be in an excellent position to choose from the available options. Having decided, you can now prepare that healthy diet. It will be of great help not only to your body but also to the rest of your environs. It will make you feel kind and more so grateful since the vast diet is at your disposal. It's now you to make a choice, and this will give you peace of mind while choosing. All these will get reflected in your body image. Many authors have tried their best to find why people are always grateful here. Many have failed, while others have concluded that there is that kind of pleasure someone derives from having a wide variety of healthy diets to choose on. Remember, these healthy diets that you have eventually chosen will support your healthy life.

Making nutritious and delicious meals are unavoidable. With a healthy diet within your disposal, you can now affirm yourself that you are in a position to make delicious meals. Meals like these are not only delicious but also are critical requirements in building up your body. Prepare them as many times as you can so that you can realize that shape.

You love having more time in your kitchen. Owning a kitchen for yourself is the first step in realizing your body image. Being in a position to have a healthy diet meal plan comes immediately after the latter. In this situation, you are only required to spend some adorable time in your kitchen just preparing that healthy diet. Affirm yourself that you can manage this behavior, putting more effort into it. Time spent on this has not gone to waste as it helps you make healthy meals. Having that right healthy diet will require lots of your time. This time you will spend it in your kitchen. Make sure that you make this affirmation your day to day routine and practice it correctly.

Feel the worthiness of your time and money spent on your health. Many people invest in their lives. The main objective here is to help improve their health. You are also supposed to do the same. Invest much in your life, and you should feel that worthiness of every input you plant in your life. Look at the money you have been investing in that health sector and make comparisons with the first time you were not affirming yourself. Is there any change? If yes, then you are worth it, your money hasn't been wasted or gone into waste. Check on time, especially the one you have invested in your life. How does the body react towards that kind of change? If everything has been positive ever since you started investing, then have an assurance that you have clicked on it, and you are worth it. Your spiritual body and external world should reflect the healthy diet that has been for so long. An improvement will add more value and worthiness to everything. Therefore, this affirmation will help you to improve so much that within a short time, your changes will realize. For you to master this, you can take it as a hobby and recite it every time that you are free then follow your heart.

You are being in a position to have a choice in choosing anything for the family. In all the aspects of life, from west to east, south to north, your family will come first. Having that basketful of a healthy diet, you will be in the right position to choose all kinds of healthy nutrition for your family.

Healthy food should be part of your family. You should be in a clear position to choose healthy food for you and your family. Your family is part and parcel of your life and providing them with excellent healthy food will be a blessing. Healthy eating leads to a relaxed mind. You should also note that this will always result in improved body image.

Your kids always appreciate new foods. Try having a change in your diet by providing a new diet. Kids still love different diets, and this will help them to improve on their body image. Eating healthy and making sure that everything is well-prepared initiate the morale of eating. Along the way, this will act as a steering wheel towards your achievements of body image. Remember, it is good to note that healthy new meals motivate you and gives you the pleasure of preparing.

Learning new things will make you heal your body. You should struggle as hard as possible to learn new kinds of stuff. New ideas might include modern diets, new cooking styles, and so on. Many studies have concluded that new things will always radiate your body. Your body will glow, and at the end of the day, you will be able to realize a good impression and improvement. Your goals will become a lesser issue since achieving them will be much easier. Your body will also feel some sort of relaxation as the process of healing continues. You will be in a position to feel juvenile, and happiness will be part of your day.

You should have the will to nurture yourself. This phrase will help you manage all the processes leading to nurturing yourself. Never lose hope in this process since it might be tedious. Concentrate on every detail that leads to the nurturing of your body image. After realizing this goal, try as hard as possible to get to bigger goals, which include shedding off more pounds of your weight. The will of nurturing will act as a driving force in your process of preparing healthy meals. According to studies carried out some years back, the intention to nurture yourself is more urging to an extent someone would wish to accomplish it first. However, for you to achieve this, then you need to play a little bit with your kitchen. Your kitchen will give you that kind of motivation and maximum pleasure to prepare that meal.

CHAPTER 9:

Positive Affirmations for Rapid Weight Loss

Affirmation for Rapid and Natural Weight Loss

1. My body is beautiful and healthy.
2. I choose healthy and nutritious foods.
3. I like to exercise and I do it frequently.
4. Losing weight is easy and even fun.
5. I have confidence in myself.
6. I am now sure of myself.
7. I feel confident to succeed.
8. From day to day, I am more and more confident.
9. I am sure to reach my goal.
10. I want to be a noble example.
11. I believe in my value.
12. I have the strength to realize my dreams.
13. I am really adorable.
14. I trust my inner wisdom.
15. Everything I do satisfies me deeply.
16. I trust the process of life.
17. I can free the past and forgive.
18. No thought of the past limits me.
19. I get ready to change and grow.
20. I am safe in the Universe and life loves me and supports me.
21. With joy, I observe how life supports me abundantly and provides me with more goods than I can imagine.

22. Freedom is my divine right.
23. I accept myself and create peace in my mind and my heart.
24. I am a loved person and I am safe.
25. Divine Intelligence continually guides me in achieving my goals.
26. I feel happy to live.
27. I create peace in my mind, and my body reflects it with perfect health.
28. All my experiences are opportunities to learn and grow.
29. I flow with life easily and effortlessly.
30. My ability to create the good in my life is unlimited.
31. I deserve to be loved because I exist.
32. I am a being worthy of love.
33. I dare to try and I'm proud of it.
34. I choose to really love myself.
35. I love myself and accept myself completely.
36. I am ready to try new things.
37. There are things I can already do; I just need to start even though I'm not ready yet.
38. I am much more capable than I think.
39. As I love myself, I allow others to love me too.
40. I accumulate more and more confidence in myself.
41. I am unique and perfect as I am.
42. I am wonderful.
43. I'm proud of everything I've accomplished.
44. I do not have to be perfect; I just need to be myself.
45. I feel able to succeed.
46. I give myself permission to go out of my role as a victim and take more responsibility for my life.
47. The past is over, I now have control of my life and I move.
48. I am my best friend.
49. I am able to say "no" without fear of displeasing.
50. I choose to clean myself of my fears and my doubts.

51. Fear is a simple emotion that cannot stop me from succeeding.
52. Every step forward I make increases my strength.
53. My hesitations give way to victory.
54. I want to do it, I can do it.
55. I am capable of great things.
56. There is no one more important than me.
57. I may be wrong but that I can handle it.
58. With confidence, I can accomplish everything.
59. I allow myself to have a lot of fun.
60. I deserve to be seen, heard and shine.
61. I deserve love and respect.
62. I choose to believe in myself.
63. I allow myself to feel good about myself and trust myself.
64. I reduce measures quickly and easily.
65. I can maintain my ideal weight without many problems.
66. My body feels light and in perfect health.
67. I'm motivated to lose weight and stay.
68. Every day I reduce measures and lose weight.
69. I fulfill my weight loss goals.
70. I lose weight every day, and I recover my perfect body.
71. I eat like a thin person.
72. I treat my body with love and give it healthy food.
73. I choose to feel good inside and out.
74. I feed myself only until I am satisfied, I don't saturate my food body.
75. I know how to choose my food in a balanced way.
76. I feed slowly and enjoy every bite.
77. I am the only one who can choose how I eat and how I want to see myself.
78. It is easy for me to control the amounts of what I eat.
79. I learn to have habits that lead me to my ideal weight.
80. Being at my ideal weight makes me feel healthy and young.

81. My body is very grateful and quickly reflects all the care I have with him.
82. My body reflects my perfect health.
83. I feel better every day.
84. Being at my ideal weight motivates me to do other things that I like.
85. The human body is moldable, and I am the (the) artist of my body.
86. Every day I eat with awareness.
87. I consume the calories needed to have an ideal weight and a healthy body.
88. Every day I like the way I feel.
89. My slender body makes me feel, agile, light (and) and strong at the same time.
90. I know how to properly calculate the portions my body needs to feel satisfied.
91. I can achieve everything that I propose.
92. No one can do this for me, only I can make the best version of me, inside and out.
93. I am the inspiration for other people.
94. I like how the clothes look on my slender body.
95. I am strong physically and mentally.
96. No one can get me out of my motivation for being a healthy and slender person.
97. Being at my ideal weight fills me with energy.
98. My metabolism is faster every day thanks to the food I eat.
99. I love my new lifestyle.
100. I am getting better and better.
101. I accept all the blessings of the universe.
102. Reality is created from my thoughts.
103. I decide to choose thoughts that will have a positive impact on my life.
104. The biggest job to do is on my own.
105. I am open to all new experiences of life.

106. I am free to think what I want.
107. I will achieve great things.
108. I will be the best to accomplish this task.
109. I value myself because I am a good person.
110. I have full possession of my means.
111. I hide all the negative things that I cannot change.
112. I love myself a lot because I am a good person.
113. I am able to climb mountains.
114. I am able to reverse any reality.
115. I totally approve of everything I do.
116. All my decisions are taken in hindsight and these are good for me.
117. I am unique.
118. I believe in myself inconsiderately.
119. I think positively.
120. Understanding is one of my biggest qualities.
121. I have all the qualities in me to reach my ends.
122. I am determined to deal with all situations.
123. I am a man capable of exceeding my limits.
124. I am a totally unique person with great qualities.
125. I am a good person and I deserve happiness.
126. All my decisions are good at different levels.
127. Serenity is an integral part of me.
128. I am the person I think I am.
129. I agree with the people around me and trust my colleagues.
130. Self-esteem is my main quality.
131. My life is plenty of confidence.
132. I am a confident person who keeps getting better every day.
133. I trust my choices and I move in that direction.
134. I erase in my life all the people who prevent me from achieving happiness.
135. I control my choices and my life.

136. I am responsible for my positive mental state.
137. I deserve a fulfilling life.
138. What I feel is healthy.
139. Trust in me is my first quality.
140. I attract good in my life.
141. I will offer everything I have given.
142. Love is present, it is enough that I believe in it.
143. I am aware that my friends love me.
144. I have a family and relatives who surround me.
145. I have a fulfilling social life.
146. I am love.
147. I make the world better every day.
148. I like family time.
149. I take the time necessary to show my entourage how important they are to me.
150. I love them.
151. I am able to take time for myself and for my loved ones.
152. Compassion is part of me.
153. I am able to give forgiveness.
154. I practice benevolence with conviction to help my entourage to evolve.
155. I am able to question myself and understand.
156. I choose to do what I like.
157. I believe in love.
158. I let my heart speak.
159. I am able to let people love me.
160. I like others and others love me in return.
161. I accept that others can love me.
162. Fusional/passion love is coming into my life.
163. The people I love me back.
164. I am able to give love to others.
165. If I give others love, they make it exponentially.
166. I am able to attract the person I want.
167. My sentimental relationships are strong and fulfilling.

168. I'm ready to fall in love.
169. I give a lot because I love this person
170. Love is in me.
171. Love is only an extension of my fulfillment.
172. Joy filled me and filled my life.
173. The people around me are filled with love and I benefit from it.
174. I'm falling in love.
175. The waves around me tell me that love is present.
176. Hidden love is a real love.
177. I love to love a person.
178. I take the front and reveal my love.
179. Like a magician I chose to give love all around me.
180. I am healthy, wealthy and clever.
181. I let go of the illness, I am not ill.
182. Thanks to my creator and everyone in my life.
183. I am grateful for all the bounty that I already enjoy.
184. Every day I grow energetically and vibrantly.
185. I only give my body the necessary nutritious food.
186. My body is my temple.
187. You can always maintain a healthy weight.
188. I deserve to enjoy perfect health.
189. Act to be healthy.
190. I respect my body and am willing to exercise.

CHAPTER 10:

Repetition of a Mantra

What are Mantras, How and for What Can We Use Them?

There are a lot of anxiety-inducing situations every day, such as an important job interview, asking the boss for a pay raise, giving a lecture in front of a bunch of people, and so on. Calm breathing often turns out to be insufficient, especially in a stressful situation. In this case, we need to apply another approach, the method of mantra.

10 Essentials You Need to Know About Mantras

1. The hidden possibilities of mantras

The strength of mantras honed by ancient Indian sages over many decades is concentrated, even in their ability to influence the physical level. "Mantras are like different doors that lead to the same end; each mantra is unique and thus leads to the same wisdom: to recognize that everything is one. That is, every mantra has the potential to unleash the veil of illusion and dispel the darkness." —Deva Premal

2. The language of mantras and their meanings

The language of mantras is Sanskrit, which is no longer considered a living language on the planet, but it is called the 'mother tongue.' We all relate to this in the same way as our language is a cellular language, a code that we understand at a very deep level. It vibrates in us something that no other language or sound can. It is a universal voice that unites us, no matter our belief system, our nationality, and our religion. You can find translated mantras, but the sounds themselves are sufficient to bring about the beneficial effects. Mantras contain deep, concentrated wisdom, meaning much more than the sum of individual words. It is, therefore, almost impossible to translate them accurately without losing some deeper meaning. Therefore, let us consider the translation as a guide and let the mantras work on their own.

3. The power of intention

As something is necessarily lost in the true meaning of translation, the power of our intention is very important. It is good to have a strong intention and a strong focus inside, but in fact, the effect that the mantra exerts on us is the most important. This is the true meaning of the mantra to every person who uses it. For each mantra, you will find a phrase called "Inner Focus," which broadly covers the intent of that mantra, but of course, you can also formulate an individual intent.

4. Keep the mantra with you all day

There are countless ways to make mantras part of our lives. I often carry a mantra with me all day. I would like to encourage you to do so! Carry the mantra with you throughout the day, and whenever you think of it, come back to it, the mantra being the last thing you think of before going to sleep. This is how you can truly commit to a mantra and the specific focus or theme that the mantra represents.

5. It's not necessary to chant the mantras aloud

Mantras do not necessarily have to be heard out loud. Understanding this can be a real breakthrough because it means you could carry the mantra on your own without actually chanting. So if there is a situation where you feel you need to sing the mantra out loud, concentrate on pushing it inward, carry it with you, and hold it in your being, your mind, your heart—this is the root of mantra practice when we connect with the Spirit.

6. Chant your mantras 108 times

108 is considered a very favorable number in the Vedas. According to the scriptures, we have 72,000 lines of energy in our body (the nadis), of which there are 108 main channels of energy or major nadi that meet in the sacred heart. When a mantra is chanted 108 times, all energy channels are filled with vibrations of sound.

7. In what position should we mantra?

I recommend a comfortable position for most mantras, one with a straight back; we can relax and yet remain alert. A position that allows us presence. Because of this, a lying position is not ideal, it is harder to sing and we risk falling asleep while doing it.

8. Contemplation

Before each mantra, let's reflect on the topic of that mantra: what does it mean in our lives, do we need it, can we develop in that area, etc.? What can we sacrifice to make this quality more fully manifest in our lives? Thinking through these steps helps to refine our focus further and deepen our practice.

9. The most important "element" of the mantra is silence

This is seemingly a paradoxical thing: the silence after singing is what our soul dives into and is reborn. This silence represents the transcendent, the eternal, the reality, and understanding or achieving this is the ultimate goal of mantra practice.

10. Importance of repetition and practice

The essence of mantra practice is not to get over it quickly and then return to our usual daily routine. The point is to practice and to integrate the mantras into our lives. Wherever we go, whatever we do, the mantras accompany us. This is the benefit of true mantra practice. It helps and supports the path of our lives. The power of mantras is multiplied by repetition and devotional practice. The more pleasure we can bring into our practice, the more pleasure we get. Like real friends, mantras can help you through times of need and stress.

How Do We Use Mantras in Everyday Life?

The method is simple! We need to talk to ourselves—of course, what we say matters. I may surprise you by saying that it's enough to repeat only three words in every situation when you feel under pressure. These three words are: "I am excited."

Yes, I know, it is not what you have expected from me. You may wonder why you should use a statement that is not so 'positive.' Harvard University published a study in the Journal of Experimental Psychology, in which scientists claim that striving to overcome anxiety may not be the best solution in such situations. Instead of trying to calm ourselves down, it can be more useful to transform stress into a powerful and positive emotion, such as excitement. Because positive feelings produce quite similar physical symptoms like anxiety, hence, we wouldn't have great difficulties switching the stress to excitement. Enthusiasm is a positive emotion; besides, it is easier to cope with. The study also recalls earlier research that mild anxiety can even be a motivator for specific tasks. So, it is worth using the energy generated by stress to increase our efficiency, instead of trying our best to suppress it. To turn fear-based anxiety into a positive feeling, repeat for 60 seconds to yourself, "I am excited." This mantra "redraws" the picture of a stressful situation into something we happen to be waiting for—which is far less exhausting than trying to calm ourselves down.

Using different mantras is very important to me, and I use them daily for my meditations or just for relaxation. You can also use them whenever you are sad, or you don't know where you belong to what you have to do with your life. They help you to see through and view yourself. If you have been to a place where people have been singing or chanting, you will know how much power and energy there is in a particular word.

One of the best-known mantras is "Aum" or "Oum." It is found among Hindus but also in Buddhism. Followers believe this mantra purifies the soul and helps to release negative emotions. This mantra is also known as a sign of the "quick eye" chakra.

If you want to reach the best result, sing AUM loudly so that its sound vibrates in your ears and soaks your entire body. It will convince your outer sense, give you greater joy and a sense of success. When singing AUM loudly, "M" should sound at least three times as long as "AU." When repeating "AUM," imagine that life energy, divine energy flows through you through the crown chakra. The breath that flows through your nose is very limited. But if you can imagine that there is a large opening at the top of your head, and life energy, cosmic energy is flowing into your body through that opening, you will undoubtedly be able to accelerate the purification of your nature, strengthen your aspiration and hunger for God, Truth, Light, and Salvation.

CHAPTER 11:

How to Practice Every Day

The first thing you need to do when it comes to managing time is to look at yourself. Look at what you're trying to get done. Look at the goals and aspirations you have. Look at how you can use your time in order to make things better. If you look at yourself and see that you need a certain amount of time in order to make sure that you get things done, you'll see that you need to have that time in order to achieve your goals. Looking at the broad picture can help.

The next thing, once you've looked at the broad picture, is to make a plan. A plan for this is the overall goal that you have and how in the world you're going to get to it. Some goals are huge, such as trying to run the marathon or getting to a goal weight, but you can achieve them. You should look at everything that you need to do in order to achieve the goal that you have. It's not something that will take five minutes to do, but if you have a plan, it'll make things easier. You want to have an exact set of steps that you'll need to do in order to get to the state that you want to be in. If you want to run the marathon, plan out how you're going to run it. Go through the exact steps, and you'll soon see the overall things that you need to do in order to get to that point. It might look daunting at the moment, but if you work on this, you'll see that the dreams that you have can become a reality if you follow the overall game plan that can help with your goals.

The next thing is to make a monthly plan. You look at exactly what you want to accomplish this month. It can be goals that are big or small but don't bite off more than you can chew. Think about what you can realistically do in order to hit a certain goal. You have to look at what you need to change in order to accomplish all of those things. A monthly plan allows you to change the way things go, and you can also change the way life goes as time passes. A monthly plan will keep you on track and motivated to keep on going with the goals that you have in mind.

Next, think of how the goal can be divided into four weeks. Dividing it down and making sure that you have a good plan in order to get to the goal by the date makes it easy. At first, it may look like hell on earth to you. You might think the idea of actually going through with this to be something on the order of trying to beat a god or something. But, in reality, you need to see that if you divide it up in a logical way that it is doable. Any goal that you have is completely doable. You need to just put it in a plan of action and stick to it. By doing it in a daily basis, you can chip at it in order to make the huge goal something that you can face.

When you make the daily plan, allow yourself time to put in that goal every day. Going a day without the goal in mind can make things hard on you. You need to leave it there for you to see. If you need to, write it on a sickly note and put it on your fridge. Every single day you'll see that you can reach the goal, and you'll feel motivated to actually work on it and not let it fall by the wayside. You want to have a strong life full of things to do, and putting the goal there each day will get you ready for you to face the hardship of the giant goal.

When you have it all planned out, it's time to actually do it. Even if you think it's one of the worst days ever, you want to have the goal there and work on it. You'll want to dedicate the amount of time that you need to in order to make sure that you reach the goal. It doesn't have to be a lot, but if you make a plan, you'll be able to get everything that you need to get done. You won't have it hanging around in your head for a long time. You'll also stay on top of things and not let the issues of your laziness take over.

Another thing that you should do is you should always get it done first. It doesn't matter if you need to wake up a tiny bit earlier just to get everything that you need to get done for it. Doing it first thing will make things that much better on you. And, if you work on the goal at first, you'll be pumped for the rest of the day. Being pumped and inspired to continue will allow you to continue to make sure that your goals are reached and you're happy.

By doing it first thing and achieving it each day, it also causes morale to be raised. When people are lazy, most of the time, they feel like crap. That might be because they don't like just sitting around, but there are other things involved with it as well. You can let you remind wander into places it doesn't need to go when you're sitting around and being idle. It could cause you to think all sorts of weird things, and that's just putting it mildly. By actually making sure that you stay focused, you'll feel better and get more done.

You should also keep yourself motivated. Some days are just draggy and most people hate them. The dog days do happen, and most people hate them. It can be a big issue for so many people since dog days usually cause people to not want to do anything despite trying. But don't let them get to you. Even if you feel like complete dirt and you just want to sit around and binge-watch Netflix, don't. Don't' do that. Laziness is like a sickness, and if you let that habit in, it'll open up the door for laziness to continue. Instead, keep working on your goals, but also have a plan for what you want to do every single day. Just make up a list of everything that you want to get done, and then just do it. It doesn't take a ton of effort to do so, you just need to have the drive and desire to continue on. It can suck for a while, especially if you're the type who is used to being lax and not doing anything. But, if you knock off the laziness for at least one day, you'll soon realize that at the end of the day, you actually accomplished more than most people. The feeling of accomplishment is remarkable, especially when you accomplish many things. If you keep yourself motivated and want to continue to work, you'll realize later on that doing that could be one of the best things you've ever done for yourself.

Another thing to do in order to help keep time better managed is to get rid of distractions. This one is probably the hardest thing for most people. It's not even the cell phone or the computer. It can be the animals that are making noise, the sound of other appliances, and even the dialogue of people. Distractions are rampant in things, and if they're not taken care of in an effective manner, they can cause a person to easily get sidetracked. Humans are fallible in the fact that they get super sidetracked and off their course easily. One little thing can usually send most people into a tizzy all day. One bad message, or even a good one from a friend, can distract you for god knows how long. You need to realize that these distractions, although nice to have every once in a while, should be eliminated from your life. When people want to talk, just tell them that you're working on something. Some might get offended, but you have to remember that this is your life. You need to make sure that you're getting everything that you need to get done accomplished. It's not that hard, and you have to remember to just keep on going and not care what people think. You're trying to reach your goals, and if a person gets joy out of distracting you from reaching your goal, then they don't deserve to be a friend to you right now. You want to surround yourself with people who support you, and if you need to eliminate them for a bit, so you don't' get distracted, it will help you out even more so later on.

A final thing is to reward yourself when you use time effectively. If you get everything that you needed to get done accomplished that day, then that's grounds to celebrate. It's not hard to do, and when you realize it you'll see you've accomplished a big feat. Don't get yourself anything too extravagant until you reach your final goal. Instead, reward yourself a little bit each day whenever you get everything that you need to get done accomplished. You will be happier, and you'll be able to use time to become more efficient as well.

Time efficiency is something everyone struggles with. Everyone seems to have the problem of staying on track and using time wisely. You will be happier, and you'll also reach your goals, which is something that feels amazing.

CHAPTER 12:

Using Positive Affirmations to Lose Weight

At the very heart of thought, power is the notion that your thoughts create your collective circumstances and conditions. Every aspect of your present life, be it relationship, finances, health, or self-image, is the offspring of your most common thoughts and the feelings, emotions, and beliefs they create.

You are not your circumstances; you create your circumstances whatever they may be, wanted or unwanted. The easiest way to create thought awareness is to accept the truth that, through their limitless creative power, your thoughts create your circumstance and therefore, by being aware of the thoughts most common in your mind, you can determine which thoughts/seeds to cultivate and care for thereby changing your reality or circumstance. To create thought awareness, look within you for your reality begins in your mind. Only by being alive to your mind can you create awareness of thought. Only by being aware of the energy created by specific, common thoughts can you change the attendant energy in specific areas of your life.

The Process of Creating Thought Awareness

The process of creating thought awareness starts with perception. Our most common perceptions are learned thoughts that lead to behaviors; how we "feel" about any given circumstance comes from our thoughts and perception of it.

To become perceptive of your thoughts is important to create time in which you can listen to your thoughts. There are many ways to do this, but the best are meditation, affirmation, and creative visualization.

On any given day, give yourself the gift of spending 5 minutes onwards with your mind, becoming aware of the thoughts, emotions, habits, and beliefs that run through it at any given time.

In these 5 minutes onwards (how much time you spend will depend on your preferences), aim to relax. Relaxation gets your conscious mind to relax, which clears the pathways between the conscious and subconscious mind, thereby making it easier to embed affirmations into the subconscious and unconscious mind.

The easiest way to relax, and covertly the easiest way to become more aware of your most common thoughts, is to practice breath and mindfulness meditation.

Breathe into a count of 4, making sure you are concentrating on every aspect of your breath as you draw it in. Hold the breath into a count of four and take note of the sensations it produces within you.

Exhale to a count of four and as you do, take note of the sensations: how air moves up your breathing canal and gushes out of your mouth or nose in a hot puff. As you exhale, imagine your hot breath, taking with it your stress, anxiety and tension; visualize this as clearly as possible, for it will help you relax deeply. Hold the breath out to a count of four and then restart the sequence and continue doing it until you feel relaxed.

Called 4-part breathing, this type of breathing activates the parasympathetic nervous system, the division of the autonomic nervous system charged with rest, relaxation, and digestion. When active, this system leads to relaxation of the conscious mind.

As you begin to relax, you can then start the process of becoming aware of your stream of consciousness and observing your most common thoughts in relation to different areas of your life.

Cultivating mindfulness, something that comes from the ability to sit with your thoughts without being judgmental of them, helps you become more aware of your most common thoughts. Awareness of these thoughts, especially as they relate to key pillars of your life, helps you determine the beliefs, habits, and mindset you need to change before you can bring about positive change in your life.

NOTE: Remember that affirmations are a transformative tool in a toolbox that has many other tools necessary for the successful completion of a project (perhaps a goal, desire, or change of belief).

Most failed cases of experimenting with affirmation turn unsuccessful because of a contrast between the affirmation repeated and one's beliefs or feelings about the subject of the affirmation.

For instance, using an affirmation such as "I am wealthy" when saying it makes you feel like a fraud because you are broke, is very unlikely to work unless you start taking action that helps you build wealth and then courting thoughts that lead you to believe yourself worthy of that wealth.

As you practice daily affirmations, keep in mind that the universe responds to the vibrations in your words (the ones you use to word your affirmations). It does not recognize the words. Simply put, how you feel about the affirmation is what determines the vibrational energy you attract into your life/circumstances.

At their core, affirmations seek to help you experience the vibrational energy/feeling you want to feel so that the universe picks up this specific feeling and attracts to it similar vibrational energies.

Affirmations, Rational Thinking, and Journaling

Affirmations, especially those created with the specific intent of changing your life, are another effective way to create awareness of thought. Affirmations aim to help change your vibrational frequency, the emotions and beliefs you attach to specific areas of your life. Without thought awareness, it is impossible to determine your current vibrational energy—let alone change it.

Before you create affirmations, it is prudent to spend some time with your thoughts as they relate to a specific area of your life. An effective way to do this is to think about the stress that comes about when you think about specific areas of your life. Doing this will reveal your most common thought patterns in relation to that area of your life; you can even go a step further and journal the thoughts in a stress diary, one of the most effective thought awareness tools.

Stress journaling allows you to log your unpleasant thoughts for a period; this allows you a glimpse of your most common stress-inducing, negative thoughts that send out a negative vibrational energy to the universe. With this awareness, you can create personalized affirmations that you believe in and that have the ability to change the emotions you attach to the specific areas of your life.

Always remember that even though affirmations are an effective tool, they do not work in isolation. When creating affirmations, it helps to know as much as you can about the area of your life you want to change. This awareness allows you to unearth the beliefs, habits, and attendant vibrational energy attached to that area of your life, all of which makes it easier to use affirmations to influence massive amounts of change in your life.

Thought awareness allows you a chance to question your most common thoughts about a specific area of your life and therefore think rationally.

Negative thoughts are often thoughts drawn from fear. When you journal them, you start seeing the underlying cause of the negativity in your life. When you become aware of what you are thinking and feeling, the process of questioning and challenging your negative thoughts becomes easier.

For instance, by looking at the negative/stressing thoughts you journaled, you can challenge the authenticity of each one of them and, by doing so, determine if the thought has some merit to it. Coincidentally, by questioning negative thoughts, beliefs, and assumptions in this manner, it will be easier to challenge feelings of inadequacy, worries and anxieties over your abilities and other people's reactions to you and your work.

On its part, journaling is one of the best ways to create thought awareness. Get into the habit of doing it every day. Journal about your day, feelings, the things you are grateful for, the things that are stressing you out, your beliefs, ideas, and whatever else you want to (a journal is personal and you are therefore free to journal whatever you want). Get into the habit of doing this and your thoughts, especially the most common ones as they relate to the specific areas of your life you want to change, shall never be a mystery ever again.

As you use the thought awareness processes we have outlined here, another important thing you should do, i.e., in addition to questioning your negative thoughts and applying rational thinking, seek to replace them with positive thoughts.

When you rationally interrogate negative thoughts about a specific area of your life, you are likely to discover that the negative thoughts have no basis in reality or truth. When you awaken your mind to this, you will gain an intuitive ability of knowing how to word and phrase your affirmations so that they change your vibrational frequency and instantly replace the negative thoughts.

As a point of note, after interrogating negative thoughts and determining their fallacy, it becomes easier to replace it with its positive equivalent. For instance, if after interrogating your thoughts towards success, you discover the fallacy of a thought such as "I will never succeed," you can replace it with a counter thought such as, "Success come easy to me because the universe wants me to succeed." As you can see, such a thought will change how you feel about your success.

CHAPTER 13:

Harnessing Positive Affirmation and Meditation for Rapid Weight Loss

I'm aware of that feeling. You are putting so much energy, such that you committed serious effort for rapid weight loss, but it's not working out as supposed. What if I tell you that there could be basic beliefs that are detrimental to your efforts? These positive affirmations are going to change everything.

You know what, when you have the feeling in the body that you've stuck at a place with your weight, you gave into the mirror and what you are seeing is quite unpleasant to sight, you feel uncomfortable in your clothing, the feeling of being frustrated, discouraged and depressed because you really put so much discipline and followed some rules so to say yet things are happening and it makes you think you should eat more and more, of course, many have cultivated eating disorder from their high school days and followed them through to adulthood, but the good news is this, several persons who have access to quality information and key points as we lay open to you in this to have been able to come over these bad eating habits.

It is funny to know that many who think they have stopped eating excessively are yet no shift or change in their thoughts and emotional experience regarding food. This then trips the body so much. It's more like moving from being weighty and graduating to the panic of being overweight. Also, unhealthy views and feeling about the body and relationship with food. You change your body image by healing them. Then, you'll love your body and build a healthy relationship with food.

These ten belief systems are keys to the fundamental unyielding energies that have been in the subconscious mind. Shall we please go through these ten sufficient affirmations? We shall see together what exactly has constituted the underlying factor that has served as a limitation to your weight loss. It could be as easy as switching your odd beliefs to affirmative, by indeed harnessing these affirmative beliefs, with this you are setting yourself up for success. It is high time you turned all the destructive, demoralizing, and limiting beliefs to affirmative ones, as you identify them and disclose them, you see things happening and changing. Alright! The highlighted affirmations are ones I have seen work people into reality of their results.

1. Affirmations Like, "I Am Healthy and Lean"

The first thing you need to have in mind is your belief and how you see your body. You are at the point between "being healthy and lean is what I want." Go ahead and declare it, not just as a wish but as a truth. Let your body system begin to digest these words. Just as you have declared and pronounced it, begin to live in the excitement and joy of the spoken truth, living in this understanding and belief is your true energy. The fact that what you say doesn't look like what you do doesn't mean you are deceiving yourself. You are only trying to establish the truth you want within you, and believing it will materialize. You no longer live in your ugly state of mind but the new one. Live in the present with the truth you profess about yourself. This is a building factor of your self-identity. When you believe in this truth, your body, one way or the other, begins to live in that reality from the inside out. May I tell you that the body has the capacity to conform to such truth?

2. I Place High Esteem to Myself than Food

There's a need to place more emphasis on yourself than food. Do well to check how frequent you treat your body and used food as compensation. We often think less of about our real needs; what about the kind of food, the measure, the style, how delicious it is, how satisfactory it will be, all these and more, this is what we really think about and engage our thoughts on at the expense of our body maintenance. This actually has been tying that span through from our childhood. When our parents buy us "special food" as a reward for doing well in school or for having a good result, these ideas have, with time, formed the basis of our belief system. At adulthood too, we feel, when we get promoted from office, or your wife put to bed or something pleasant happens, we seem to eat excessively and use food as a tool of celebrating such successes, even to the detriment of our health most times. Going this way with an unhealthy relationship with food is so detrimental.

3. Affirmations like, "I love my body"

It's therefore required of you to grow beyond the relevance of food to the relevance of the body. You are eating for your body to structure well and you aren't building your body for the food. So, it is food for the body and not the body for the food. Just declare to yourself that "I love myself and the fat should leave." When you look in the mirror and you hurriedly and sluggishly put it down, you, therefore, make some words and perhaps statements to yourself. The question then is, can you say to your intimate pal that you cherish so much what you just told yourself while gazing at the mirror? Your body systems are all ears and quietly listening to your confessions on them. I think it's time to tell yourself to love your body.

This junk circulates through our experiences; what if I choose to love my body and see it in a way I don't like? Does it not mean I'm just flattering myself or does it mean I just need to love my body even when I know it isn't going to change or make any effect? I don't care what happens to my body, I just got to love it though. This is not the idea, the idea truly is, where there is love, there is growth, there's development, there are greater tendencies of change. When your body is shown some love, it is inspired to change. But when you think otherwise by being shameful and self-humiliated, you then think of overreacting.

4. Affirmations Like, "I Have My Ideal Weight"

Go back to that mirror and guess what? Say to yourself, "this is the way I am and I'm going to love it like this now, I will surely harness the potency of love to enhance, support and evoke the necessary change in my body." Claim to yourself, saying, "I am my ideal weight. Hoooooo!" "How long and far will I go about saying what I am not?" No, that's not the thing, you just have to build for yourself what you want. You know what? You really need to believe it to see it; if you don't believe, you can't see.

5. Affirmations Like, "I Am Super Comfortable in My Clothes"

I feel good and nice in my clothes. It sounds awkward and impractical, isn't it? The question that pops up your mind is; "how do I claim to feel good and nice when the clothes on me are not fitting, in a dress that's not my size?" The real deal is, you just got to prefer the size you aim than the weight you are now. In dressing your truth out to the physical, here is a link I can relay to you in getting clothes suiting and sweet for your size. You just need to create the feeling of fitness on clothing, otherwise, every clothes will appear not fitting you.

6. Affirmations Like, "I Wave Away Foods That Are Unhealthy for Me"

One of the wrong styles of eating or poor relationships with food is by checking how many foods you say yes to that are practically unhealthy. What if you had said no so easily? It's just the truth to say no to unhealthy food. Be intentional about it and have no regret saying it because it's going to end in good news. Don't waste money on foods that are destructive to you, invest in affirmations instead.

7. Affirmations Like, "I Am Glued to Foods and Materials Enhancing My Body"

At this, we are wrestling psychologically with two things. The old self and the new self, the old belief and the new belief, the old feelings and the new feelings, the old life and the new life, the old relationship and new relationship with food. All these are stages with the need to leave for the other. You don't have to feel a sense of denial, in the first place, what the sense of denial when you are on the path to making life good or possibly better for you.

8. Affirmations Like, "I Am Satisfied with the Necessary Amount of Food"

This is so lovely, as it regulates and exposes you to how much you have been eating and how much you should eat. Many people only stop eating when they're finished, not when they are satisfied; some just need to eat to the fullest before getting hands off the food. It doesn't work this way as it an unhealthy style of eating. This is it; say, "I had enough," "I'm done," "I feel satisfied."

9. Affirmations Like, "I No Longer Take the Protection of an Extra Weight"

Alright! Now we are hitting the nail on the head. Let it just count and appear to your senses that extra weight has nothing doing with you being protected. Come up real to the world that you don't need a protection, you've got confidence and live from the inside world within you to keep you motivated and firm.

10. Affirmation Like, "I Gaze Through the Mirror and I Can See a Healthy and Fit Body that is Pleasing Me"

It's just about you not waiting any longer but start practicing it now. Saying to yourself when looking through the mirror that I see a healthy and fit body. Can you imagine your dream body? The body that wants to emerge? The body that wants to reveal itself to you? Can you gaze through the mirror and see your incumbent experiences and see your potentials there? Just visualize it this way; what would you like? What would your legs look like? What about your arms shape and size? What will be the extent and measure of your feelings? Start expressing them now as if it's happening now. Don't wait for other people to show yourself some hits of appreciation. It must always come from you, even when others aren't.

CHAPTER 14:

Rapid Weight Loss through Affirmation

Affirmations are a pillar of New Age reasoning. Louise Hay's book "You Can Heal Your Life," which has numerous affirmations that purportedly have permitted individuals to change their lives through affirmations and representation, gives us an incredible asset in the journey for rapid weight loss. Affirmations, regardless of whether you have faith in them or not, generally appear to work.

What are affirmations? They are basic proclamations that you rehash to yourself, for all to hear, glancing in a mirror if conceivable. They are current state proclamations beginning with "I"—for instance, "I get in shape rapidly and easily." After some time, they tend to 'work out as expected' with stunning recurrence.

Beset up to feel somewhat senseless from the start—even somewhat 'counterfeit,' if you like. Try to continue saying them, paying little heed to how it feels. Luckily, you don't need to have confidence in affirmations with the goal for them to assist you with getting thinner, or change whatever else that you have to change about your life. They are truly important apparatuses. Regularly, affirmations can assist you with getting over an inability to think straight and quicken or kick off your rapid weight loss journey.

The puzzle is the reason they work. Our best estimate is that they are like hypnosis—aside from, obviously, that you 'entrance' yourself, and you remain in charge of the whole procedure. Affirmations most likely detour the cognizant mind and talk straightforwardly to the psyche, which is significantly more successful at 'completing things' than the regular cognizant mind. A significant number of our obstructions to weight loss likewise begin in the intuitive mind. The intuitive, in this manner, is the main spot wherein they can be changed and improved.

Past that, why affirmations work is impossible to say. There are numerous philosophical clarifications, no doubt. For instance, numerous individuals attest that considerations and convictions are the most remarkable thing on the planet, regarding human inspirations, capacities, and activities. There is a well-known expression that addresses that; it is ascribed to Henry Ford. The statement is as per the following: "Regardless of whether you feel that you can or that you can't, no doubt about it." That is, if you feel that you can do something, you are in all probability right, and you will succeed. If you figure you can't, in any case, you're correct once more. That conviction will prevent you from succeeding.

The majority of the purposes behind individuals' weight issues are mental or mental. They can be categorized as one of two classifications, in any case. A few of us have mental issues that cause it to appear to be more secure to convey additional weight. For instance, women who have been mishandled in the past may have a sense of security, and undetectable, if they are overweight. Men don't take a gander at them in a similar way. The women feel genuinely greater and progressively ready to take care of themselves. All that is fine, as it were. However, it comes to the detriment of one's physical well-being. If your mental need to keep weight on is inconsistent with you should be truly solid, something needs to change. Something needs to 'give' in short. Affirmations can help you over that bump.

The second mental explanation behind individuals' weight issues is less deep, yet no less risky. This reason is the improvement of unfortunate propensities, which are, obviously, very simple to create given the prevalence of cheap food and bundled nourishments, and the high-fat nourishment that most eateries appear to be set on serving us, regardless of whether we need them or not. Affirmations are extremely powerful in helping individuals' bread ruinous eating propensities. For instance, you could certify, "I oppose unfortunate nourishments" or "I pick chiefly crisp, sound food sources." Odds are, you will before long get results. These might be unpretentious from the outset—you may falter before getting that chocolate bar—yet rapidly, new propensities will be framed, and you will have the option to oppose undesirable nourishments all the more emphatically.

An expression of alert, however, affirmations ought to consistently be stated in the positive. Try not to state, "I don't eat shoddy nourishment," for instance. Expression them emphatically, "I eat" or "I pick"—and state them in the current state. That is the ideal method for ensuring that your affirmations will address your intuitive mind rapidly and successfully and that you can start building up more advantageous eating propensities.

The Psychology of Weight Loss

You might be amazed to discover that various popular individuals, one after another, experienced issues keeping up a solid weight. Be that as it may, they had the option to overcome their concern because of an as good as ever, sound perspective on eating. You may not understand it. However, there is a sure brain science grinding away in fruitful weight loss. It is nothing unexpected, at that point, that the magazine Psychology Today has investigated the issue inside and out. Quite a while back, the magazine posted an article on its site enumerating the encounters of Diane Berry, an attendant medical professional who considered women who had shed in any event 15 pounds and had kept up their weight loss for a normal of seven years.

The women shared some significant things in that manner. For example, they all accomplished their weight loss through Weight Watchers or

TOPS, which implied that they had a firm encouraging group of people as they attempted to keep up their weight. The gatherings were profoundly significant because they figured out how to perceive that they were positively not the only ones in their battles with weight. The women were likewise very abnormal because up to 90 percent of people who have shed pounds wind up returning it on inside five years.

Another normal attribute of these women is that they seemed to experience a significant state of mind move as they made the change from fat to thin. From all signs, they gave off an impression of being discouraged when they were substantial be that as it may, as they endeavored to get in shape, their disposition lit up.

For these women, smart dieting turned into a propensity—a propensity they would not break. They perceived the gigantic job that brain science plays in rapid weight loss. They would not yield to negative sentiments of dissatisfaction and forswearing and picked a positive way. The women also made it a point to gauge them consistently so they could outline their advancement.

What's more, they perceived that keeping up with weight loss would be a lifetime battle. They realized that they couldn't endeavor a weight loss program at that point set it back on the rack. They needed to learn new eating designs that they could proceed with throughout every week. At times, they compared their battle to that of a drunkard. As it were, they perceived the gravity of their concern and found a way to address the circumstance.

Maybe the most intriguing part of these women' encounters was the way that their weight loss came in spurts. Now and again, they recaptured their weight, yet they didn't let that prevent them from their last objective. They essentially saw their misfortunes as difficulties that they expected to survive. This might be the key mental quality that isolates effective dieters from fruitless ones—diligence. Generally, these women had the option to change their characters positively to accomplish their long-haul weight loss objectives.

Another fascinating part of this examination was that it indicated that the women who had experienced rapid weight loss change were cheerful. This shows the gigantic mental effect that weight loss can have on a person. When an individual is liberated from the weight of additional weight, the person is better ready to address the difficulties of life head-on. The dieter profits by uplifting feedback, as family members, companions, and associates salute that person for the weight loss. Right now, weight can be a serious invigorating encounter and can prompt a progressively idealistic point of view.

It must be noted here that the brain research of weight loss is an entangled issue. There is no single fixing that can transform a husky individual into a slender one. Nonetheless, perceiving that there is a mental part to effective weight loss may, truth be told, be a large portion of the fight. When an individual perceives that the person in question is occupied with a mental battle, the individual in question is better ready to do fight. By retraining oneself to look for sound ways to deal with diet, one can, as a result, form oneself into another individual—one that never again lives to eat, yet essentially eats to live.

Accomplishing Rapid Weight Loss through Affirmations

One of the most significant bits of putting on perpetual weight loss has nothing to do with the nourishments you eat or the activities you do. It has to do with your mindset. A few people can get in shape successfully, and afterward recover everything. In contrast, others, the individuals who have rolled out the correct improvements to their lives to get in shape, can remain slim for the remainder of their lives. The significant distinction between these two individuals is that one individual is accomplishing rapid weight loss through affirmations, frequently without acknowledging it, while the other isn't. One of the most useful assets for getting more fit is through a rapid weight loss through affirmations session.

Affirmations are an idea or an explanation that we state to ourselves, which profoundly affects how we act or feel. Contingent upon its positive or negative nature, the mind at that point demonstrations appropriately, which can prompt either a positive or negative effect on our lives. Hence, if you need to accomplish weight loss through affirmations, you have to realize how to use these methods to give you the mindset of a thin individual. Weight loss through affirmations is an underused and understudied procedure. However, the impacts can be significant.

To accomplish weight loss through affirmations, we should initially conquer our negative considerations since it is a significant supporter of our general mindset. We should relinquish these considerations as these musings are significant protection from our weight loss through assertion treatment. Rather than speculation 'I am fat' or 'I will never be thin again' have a go at deduction 'Today I have to prevail with regards to losing some of the overabundance fats' or 'I look slenderer.' These sorts of articulations prompt positive and productive outcomes.

CHAPTER 15:

Weight Loss Affirmations

Affirmations are verbal statements that help us to affirm something we believe. So often we say negative affirmations to ourselves without even realizing it. Recognize those negative thoughts and replace them with the positive affirmation that we have listed below. Repeat these to yourself on a daily basis. Write them down on a piece of paper or have notes with them on them that you leave throughout your house. Remember to practice your breathing exercises that we have learned through the other mindset exercises and keep an open mind as always.

Affirmations to Lose Weight Naturally

Losing weight is more than just looking good to me. I understand that I need to live a healthy lifestyle to feel better all of the time.

I know how to lose weight, and actually, I choose to do this in a natural way because it helps me be healthier. I know exactly what I need to do in order to get the things I deserve from this life.

I am capable of reaching all of the goals that I set for myself, and I am the one who decides what I do next with my life.

I recognize that it's important for me to be patient throughout this process. I am able to wait for the results because I know that I will get everything that I want in the end. I do not punish myself because I don't achieve a goal as fast as I had originally hoped. I nourish myself throughout this process. I constantly look for ways to encourage myself and build my self-esteem because I know that is what is going to help me feel the best in the end. I am able to control my impulses. I know how not to act on my greatest urges. I recognize the methods that will help me to enable myself to work harder in the end. I am happy because I know how to say no.

I am able to turn away when I'm confronted with an impulse. I am stronger than the biggest cravings that I have. I am proud of my ability to have a high level of willpower. I trust myself around certain foods and recognize that what tempts me does not control me.

I look to the things that I already have in my life instead of only paying attention to things that I don't have.

This is the way that will help me better achieve everything that I desire. I do not allow distractions to keep me from getting the things that I want. I am able to stay focused on my goals so that I can create the life that I deserve. In the end, even when I am tempted by something or somebody else, I know how to push through this urge and instead focus on my goals. I will wait for everything. Love is coming to me because I know that, when it does, I will feel entirely fulfilled. I am enjoying the journey and the process that it takes to get the body that I want. I recognize that small milestones are worth celebrating.

I do not wait for one big goal to be reached in order to be happy with myself. I look for all the methods needed in order to achieve greatness in this life. I understand that a temporary desire to eat something unhealthy is not worth giving up all of my goals. I know how to distract myself from my biggest cravings so that I can do something healthy instead. I recognize that doing something small is better than doing nothing at all. Even on the days that I don't want to go to the gym, I do something at home to work out so that I can at least accomplish something minor.

Just getting started is the hardest part for me, but I know how to work through those feelings now. I am emotionally aware of what might be holding me back so that I don't allow myself to be tempted by distractions.

I control my feelings and my urges so that I don't do anything that I regret. I am happy because I am knowledgeable about the things that make me who I am.

I am forgiving of myself when I do act on an impulse. I don't punish myself or deprive my body of the basic things that it needs just because I did something wrong. I sacrifice certain things that I want but never to a point where I cause punishment or torture on myself. I am successful because I am dedicated. I have strong willpower because I am successful. I move through my life with gratitude and always look to appreciate the things that I have around me. I can pick myself up when I'm feeling weak.

I appreciate even the hard parts of my life because they create the person that I am. I am an important and powerful person. I have control over my body, and nobody else does. I recognize my weaknesses, but in the same breath, I am very aware of my strengths. I balance my life with these things. I empower my strengths and thrive when I am in an environment that helps me grow. I recognize my weaknesses, and I always look for ways to turn them around in order to live more happily and healthily after. I cook meals for myself because it makes me feel healthier and stronger in the end.

I am going to get the dream body that I want because I am able to recognize things that might be healthy or unhealthy for me. I move my body at least once a day. I always feel better after I agree to a workout rather than if I try to avoid one. I am able to give myself rest when I need it. I don't push myself when I'm too stressed out because I know that this isn't going to help me get the things that I want.

I am able to always find motivation and passion within myself. I set my own goals, and I set newer and bigger ones after I achieved ones that I already completed. I do not procrastinate with my goals. I know exactly what I have to do every single day to reach these goals, and I always look for ways to go above and beyond as well. I am constantly improving the methods that I use to live a healthy lifestyle. I self-reflect productively so that I can find real solutions to any issues that I might face. I don't let what other people think take over how I see myself. I am not afraid of judgment from other people because I know that not everything negative that somebody thinks about me is something that is true.

I make the right decision for my body. I understand that even if I make wrong decisions sometimes, they all play a vital role in making me the person that I am today. These struggles are something that I had to undergo in order to become the powerful individual that I am.

I am constantly losing weight because of all this dedication and passion. I feel lighter, happier, and healthier. I am free. I am pure and clean. I am collected and calm. I am peaceful, and I am happy. I heal myself through my weight loss. I take everything bad that I did to my body in the past and turn it into something good, as I exercise and make healthy choices. I am always getting closer and closer to the things that I want. I'm focused on pushing through my biggest setbacks in order to achieve the things that I deserve. I do not sit around and fantasize about what I want anymore. Instead, I know exactly how to get this. I believe in myself because I know that this is going to be the most important part of my journey. I trust my ability to actually lose the weight, and I'm not afraid of what will happen if I don't. I know how to say these affirmations to myself when I feel better.

Other people like being around me. Others recognize my hard work. Others know that I deserve to have good things in my life. When I listened to my body, I am able to thrive. I recognize the things that my body tells me in order to get the best results possible.

I feel good, and I look even better. I look great, and I look incredible because of this. Not only does losing weight help my body to look better, but it also helps my soul, and that is something that can show through so easily to other people. I choose to do things that are good for my body. I value myself, and I have virtue in all that I do. I add value to other people's lives as well. I motivate myself, and therefore, I know how to motivate other people.

I am not afraid of anything. The worst thing that can happen to me is that I stop believing in myself. I will always be my best friend. I will always know how to encourage myself and include confidence in everything that I do. I love myself, and I am proud of the body that I have. I am perfect the way that I am, and I am beautiful. I am happy, I am healthy, and I am free. I am focused, I am centered, and I am peaceful. I am stress-free and thankful. I have gratitude and love. I am attractive, and I am perfect. There is nothing that I need to punish myself for. I accept everything that I am. I love myself. I am healthy. I am happy. I am free.

CHAPTER 16:

How Do I Pick and Use Affirmations for Rapid Weight Loss?

Choosing affirmations for your rapid weight loss journey requires you to first understand what it is that you are looking for, and what types of positive thoughts are going to help you get there. You can start by identifying what your dream is, what you want your ideal body to look and feel like, and how you want to feel as you achieve your dream of losing weight. Once you have identified what your dream is, you need to identify what current beliefs you have around the dream that you are aspiring to achieve. For example, if you want to lose 25 pounds so that you can have a healthier weight, but you believe that it will be incredibly hard to lose that weight, then you know that your current beliefs are that losing weight is hard. You need to identify every single belief surrounding your weight loss goals and recognize which ones are negative or are limiting and preventing you from achieving your goal of losing weight.

After you have identified which of your beliefs are negative and unhelpful, you can choose affirmations that are going to help you change your beliefs. Typically, you want to choose an affirmation that is going to help you completely change that belief in the opposite direction. For example, if you think "losing weight is hard," your new affirmation could be "I lose the weight effortlessly." Even if you do not believe this new affirmation right now, the goal is to repeat it to yourself enough that it becomes a part of your identity and, inevitably, your reality. This way, you are anchoring in your hypnosis sessions, and you are effectively rewiring your brain in between sessions, too.

As you use affirmations to help you achieve weight loss, I encourage you to do so in a way that is intuitive to your experience. There is no right or wrong way to approach affirmations, as long as you are using them on a regular basis. Once you feel yourself effortlessly believing in an affirmation, you can start incorporating new affirmations into your routine so that you can continue to use your affirmations to improve your well-being overall. Ideally, you should always be using positive affirmations even after you have seen the changes you desire, as affirmations are a wonderful way to help naturally maintain your mental, emotional, and physical well-being.

What Should I Do with My Affirmations?

After you have chosen what affirmations you want to use, and which ones are going to feel best for you, you need to know what to do with them! The simplest way to use your affirmations is to pick 1–2 affirmations and repeat them to yourself on a regular basis. You can repeat them anytime you feel the need to re-affirm something to yourself, or you can repeat them continually even if they do not seem entirely relevant in the moment. The key is to make sure that you are always repeating them to yourself so that you are more likely to have success in rewiring your brain and achieving the new, healthier, and more effective beliefs that you need to improve the quality of your life.

In addition to repeating your affirmations to yourself, you can also use them in many other ways. One way that people like using affirmations is by writing them down. You can write your affirmations down on little notes and leave them around your house, or you can make a ritual out of writing your affirmations down a certain amount of times per day in a journal so that you are able to routinely work them into your day. Some people will also meditate on their affirmations, meaning that they essentially meditate and then repeat the affirmations to themselves over and over in a meditative state. If repeating your affirmation to yourself like a mantra is too challenging, you can also say your chosen affirmations to yourself on a voice recording track and then repeat them to yourself on a loop while you meditate. Other people will create recordings of themselves repeating several affirmations into their voice recorder and then listening to them on loop while they work out, eat, drive to work, or otherwise engage in an activity where affirmations might be useful.

If you really want to make your affirmations effective and get the most out of them, you need to find a way to essentially bombard your brain with this new information. The more effectively you can do this, the more your subconscious brain is going to pick up on it and continue to reinforce your new neural pathways with these new affirmations. Through that, you will find yourself effortlessly and naturally believing in the new affirmations that you have chosen for yourself.

How Are Affirmations Going to Help Me Lose Weight?

Affirmations are going to help you lose weight in a few different ways. First and foremost, and probably most obvious, is the fact that affirmations are going to help you get in the mindset of weight loss. To put it simply: you cannot sit around believing nothing is going to work and expect things to work for you. You need to be able to cultivate a motivated mindset that allows you to create success. If you are unable to believe that it will come true: trust that it will not come true.

As your mindset improves, your subconscious mind is actually going to start changing other things within your body, too. For example, rather than creating desires and cravings for things that are not healthy for you, your body will begin to create desires and cravings for things that are healthy for you. It will also stop creating inner conflict around making the right choices and taking care of yourself. In fact, you may even find yourself actually falling in love with your new diet and your new exercise routine. You will also likely find yourself naturally leaning toward behaviors and habits that are healthier for you without having to try so hard to create those habits. In many cases, you might create habits that are healthy for you without even realizing that you are creating those habits. Rather than having to consciously become aware of the need for habits, and then putting in the work to create them, your body and mind will naturally begin to recognize the need for better habits and will create those habits naturally as well.

Some studies have also suggested that using affirmations will help your brain and subconscious mind actually govern your body differently, too. For example, you may be able to improve your body's ability to digest things and manage your weight naturally by using affirmations and hypnosis. In doing so, you may be able to subconsciously adjust which hormones, chemicals, and enzymes are created within your body to help with things like digestive functions, energy creation, and other weight- and health-related concerns that you may have.

We are going to explore more than affirmations you can rely on to help you lose your weight, increase your health, and feel better overall. You can use these affirmations as they are, or you can adjust them to match what you need for your own belief system.

If you do rewrite them, make sure that you are creating ones that directly reflect what you need to hear so that you can change your beliefs to ones that are more supportive and less limiting.

Affirmations for Self-Control

Self-control is an important discipline to have, and not having it can lead to behaviors that are known for making weight loss more challenging. If you are struggling with self-control, the following affirmations will help you change any beliefs you have around self-control so that you can start approaching food, exercise, weight loss, and wellness in general with healthier beliefs.

1. I have self-control.

2. My willpower is my superpower.

3. I am in complete control of myself in this experience.

4. I make my own choices.

5. I have the power to decide.

6. I am dedicated to achieving my goals.

7. I will make the best choice for me.

8. I succeed because I have self-control.

9. I am capable of working through hardships.

10. I am dedicated to overcome challenges.

11. My mind is strong, powerful, and disciplined.

12. I am in control of my desires.

13. My mindset is one of success.

14. I become more disciplined every day.

15. Self-discipline comes easily for me.

16. Self-control comes easily for me.

17. I achieve success because I am in control.

18. I find it easier to succeed every day.

19. I see myself as a successful, self-disciplined person.

20. Self-control is as natural as breathing.

21. I have control over my thoughts.

22. I have control over my choices.

23. I can trust my willpower to carry me through.

24. I can tap into self-control whenever I need to.

25. My self-control is stronger than my desire.

26. I easily maintain my self-control in all situations.

27. I see things through to the end.

28. I can depend on myself to make healthy choices.

29. Healthy choices are easy for me to make.

30. It is easy for me to control my impulses.

31. Self-control is my natural state.

32. I will keep going until I reach my goal.

33. I am starting to love the feeling of self-control.

34. I have unbreakable willpower.

35. I have excellent self-control.

36. I am a highly self-disciplined person.

37. I succeed with every goal I create.

38. I am a highly intentional person.

39. Every day, my self-control gets stronger.

40. I am becoming highly disciplined.

41. I am successful because of my self-discipline.

42. I am a strong, capable person.

43. I am dedicated to achieving my wellness goals.

44. Self-control is one of my greatest strengths.

45. I am in complete control of this situation.

46. I can do this.

47. I am self-aware and capable.

48. I can move forward with self-control and gratitude.

49. I always do what I say I am going to do.

50. I show up as my best self, and I achieve my dreams.

51. I have the willpower to make this happen.

52. I can count on myself to make the right choice.

53. I trust my strength to carry me through.

54. I am becoming stronger every day.

55. I make my choices with self-discipline.

56. I have the discipline to see this through.

57. I make my choices intentionally.

58. I am committed to my success.

CHAPTER 17:

What Are Beliefs, Patterns, and Blocks of Hypnosis Therapy to Weight Loss?

In case you are beginning the walk on hypnotherapy, you must ask yourself some questions that can be at the brim of your mind. Hypnosis has been recommended for almost everything, like stopping smoking up to losing weight. A lot of study shows that hypnosis is a commanding tool for self-development. Hypnotherapy helps people to adopt a new way of life and their beliefs. With hypnosis, you can reframe old theories like smoking will be difficult and painful to substitute them with current and assisting expectations.

Hypnosis Work on Reshaping Assumptions

Hypnosis is a vastly relaxed mind state where the psychological state is where we bypass the critical awareness. Hypnosis allows you to adjust your insentient thinking process to assist you in achieving certain goals. For instance, if you want to use hypnosis to lose weight: your mind will have a lot of perceptions when it comes to weight loss. You may end up thinking automatically that losing weight is not possible. Thus, you won't be able to abandon your favorite dishes and create time for exercise. Such perceptions created by the mind will definitely change your conscious, and you won't be able to know that it is happening. Most of the time, your perception will set you up to fail. This will lead you to bad behavior like negative personal talk, smoking, and eating too much. Using hypnotherapy, you can start to alter and update the negative perceptions. This will give an explanation of why the study toughly proposes hypnosis works for conditions such as enduring pain, abuse of drugs and losing weight.

When you teach your mind to have different thoughts about the encounters, then you can easily dismiss the negative opinions that mostly lead to personal incapacitation. Hypnosis gives you positive energy to have another option about your insensible beliefs. That is how hypnotherapy operates. Hypnosis has been here, fascinating people for many years. In the 19770s Austrian physician did an experiment placing patients into a dream-like state. After then play music, dim the lights, and apply reduction procedures. He had eccentric perception thoughts to know what happens in the dreamland, such as he infused patients with undetectable compelling liquids. The physician was wrong with his conclusions and spark gathered curiosity in the knowledge of hypnosis.

Making choices on food can't be an issue due to it being in plenty. People in the city will have access to many restaurants, food joints, groceries, and cafes. This definitely will give a lot of temptation and eat whenever you feel hungry or when you sense a delicious smell. There are major topics that you need to be aware of when you want to have a positive impact of hypnosis to reduce or lose weight.

Every belief will have a connection with food. Food has been considered to be vital to all living things, but it's very key to human beings. It has collective implications and some rituals surrounding it. This is a bull's eye point in life. Despite your environment, occupation, upbringing or your habitat, food has a big role in your day-to-day life. Such a statement makes sense when you think about it, and in the modernized world, food is essential and is taken three times a day. Most people control their feeding habits by coming up with excuses such as "I am eating to survive." Nevertheless, such statements are just exceptional and not a rule.

Most traditions take food as the central point of celebrations such as weddings, birthdays, engagements anniversaries and many more. Most of the occasions are revolving around food. There is various importance of food according to the traditions within it. Like in African traditions, it's considered a ritual and also a collective role. For you to understand a discipline with food, you have to get it right about the culture they grew up in. You have to really explore for you to get to know a person's culture and what influence it has on food. When you are using hypnosis to cut your weight, you are advised to have a three to six-months program. You can even extend it one year if you find it necessary for you as this is essential to handle your food issues.

Losing Weight

Weight loss can be a hectic procedure and has not been made at ease by the conflicting, risky advice out there in the biosphere. You can be blasted with TV programs advertising images of food, and these activities can make you be tempted to lose concentrate on healthy living. There are pills that bring about weight loss that will restrict you from what you are eating and what you are taking. You won't be astonished by how you have established negative perceptions around what you eat. Hypnosis, when it comes to losing weight, is the best technique for stimulating theses mentalities and flashes of enticement that will assist you in having a better life.

Hypnotherapy for the loss of weight is to make you have confidence about your body, have positive perceptions about eating, and assist you in reducing your weight responsibly without having negative emotions about your well-being. A hypnotherapist can help you have a positive association with exercise and food when you have an insensible mind. This is a very critical method as it will help in healthy weight loss and a long duration of managing your weight. Many people want to reduce weight, not considering if they are overweight or not. Study shows that a lot of people are not proud of their body size and shape irrespective of whether they need to drop mass.

Confidence of the Body

It is very important for you to lose mass due to health purposes if you are overweight, you are allowed to feel bad about wanting to reduce your mass. Shape and size of the body are compatible with beauty; thus, a lot of people are in a hurry for solutions about mass loss. You will be likely to try to take mass loss pills or going to the gym just to try and cut your weight. When you have decided to do that, you have to ask yourself if you are happy and want to go on with the process for the rest of your life. From this point is where hypnotherapy for mass reduction can assist. For you to have changes in your body, you also have to change your mind. There are queries you have to ask yourself, like why are you not happy with your body, and why are you not reducing your mass? Hypnotherapy for mass reduction has increased popularly, and people worldwide are getting it a positive process assisting in enhancing a healthy mass in the coming times ahead. During such moments of the hypnotherapy sessions, you will get to know that you have to adjust your negative characters and feeding designs with the positive ones as directed by your hypnotherapist. During hypnosis for mass reduction, the following will happen:

- You will be guided by your hypnotherapist to a state of profound relaxation.

- After your body and brain are cooled down, your hypnotherapist will now have the ability to study your insensible brain.

- Soothing, cautiously articulated scripts can be castoff to discover a consumer's explanations for feeding a lot and give other ways of thinking through therapies. You have the room to refuse any recommendations you don't want and aren't happy about it or haven't been guided by your hypnotherapist.

Techniques Hypnotherapy Use for Rapid Weight Loss

Every case is not the same as everyone got their own reasons as to why they want to reduce in mass; there are some recommendations that you might come across:

- You must envision your body the way you want, or to the level of fitness and health, you want to attain.
- Just try to think of how you will feel with your new appearance and health.
- Think about how to be there effortlessly.
- Have a look at how you are improving daily.
- Think about how energized and confident you will feel.
- When you get to know that with more exercise, It's the more you will be exercising, and it will be much easier.

The methods have been put up to encourage and inspire you and assist you in taking charge of your choices.

When you have negative thoughts about some foods being unhealthy, hypnotherapy for food addiction can be of help to cut out such negative thoughts.

With the help of weight reduction hypnosis, you can enjoy the taste of healthy meals and stop craving for fatty and sugary foods. Hypnosis for mass loss will assist you in adopting a healthier life pattern and happier mentality by tackling the deep feelings that bring about the creation of your feeding habits.

Your Probable Mass Loss Blocks

Many people are trying and failing to lose weight for a number of whys and wherefores. Reasons which can also be referred to as "secondary gains" are most of the time insensible, thus being difficult for you to overwhelm them. When you have focused on reducing or cutting your mass, you must look at the belief that has kept your mass for that period. Most of us have beliefs where we think about ourselves, value and what we want as humans. Insensible characters will take away your emotional opinions towards yourself.

A clinical hypnotherapist, Amreeta Chapman, explored the hurdles humans can experience when trying to cut mass. Most of you will gain comfort when you don't make any change, thus feeling secure just being the way you are. You may want to reduce mass, but the insensible things are baring you from making them happen. Hypnotherapy for mass reduction helps to solve such reasons, thus making patients have a break from hurdles that prevent you from reducing mass over a period of years.

Comfort Eating

When you are still an infant, you will associate eating with the help of your mother. A lot of professionals have been able to prove that the association never gets over; thus, when life gets stressful, you can look back at the previous days of full dependence. From this point, emotional eating can be hectic. At times, you can get yourself going for a chocolate bar after a tiresome day or having a takeaway when you are all alone and sad; this can make you a relaxed eater. When you are a comfort eater, then there will be some difficulties in cutting your weight as you will have been compatible with food and without it, you can't be able to handle your sensations.

Hypnotherapy will assist you in addressing this, make you learn how to handle negative sensations in a way that won't bring about comfortability in your feeding. The greatest change you can have is being less bothered about feeding. You can still have fun but teach your body to eat only when you are hungry and not when the brain feels like it and want to appease those feelings. Hypnotherapy has assisted so many people in stunning their passionate eating.

CHAPTER 18:

Sharp Your Mind to Shape Your Body

Perfect Mind, Perfect Weight

Perfect thoughts and ideal weight." The term may seem like a fantasy to you. Which is the ideal mind or ideal weight? They're the realistic conditions you'll be able to utilize as you pursue fat reduction. "Realistic?" You inquire. "How can anything be 'ideal,' let alone my burden and my ideas about my burden?" Well, recall what we said about the strength of believing and belief. Is it serving your curiosity to desire or hope to anything less than perfection on your own? Indulge us for some time as we clarify why you're able to think your mind and burden because "perfect."

Perfect fat is your weight that's ideal for you. It's the weight that's attainable and consistent with everything you need and precisely what you're ready to give yourself and accept yourself. More to the point, your ideal weight provides you with the healthy entire body, the human body which goes effortlessly, and also the one where you are feeling great about yourself and joyful. And what're ideal thoughts? You presently have a mind. It's flawless. But there can be a few ideas in that ideal thought of yours who are providing you with undesirable outcomes. There can be something that you keep in your mind, possibly habits or routines, which provide you with undesirable outcomes. However, you may use your ideal head to match your ideas to offer you precisely what you desire. It's possible to use your head to accomplish the bodyweight that you desire.

In the Twinkling of an Eye

Your current body is the consequence of your ideas and beliefs. You've behaved out these ideas and beliefs by your lifestyle, which generated your current weight. You haven't made any errors, regardless of what you may be thinking of yourself; instead, you've just experienced undesirable outcomes. These undesirable effects are an immediate effect of misaligned ideas and beliefs about yourself, which are very patterns of behavior or lifestyle. The Rapid Weight Loss Hypnosis is all about utilizing your perfect thoughts.

To align your ideas to provide you with the results you desire. You honestly can use your head to accomplish the bodyweight you desire. Let's take a look at a few of the learning that has occurred in your life, which has let you know where you're now together with your body weight. Do you wake up one afternoon, and you had been using the additional pounds? Or could it be a slow accumulation with time? Or perhaps you've understood nothing else as early youth. Whatever the situation, there are lots of factors that made your body:

- Food options
- Eating customs
- That the self-critic in you
- Economic history
- Psychological history
- Impact of household
- Impact of buddies
- Cultural heritage

These and several other variables were discovered in your life and eventually became the beliefs, which subsequently became routines of activity that generated your body. In other words, consider what you did understand about your youth about eating and food.

- What kinds of grocery stores did your household buy?
- What foods did your kids cook, and were they typically ready?
- Can you eat only at home or often grab food?
- Have you been served fresh, healthy, high-calorie foods, or can you eat mainly processed and extremely processed foods, fried foods, and "junk" foods?
- Was there aware focus on nutrition, or has been there any irresponsible disregard for that which your household ate?
- What did you find out about eating mindfully?
- Were you educated that healthful food options led to healthy bodies?
- Did anybody teach you how you can understand what's healthy food and what's not?
- Are your meals selections based on which tasted or seemed high or priceless?
- Can your loved ones or college instruct you about healthy lifestyles and audio nourishment, or has been the "nutrition education" through TV advertisements and food makers' advertising?

What exactly did you learn as a kid? What're your beliefs about eating food, along with your entire body? Analyze your own socioeconomic or socio-cultural roots and see if they had an effect on the way and what you've learned to consume. Over thirty-five Years Back, sociological research pointed out weight issues in the working and lower class according to their intake patterns of what's been known as "poverty-level foods," like hot dogs, canned meats, and processed luncheon meats.

Cultural groups also have been analyzed to understand their nutritional patterns and meals, like eating with lard or ingesting a diet of fried and high-fat foods, which can lead to higher body fat loss. These influences can readily be accepted because they're "regular" into the category, of course. Then let's take a look in the teen years. During adolescence, are there some changes in your weight loss? Just as a boy, have you been invited to pile more food on your plate? "Look at him eating! Certainly, he will develop to a large guy!" (There's a telling metaphor) Or are you currently admonished to eat? When you're a budding young woman, did a Smart girl take you under her wing and then discuss with you that the marvel of menses and the wonderment of body modifications, such as the organic growth in body fat with all the evolution of breasts and broader hips?

Were you conscious during puberty which unless the body improved body fat by 22 percent, it wouldn't correctly grow and create menses? Or was that "hushed up" within an awkward improvement? It was likely during adolescence which you heard there's a stigma involving obese individuals. Ponder the encounters and influences which are forming your body. In high school, the athletes at college sports have always been a healthful weight and are the cheerleaders and homecoming queens.

What ancient beliefs regarding your popularity and self-image could have formed from your social interactions in high school? What did you understand about physical activity, and what customs did you produce? Have you been introduced to physical activity as part of a healthy lifestyle, through family or sports outings of walks or hikes? Or was that the blaring TV a regular fixture, enticing everybody to the sofa? Next is a matter which most people have never been aware of throughout their development.

As you're growing up, has been that the attention of self-care based on trendy clothes, makeup, and hairstyles, or about healthful food, routine physical activity, along with spiritual and intellectual nourishment? What about today? Spend a couple more minutes writing down the aspects that appear to be accurate for you in the past couple of decades. What influences and experiences formed the ideas, which turned into the beliefs that turned into your body?

After high school, you moved away from the house. Suddenly you're no more captive to your family lifestyle. Can you be aware of your options, or can you start eating with blow off? If you input into a close connection, just what compromises or arrangements about foods and physical activity did you input into too? Most associations develop from similar pursuits, including food preferences and eating styles. In the end, the relationship comprises eating routines and tastes, which are a consequence of compromise.

Have your connections encouraged smart food choices and healthy eating? Maybe you've experienced pregnancy. Can you learn the way to get a wholesome pregnancy and then nourish a healthy infant within you? Or did you put in pounds? After giving birth, how did your lifestyle assist you in recovering your typical fat or suppressing it? If you were more active in the league or sports games, did your livelihood or family duties take priority and eliminate these physical fitness tasks from your regular? Can you correct exercise and diet so, or even did the fat begin to collect? Did an accident, injury, or disease happen that disrupted a standard physical action that has been supportive of healthy fat?

Because you can see, the way you got to where you're now was no crash. You heard from the folks about you—or you also consumed out of the surroundings—the best way to create food decisions, the way to eat, and the way to look after yourself emotionally and physically. Whether the thoughts you heard were tremendous and healthy or not so high and not as healthy, they became your own beliefs, and eventually became you and the own human body because it is now. Bear in mind, and you didn't do something wrong; however, you need to experience the outcomes of eating and living, which have been consistent with your ideas and beliefs.

Through time, what's been your answer to individuals and their opinions about your weight loss, bad or good? Can you go out and purchase a fantastic pair of sneakers, or do you consume to facilitate psychological distress? Maybe you even heard the latter response on your youth.

Did your mom ever provide you with a plateful of food to comfort you when you're miserable? These are learned answers, and they may be unlearned and replaced with new answers and routines to make your ideal weight. Just ask, "Just how long does this happen?" We inform you, "In the twinkling of an eye," For the minute that you understand that you need it sufficient to get anything to possess it, it's completed. You've just altered the management of highly efficient energy in you, which will be directed at figuring out how to attain the outcome which you need: your ideal weight.

Your Perfect Mind Relearning

It's simple to comprehend how you got or "heard" to contemplate over your ideal weight. And it'll be simple to create new decisions, to relearn new routines, and also to make new and much more healthful habits. How can we learn? We understand by mimicking another individual, analyzing books with different tools and practicing the activities that create the outcomes we all seek. The best and lasting learning entails repetition and practice. The best way to practice is essential. Pretend for a minute that you're a violinist. You're searching for a grand symphony operation in New York.

The critical thing is that you're giving your focus on practicing correctly.

Heal Your Relationship with Food

As you can see, the desire to reduce sugar is not easy. It becomes not only our habit, but we also become physically dependent on it. It disturbs our health and even our overall functioning as individuals in the society.

A Simple and Magical Solution Does Not Exist

Yes, there are foods that are healthy and which can replace sugar, but it takes discipline and a change of lifestyle.

In the morning, after a night when you don't eat, your blood sugar level is the lowest and we should eat a meal that provides a constant increase of sugar to avoid hunger attacks. It is best that this meal contains a combination of protein and complex carbohydrates (bread, pasta) because they are digested slowly.

This is about enough for me to start the day. Fruit also causes relatively rapid rises in blood sugar, and therefore it might be better to eat it in the afternoon after lunch, but with a gap as it is quickly digested and absorbed best on an empty stomach. This will help in the afternoon when our energy is lowered, and will not have such a yo-yo effect on blood sugar as chocolate or ice cream.

CHAPTER 19:

Overcoming Negative Habits

Fortunately, most of our days have a sort of "groove." Actions in a plan that you perform with little thought are performed almost automatically. Otherwise, our lives become tediously complicated, and we spend a lot of time figuring out how to tie our shoes, prepare our meals, go to work, and more. In this way, we can carry out our daily routines with almost no thought and focus our attention on more demanding activities. Repetitive work in life becomes a habit.

Habits can also be undesirable, and these grooves are deeply rooted in today's patterns. They are against us because they waste our time. For example, if you know that you have a limited amount of time to get to work after waking up in the morning, you'll notice that in the middle of breakfast you'll find the morning paper at the table, pick it up, and usually spend the next hour studying. Spend In the daily news, you could spend a good deal of the rest of your time explaining delays or looking for new jobs.

By the way, in our discussion of habits, we call them "desired" or "undesired" rather than "good" or "bad." The words "good" and "bad" have moral implications. These mean certain decisions. In the example cited in the paragraph above, reading a newspaper is not morally "bad," but not desirable at this time.

The terms "desired" and "undesirable" are the terms "ego," meaning self-determination, not decisions made externally. As with psychoanalysis, our goal is to push material from the "conscience" camp into the "ego" realm.

In many cases, you may even say that removing unnecessary habits requires more than a simple choice. You may want to consciously discard your habits, but fulfilling a wish is a very different matter. There are several reasons for this. First, habits are inherent in their definition and are deeply rooted in their behavior, so they are reflected without thinking. Just thinking "I don't do" does not necessarily affect us deep enough to stop unwanted behavior.

The longer the habit we have with us, the more often we do it, the more secure it will be, and the harder it will be to wipe it off. Please quit overeating. It is not uncommon to start eating without knowing it when already taken a full meal or when absorbed in conversation or work. Such behaviors are driven into individual behavioral patterns dozens of times a day, daily, and over ten years, actually becoming a second cortex that is as natural as breathing (ironically, overcoming eating habits are becoming increasingly difficult for people).

Such habits have physical-neurologic-foundation. The neural pathways in our body can be compared to unpaved roads. This road is smooth before vehicles drive on dirt roads. When a car first rides on the road, its tires leave marks, but the ruts are flat. Rain and wind can easily pass by and smooth the road again. However, after 100 rides with deeper and deeper tires, rain and wind make little impression on the deep ruts. They stay there.

The same applies to people. To expand the metaphor a little, we were born with a smooth street in our heads. When a young child first buttons a jacket or ties a shoe, the effort is tedious, clumsy, and frustrating. More trials are needed until the child gets the hang of it, and a successful move becomes a behavioral pattern.

From a physiological point of view, these movement instructions travel along nerve paths to the muscles and back again. The message is sent to the central nervous system along an afferent pathway. The "I want to lift my legs" impulse continues in the efferent pathway from the central nervous system to my muscles: "Raise my legs." After a while, such messages are automatically enriched by countless repetitions and automatically sent at electrical speed.

Return to the car and the street. Suppose the car decides to avoid a worn groove and take a new path. What will happen is that the car will go straight back into the old ditch. Like people trying to get out of old habits, they tend to revert to old habits.

Still, we haven't developed any unwanted habits. We learn them, and we can rewind the learning. It can be unconditional. And here, self-hypnosis takes place, pushing the individual out of the established habit gap in a smooth manner of new behavior.

The advantage it offers compared to simple willpower trial and error results from an increase in the state of consciousness that characterizes the state of self-hypnosis. A further extension of the unpaved road analogy is that the hovercraft slides a few centimeters above the road, over a rut or habit. Regardless of the habit of working, the implementation process is the same. Only the verbal implant and the image below are different. To encapsulate the induction process, count one, for one thing, two for two things and count three for three things:

1. Please raise your eyes as high as possible.
2. Still staring, slowly close your eyes and take a deep breath.
3. Exhale, relax your eyes, and float your body. Then, if time permits, spend a little more time and introduce yourself to the most comfortable, calm, and pleasant place in your imagination.

Now, when you float deep inside the resting chair, you will feel a little away from your body. It's another matter, so you can give instructions on how to behave.

At this point, the specific purpose of self-hypnosis determines the expression and image content of the syllogism. It provides suggestions for discussing different habits that can be followed as shown or modified as needed. This strategy can help overcome the habit of overeating.

Overall, we are a country boasting abundant food. Most of us (with the blatant and lamentable exception) have enough money to make sure we are comfortably overeating. As a result, many of us get obese. So, the weight-loss business is a big industry. Tablet makers, diet developers, and exercise studios will not confuse customers who want to lose weight.

It is said that every fat person who has a hard time escaping has lost weight. Unfortunately, too often, the lean man spends his life, nevertheless never succeeding in his escape. Despite the image of a funny fat man, everyone rarely enjoys being overweight—most people become unhappy, rarely so confident, and less than confident and ruining their lives. Obesity seems to creep on only some of us, and by the time we notice it, it is a painful habit to overeat or eat, like the excess weight itself.

Self-hypnosis can help this lean man release his bond of "too hard" and start a new life. An article in the International Journal of Clinical and Experimental Hypnosis (January 1975) reports on such cases. Sidney E. and Mitchell P. Pulver, cite family doctors, study hypnosis in medical and dental practice.

Dr. Roger Bernhardt, while mentioning one of his overweight patients, said that "I brought the patient to the hospital for about a year and a half ago. She went to many doctors to cut back. She said she was rarely leaving home because she was extremely obese; she was relaxing and avoiding people. She came in for £380. I started Trans in my first session. She continued on a diet and focused on telling her she would like people when she lost weight. She came for the first three or four sessions each week, after which I started teaching her self-hypnosis. Now, this woman lost a total of £150, but beyond that, she became another person. She was virtually introverted and rarely came out of her home. She dared to do a part-time job in cosmetics. She hosts a party to show off her cosmetics and hypnotizes herself before the party. She became the state's second-largest saleswoman and earned tens of thousands of dollars."

Simply put, here are the therapies you should use when using self-hypnosis for weight management. After provoking self-hypnosis, mentally recite the syllogism. "I need my body alive. To the extent I want to live, I protect my body just as I protect it."

In the case of a tie mate picture, one can imagine himself in two situations where he is likely to overeat: between meals and at the dining table. With his eyes closed, he imagines a movie screen on the wall. He is on the screen himself, in every situation he finds when he is reading, chatting with others, watching TV, or having trouble calorie counting.

Instead of reaching for popcorn, potato chips, or peanuts as before, he is now simply focusing on the conversation, the television screen, or the printed page, perhaps except for a glass of water, and I congratulate you on being unfamiliar with anything at the table.

The second scene that catches your eye is the dining table. Do you tend to grab this second loaf? Instead, put your hand on your forehead and remember, "Protect my body." Looking at a cake, a loaf, a potato, or a cake raises the idea, "This is for someone. I'm good enough." With the fork down, take a deep breath and be proud to help one-person flow through the body.

Then, imagine a very simple and effective exercise method that simply puts your hand on the edge of the table and pushes it. Better yet, stand up from the chair and leave the table at this point.

Here's another image I'd recommend to a self-hypnotist. If you introduce yourself to the screen of this fictional movie, you will find yourself slim. Give yourself the ideal line that you want to see to others. Cut the abdomen and waistline to the desired ratio. Take an imaginary black pencil, sketch the entire picture, and make the lines sharp and solid. Hold the picture because you can keep this one, you can lose weight.

Then get out of your hypnosis and repeat it regularly every few hours. Exercise is especially useful during the temptation to be used as a comfortable, calorie-free substitute for fatty snacks or as an additional serving with meals. It would be a good time to practice it just before dinner.

CHAPTER 20:

Stop Sugar Cravings Hypnotic Session

While on your weight loss journey, you may notice that you are craving sugar more than you normally would. This is completely normal, especially when you are suddenly cutting out sugar when you have formerly been consuming large amounts of it throughout the day. Sugar is an addictive substance. And like all addictive substances, it can be beaten through the power of the mind. All you need is to reprogram your conscious and subconscious mind to be stronger and more resilient against such cravings.

You are taking the first positive steps towards beating those cravings right now. But before we can begin, make sure that you are sitting comfortably. Give yourself a moment to get nice and comfortable in a chair. Keep your eyes open at this point. You will be closing them on, but only when we will be getting deeper into the hypnosis.

Now take in a deep, refreshing breath. Imagine that the air you are breathing in is bringing in a feeling of safety and security. Hold the air inside for a couple of seconds, so then those feelings of safety and security can move through your body. Then, as you breathe out, imagine that the air leaving your body is carrying away any feelings of tension or impatience. Impatience or lack of attention is two of the most common issues many people have when taking part in hypnosis. By imagining that your exhalation is helping to carry those feelings away, you are helping your mind feel more comfortable powering down and taking this time for yourself.

Do this a couple more times and then just breathe normally. Turn your attention to your body. Find the areas where you feel completely comfortable and relaxed. Really focus your mind on those areas of your body. Now imagine that you have mentally taken hold of those feelings, like you have gently scooped them up in your arms. Now imagine that you are releasing that feeling across your body. Notice how it is starting to spread, so then you feel completely relaxed from head to toe.

Feel the lines on your forehead relax. The skin on the top of your head is relaxing. Feel that sensation moving down your face. Around your cheeks and your mouth. Around your eyes. As your eyes start to relax, you can gently allow the lids to close. Just shut the rest of the world out now. All you need to focus on is your body becoming more comfortable. Becoming more relaxed. Feel how your jaw is starting to loosen slightly. Maybe your mouth even drops open a little. Your entire head is just completely relaxed.

And now those calming sensations are just moving further through your body. Over your shoulders. Just allow them to drop so they're nice and loose. Feel how your arms are becoming heavier. All the little muscles in your hands and your wrists gently relaxing. All the tension just floating away. And now further down into your chest. Notice how the rhythm of your heart is slowing as your whole body becomes more peaceful. Notice the rise and fall of your ribs as you naturally breathe in and out. The muscles and bones rising on the in-breath and then lowering and gently releasing on the out-breath.

Now move down to your stomach. Feel it rise and fall with the breath. The muscles tighten as the air enters the body. And then relaxing as the air leaves. Notice how relaxing this natural sensation feels. Just the air flowing through you. Natural and life-preserving. A wonderful feeling.

Moving down further now to your hips. Feel them loosen and sink a little deeper into the chair. Now down to your pelvis and your thighs. Feel the muscles becoming heavy as they sink deeper and deeper into the chair with each passing moment. Fully experiencing the feeling of total comfort and relaxation.

Feel the tension leaving your knees as they start to relax. And now further down to your calves as they start to feel warm and comfortable. And further down still now to your feet. Notice how comfortable they feel resting on the floor. How they are rooted to the earth. Almost like calming energy is being passed into your body from the ground.

Do a quick scan of your whole body now. Take in the feeling of relaxation all the way through you. If you notice any tension or discomfort you may have missed, that's okay. Simply imagine that the air you are breathing in is traveling to those tense areas. And then the air is carrying that tension out of your body as you breathe out. Notice how by imagining this in your mind, the tension is slowly starting to leave your body. You're now totally free to feel completely relaxed.

We will now start to count down from ten to one. And when we hit one, you will fall into a deep state of perfect relaxation. A state where you will be able to take in everything that I am telling you as it enters your subconscious mind. Remember, you are completely safe and secure in this hypnosis. Now is a great time to feel relaxed and completely at peace.

Ten. Sinking deeper into your seat now. Nine. Breathing becoming more shallow and deeper. Eight. All your muscles becoming loose and heavy. Seven. Six. Five. A wonderful feeling of comfort washing over you. Four. Feeling heavier now. Three. You feel so warm and secure. Two. A feeling of safety and securing gently washing over you. One. Completely relaxed now. Your entire body and your mind completely free of tension or intrusive thoughts. Just completely relaxed.

Now that you are relaxed, you can start thinking about why you have taken this hypnosis session. You want to beat your sugar cravings. Having an addiction or a regular craving for sugar is completely normal.

Many people have these cravings, quite often without even directly knowing that it is linked to sugar. The worthy update is that it is very easy to beat.

Whenever you have a craving for sugar, try eating a fruit that has a high natural sugar level, such as an apple or an avocado. This will help you keep those cravings at bay. And if you have sugar in your tea or coffee, try using a low-fat honey instead to keep your drinks sweet.

But aside from the practical fixes, it's important that you have the right mindset. So, I want you to envisage that you have in your hand a bag of sugar. You open the bag and start to tip the sugar out of the bag onto the floor. You look down and see that you are, in fact, not pouring the sugar onto the floor. Instead, you are pouring it down a large waterfall. You watch all the white grains slowly starting to disappear as they hit the water.

As you watch this happening, you feel a positive feeling washing over you. Being able to turn your back on sugar like this is making you feel good. You feel strong and confident. You feel like you have good willpower and that you would be able to resist having a sugary drink or a snack in the future.

Tell yourself, "You are more than your cravings. The foods and drinks you desire do not make you who you are. They also don't make you weak or bad at losing weight. Remember that everyone has cravings like this. And also remember that they can be beaten."

Say to yourself, "I can beat my cravings. I do not want to have any sugary drinks or snacks. I have complete control over what I put in my body and I only want to consume things that are good for me. I know that if I resist it that I will be able to beat it. Having a positive mindset about my cravings is all I need in order to beat them. I know that I am strong enough to resist."

You know that you can beat your cravings. The power to beat them is within you. All you have to do is unlock the confidence and the strong will deep inside you in order to do it. I believe you can do it.

With each day that passes, you are moving closer and closer to your ideal body and ideal weight. Do not let sugar cravings derail this journey for you. You know that you deserve to have the results you want. All you have to do is beat these sugar cravings until they never bother you anymore.

Now, start to imagine that a warm energy is coming through the ground. As it comes through the ground, it will enter into your body through your feet. As I count from five down to one, it will spread through your body, giving you confidence and a new strong will to hold off your sugar cravings. Once I reach the number one, you will open your eyes and fully embrace this new feeling of mental toughness and positive mental attitude.

Five. Feel the energy coming through your feet up into your legs now. A feeling of confidence and strength. You know that you can beat your cravings as long as you put your mind to it.

Four. The energy is now moving up into your pelvis and your hips and stomach. It's a warm, soothing energy that is starting to swirl around you. With each number, you feel more comfortable with your cravings. More confident that you will have full control over them from now on.

Three. The energy moves up again to your chest. Feel it fill your heart with a wonderful feeling. You feel so happy that you have been able to take this positive step towards beating your cravings for good.

Two. The energy now flows through into your arms and your hands. Wiggle your fingers a little as you feel the energy swirling around you. Tell yourself, "From now on, I will not be a slave to my cravings. From now on, my cravings will do what I tell them to do."

One. Feel the energy reach your head. It swirls around until it reaches your brain. And as you picture the energy lighting up your brain, you open your eyes. Smile as you take in a nice, deep, refreshing breath; slowly breathe out now as you begin the following step of your weight loss journey, knowing that you are now more confident than ever that you can beat those sugar cravings for good.

CHAPTER 21:

Rapid Weight Loss Hypnosis Sessions

Start by taking a deep breath in... then, let it out slowly. Make sure that you are seated comfortably and that you are somewhere safe where you can relax for twenty minutes or so. During this session, you will ignore all daily noises like the telephone ringing, traffic sounds outside or any other sounds except for sounds of alarm. If you hear an alarming sound, you will immediately come out of the trance state with no residual sleepiness.

Relax... take another breath in... and out. Let go of all of the stress that you are holding onto. Relax... breathe in... and out.

Start by relaxing the muscles in your feet and legs. Think of each muscle one by one and let them all just let go and relax. Feel a warmth spreading from your toes up to your calves... feel the warmth go to your thighs and as it moves across your body, feel each muscle group that it reaches completely let go and relax.

Relax your stomach muscles... and moving up to your chest and shoulders. Feel the warmth move up your body and relax... breathe in... and out... now your neck muscles are feeling warm and relaxed. Feel all of the muscles in your face relax completely.

Imagine yourself at the top of an escalator. As you step onto the escalator, you realize that you are passing numbers on white signs on the way down. The first number is 10. As you pass each number, you will fall deeper and deeper into a relaxed state. Take another deep breath in... 9... the escalator is moving you slowly forward and down... 8...

you are becoming more and more relaxed each time you pass a number... 7... relax your body completely and let go of everything... 6... you reach the halfway point of the slow-moving escalator... 5... you are very relaxed now... completely relaxed... 4... you feel as if you are floating down the escalator becoming more and more relaxed... 3... you can see the bottom and when you reach it you will become even more deeply relaxed than you are now... 2... you reach the bottom of the escalator... 1... breathe in... and out... very relaxed now...

With each of the suggestions that I give to you, you will become more deeply relaxed than before. Each of these suggestions will stay in your subconscious and they will be used to influence your behavior when you awake... continue to relax as each suggestion is given...

You no longer have to eat too much food to feel the good feelings about yourself that the food provides... your feelings are good as they are...

When you feel an emotion, your response is to eat. However, you don't need to do that. When you feel anxiety, you should slow down and try to find the cause. You don't need to overeat to solve anxiety. Overeating will not solve the problem; it will only make it worse. If you feel depressed, that means that it is time to spring into action. When you feel frustrated, what you have been doing may not be working and instead of eating, try something else. If you feel stressed, you will not become less stressed by eating. Instead, try to relax and take things one by one as they come. If you feel the emotion of loneliness, try to surround yourself with people instead of food.

Eating will not satisfy these emotions. When you feel these emotions, your response will be to do something other than eating. In the future, you will find it easier to understand these emotions and you will not feel compelled to eat. Your feelings are there to guide you through life and each one means something different. Your response to these will no longer be to eat. Instead, you will allow each emotion to happen and then take action.

In the future, you will be free from the cycle that you have fallen into in the past. Eating will not solve any problems, even temporarily, and will only make you feel worse. Eating should only be done when you are hungry and you should eat until you are no longer hungry. When you find yourself tempted to make large portions, you will have the willpower to say no and you will be very satisfied with the amount you have.

When you have other emotions, they are not hunger. Those are simply emotions and eating will not make them go away. You will remember these things when you awake. As I count up from 1 you will start to feel more awake, but still remembering all the suggestions given... 2... you are coming up... 3... you are starting to feel less relaxed and more alert... 4... when you awake at the end of the count, you will feel refreshed and ready to continue your daily activities... 5... you are more awake now... 6... 7... 8... 9... you will wake up completely refreshed on the number 10...

Self-confidence is essential to progress well in your life. Not enough confidence prevents you from going to the maximum of what you can do and from developing fully. But too much self-confidence, pretension, will shut your doors. Therefore, self-confidence is good as long as you don't go to extremes: be honest with yourself and trust yourself. How to successfully achieve this goal? With only a little practice.

Nothing is sexier than a woman who radiates confidence!

CHAPTER 22:

Rapid Weight Loss without Diet

How often did you try a diet? We don't remember how many ways we struggled to lose weight. As an "ordinary" girl, during the 47 years of our life, we have tried to lose weight for a long time. Sadly, we do not belong to the metabolism of people who allow them to eat anything without gaining weight. While we enjoy food and drink, my body turns any extra calories into fat. But-and here is the good news-we have handled my weight effectively over the years. We are 1, 75 meters tall and weigh about 60 kilograms (its 5 feet 9 inches, 132 pounds for the United States). If we can, you can, too. You can. My secret: Forget about all diets and please your soul and body.

My qualification: You might tell me about my credentials for the subject "weight loss without diet": we're not a food expert. We served as a professional journalist for newspapers and radio in Germany for a decade, but we are now specialized in information collection and processing. We have also been struggling with weight problems for many years. When we grew up, we passed a two-year "Anorexia nervosa" phase, although we were not correctly diagnosed and treated as such at this stage. Fortunately, it didn't last long enough. When we were divorced at the age of 29, my binge eating disorder reappeared. This period we received a lot of supportive psychotherapy.

So, from a layman, we dare say that diets make you fat.

There are exceptions, of course, if you are super-rich and can afford your chef or diet caterer, this rule may not apply to you. However, for the average person who follows a diet, it is too restrictive to succeed for a long time. Who needs to weigh every bit before eating? What wants to eat what a diet tells you exactly? A diet does not leave space for urges and appetites, so a diet makes us continuously feel dissatisfied and restrained.

I firmly believe that a slim body can only be a satisfied, well-nourished body. Our bodies convey in cravings their desires. When a strawberry thought makes my mouth water, we suppose that my body needs a strawberry, and only a strawberry can give me the satisfaction that makes me feel good and better.

The body gets used to a low-calorie intake if you adopt a diet. Once you start eating normal again, your body packages happily, and all your effort is lost. This is particularly true for any fasting or crash diet: once we fasted for three weeks absolutely and lost our weight. Nonetheless, my slim body lasted just one week. When we began again to eat, my body jumped at all the calories it was denied-a very frustrating experience, not to mention the exhausting mental fight for three weeks to refrain from eating.

According to my experience, you have to understand why your body looks like it before you lose any extra pounds.

There are many explanations for overweight, but we dare say: the bulk of overweight we bear is ingrained in our subconscious. Explanations for overweight: We prefer to pile on pounds if we take life too hard. Will you put on your shoulders too much responsibility? Do you like to do more than you could? Or are you suffering from depression without it being realized?

We have to dig within ourselves if we want to shift our weight. Perhaps you have just too much enjoyed the culinary pleasures of life and thus put in additional pounds. On the other side, why do you need food or drink to relax?

It may sound transparent and pseudo-psychological now, but we were there, and we know what we are talking about. If you have been seriously struggling with your weight for many years, you must seek the help of a good psychotherapist or get psychological assistance in all ways. A friend's sympathetic ear cannot be underestimated.

Only when you find out what makes you fat will you lose weight.

I think one of the main factors for accumulating pounds is the multitude of chemicals that are incorporated into fresh food. First and foremost, there are the different glucose and malt syrups that go straight into your blood from your mouth into your hips.

Then all the preservatives make the digestive system have cable. Only consider the essence of a preservative: its purpose is to prevent bacteria from spoiling food. Sadly, our digestive system also works with bacteria. We cannot believe that food swamped with preservatives can easily be digested or provide our bodies with enough nutrients.

If you like overeating, you eat a lot of unhealthy fats. Have you ever checked what type of oil a restaurant kitchen uses? We dare to say that anyone who wants to stay healthy ought not to eat fast food or restaurants every day.

Another source of overweight can be an undetected digestive system infection with the yeast. Yeast infections are now common, and you can easily catch them in any public place. They're really difficult to get rid of. Candida albicans tend to penetrate the digestive tract and absorb food from our food. This can lead to regular food cravings and binge eating.

How to stay slim or lose weight: after this, let me show you how we keep my weight free of diet, and we are fond of eating and drinking. For all people who claim that there are foods that make you lean, we would like to say this (it's hard to gain weight eating just leafy and green beans, of course, but who wants to live like that?): The only food that doesn't get into your mouth does not make you fat.

If you want to lose weight, minimize the amount that you eat—but don't deny anything to yourself. Bring your appetites and cravings, whether it's chocolate or French fries. Don't overeat this sinful pleasure. Stop following a little slice of cakes or some French fries. The stomachs are habituated creatures: once you are used to smaller portions, you are comfortable with less. Permanent loss of weight is always a slow process, so you should be ready to eat less for a long time.

1. **Move:** Exercise. If people ask me how we can stay slim over the years, we answer: we don't overeat, and at least three days a week, we go to the gym. There is no option for exercise at all. Our bodies have to function well. Use increases the heart rate, which gives our cells more oxygen and nutrients. The workout increases our metabolism and hormone production. You feel good and comfortable after a good workout. What kind of exercise you do doesn't matter; it's essential to move your body and pump your heart. We never thought of me as a sportsman, but we like to exercise in the gym because we feel so good afterward. Fortunately, exercise is very addictive: after the workout, you start to enjoy the great feeling.
2. **The magic of love:** the simplest way to lose weight is to fall out of love. Usually, if we fall in love, we lose a few kilograms without notice. This way of losing weight cannot be programmed, unfortunately, though you can fall in love with yourself. When was the last time you got mimicked? How did you say to yourself how good you were the last time? Have you ever looked at your bare breasts and told yourself how gorgeous you are? Remember: Gender is one of the best slimming and slimming practices. If you are lucky enough to live with a girlfriend, do all you can to spice up your sex life. Many publications are available. Just check what works for you. There's no cause to worry if you're alone. Sexual activity with

your self can always be a healthy and slimming workout, anywhere. You know best, what turns you on. Be your very best friend and lover.

3. **Avoid sugar and pure carbohydrates:** without the natural fiber, the blood flows directly from your belly to the sugar, white flour, rice, and other cereals. They increase your blood sugar levels so that you boost until the sugar is consumed, and you get a drop-in energy. Then you need some more sugar to raise you. DA diet rich in sugar and empty carbohydrates keeps you eating all day without ever being satisfied and full. The occasional ice cream, cookie, or cake, of course, belongs to the pleasures to be enjoyed—but not regarded as a natural part of a healthy diet.

4. **Drink plenty of water and eat plenty of fiber:** keeping your digestion together with exercise. You never complain of constipation if you eat enough food and drink water at the same time. Healthy bowel movements are essential to feeling good. If your food stays in your body for too long, waste builds up. If you eat food, don't forget to drink water: fiber without liquid clots, the digestive system.

5. **Take lactobacillus:** the bacteria in your bowel help break the food and feed your body, so it doesn't have to build up fat. You never complain of bloating or excess gas when you take lactobacillus in one form or another every day. Lactobacillus is now present in many ways and is extremely helpful for all types of problems. Take capsules if you don't like eating curd or other dairy products.

6. **Avoid high foods:** it is, of course, good to have a meal of five or six times at parties or just when you feel like it. Without indulgences, what would life be? However, it is better to keep your meals small and eat them more often daily. Stretch the calorie intake and don't eat too late throughout the day.

7. **Stop hunger pangs:** don't wait until you're thirsty, keep on eating. When your stomach grumbles and you need something to eat, you tend to eat too fast. It takes about 20 minutes for our

brain to realize that we filled our stomachs, and it helps to eat slowly and to chew carefully.

8. **Satisfy your cravings:** try to satisfy this urge when something is making your mouth water. Your body tells you what it has to do. Cravings are one of the manifestations of our bodies. As stated earlier: If you want to eat strawberries (or a chocolate bar or hot dogs) in any way, follow your will.

9. **Minerals and Vitamins:** make sure that you have enough vitamins and minerals on your doctor's advice by taking supplements.

10. **Then, the obvious thing:** don't drink too much alcohol, eat plenty of fruit and vegetables, and rest enough. If you cannot sleep properly, you may have anxiety and a hormonal imbalance, feel fatigued or depressed. Go to the doctor and get assistance. Consult online and ask your doctor about your symptoms.

CHAPTER 23:

Create Reasonable Goals

Manage Your Expectations

It's good to want to push yourself to be the best that you can be and strive to be a brand new person. Having huge expectations for yourself can help you create and achieve your goals. It's healthy to believe in your power to have enormous success. It's okay to want dramatic changes, but keep in mind that you need to be realistic with yourself. Take this process day by day if you have to, but know that you will get results eventually, but how long and how much those results require will vary based on what you experience along that journey and how well you respond to hypnotherapy. Everyone will react to these changes differently, and it doesn't make anyone better or worse than anyone else.

It's okay to take it slow. Work at your own pace and be fine with the pace that you are working at. Don't compare how fast you are losing weight to how fast other people are losing weight. Some people may be able to lose two or even three pounds in a week while you may struggle just to lose one. That doesn't mean you're not doing well. Comparison can be deadly for diets, so focus on your own progress instead of desperately trying to keep up with other people. Your body is unique, and your pace is all your own. Take pride in your pace, no matter what that pace is because any progress is better than what most people accomplish, so that's something to celebrate!

Because repetition helps people absorb information, I'm going to reiterate once more that you shouldn't expect instantaneous changes. This is going to be a lifetime pursuit. This is not a diet that has a beginning and an end. We are programmed to believe that weight loss routines have an expiration date, and for that reason, diets often fail. An end date suggests that you can go back to how you were before. The point of this is not to return to the person you used to be. The point of the changes I endorse is to make it so that you don't want to go back to behaving how you used to behave. Hypnosis allows you to make changes and normalizes them to your brain so that those changes become habitual, and you're able to do them consistently.

Be aware of your body's limits. Some people just aren't going to be able to start running miles at a time. Some people will never be able to do that. Your body has limits, and there's nothing wrong with having limits. You can expand upon your limits, but make sure you don't push yourself too far, too soon. If you hurt your health or injure yourself, you're going to have more trouble staying active and eating right, so take care of your body. It's the only one you have, and if you neglect its needs and push it more than it can handle, you're not being reasonable with yourself.

Don't force yourself to do things that only feel like a chore. You need to create expectations that will make your life not just bearable but pleasurable. Most importantly, stop grumbling about the changes you need to make. They are hard, but negativity only creates more negativity. If you can find the positives, you will feel better about your entire situation and be able to keep up with all the plans that you have made. If you ever start dragging your feet during this process, make some changes that put some pep in your step.

Be flexible. Any plan worth having should have enough wiggle room that you can take detours on the way without your whole plan being derailed. Like you need to be open to the changes, you need to be open to how you'll have to adjust what you are doing based on your circumstances. Weight loss takes months or even years, so your needs now may not meet your needs in the future. If you get sick, for example, you may have to put exercise on pause and shift your diet for a while. This is just a bump in the road, and if you're flexible, you can endure it.

Lots of bumps in the road may make you feel disheartened. Be prepared for obstacles. They're going to happen. Lots of them. You'll have bad days that make you feel like you'll never get back on track. You'll overeat sometimes, and you'll fall off track with your exercise regime. Sometimes, you'll just feel bad. You'll be upset about your lack of progress. You'll be desperate to hurry up and get the weight off already. Tragedies, like a death in the family, may impact your emotions and make it harder to keep true to your diet, but these obstacles are all part of life, and learning to handle them and your weight at the same time is how you create lifelong change.

Be merciful with yourself. Don't be too harsh on yourself for mistakes or the way you handle the obstacles you face because you probably wouldn't be that harsh with anyone else. If you wouldn't be as hard on your best friend as you're being on yourself, you need to be gentler with yourself. Treat yourself as you would treat the people who are most dear to you. Practice positive self-talk and expect that the people in your life talk positively about you as well.

Don't expect magic. Even with hypnosis, you're going to have to put in a lot of work. If it starts to feel too easy, push yourself a little more. Don't let yourself get complacent with your weight loss. Continue to push your mind and body towards where you want them to go. Your expectations will outline your progress. Maintain your expectations for yourself because expectations are what will show you whether you've made progress or not. Always keep your expectations in mind so that you can remind yourself of what you want and why you want it. Celebrate your progress as it happens, and the weight loss will feel magical just because of how good it makes you feel.

Good Goals Are Hard to Find

Goals help you get where you want to go better than anything else. You need them to navigate the curves of life. If you want to get anywhere in life, it helps to have a clear plan of where you want to go. If you get in the car and drive aimlessly, it's going to be a lot harder to find the destination you are yearning to find. Hypnosis is hard if you don't know what you want; however, if you know where you'd like to be, suddenly, hypnosis becomes like a GPS. All you have to do is enter where you'd like to go, and your hypnotist will guide you to the location. You'll still have complete control of the car, and only your goals will guide the session.

Making goals is a big deal because most people fail to make goals at all, which is detrimental to their progress. A Harvard Business study showed that only fourteen percent of people even make goals. Further, those with goals are ten times more successful at accomplishing what they want to accomplish than those who do not make goals. Thus, the feat of simply making goals is a huge step that brings you just a little bit closer to making your aspirations come true. Accordingly, be clear with yourself about what you want so that you know exactly what to work towards.

Make incremental goals. Incremental goals help you from feeling overwhelmed. When you're overwhelmed, you shut down and become unable to make any progress. Thus, don't let yourself get overwhelmed by making a series of small goals to build up to your bigger goal. Use these goals to propel yourself forward. Incremental goals serve as mile markers that mark the progress you've made. You can celebrate those little victories and use them as motivation to keep going. Always keep the larger goal in your mind but focus on the smaller goals as you get to them.

Your goals should make you feel energized, and they should be measurable. A goal of "being the weight that makes me happy," isn't going to give you much direction and will do little to push you forward. When your goals are too abstract or vague, they will quickly lose steam, and you won't have the energy to complete them. Be sure to have ways to quantify your goals so that you can see how much closer you are to your objective. Your goals should excite you throughout your journey and make you excited to complete them. If that motivation is ever lost, you need to reevaluate.

The quality of your goals matter. Be clear about what you want. Don't make half-hearted goals. Half-hearted goals aren't going to satisfy you, and they aren't going to give you any direction, either, making them useless. Even if your goal is measurable, if it is not achievable or won't challenge you at all, it is not a quality goal. Find goals that you can invest fully in. Find goals that make you motivated to work hard for a long time to come.

No matter what your goals are, write your goals down. Only three percent of people make written goals, but those people are three times as successful as those who have goals but have not written them. This statistic shows how powerful it is to write your goals down. By writing them down, your declaring your dedication to those goals, and you feel more motivated to keep up that goal when it's preserved on a piece of paper. When you write something down, you commit to it, and you feel accountable for that objective you've written down.

Create a timeline for your goals. By January 15, a whopping ninety-two percent of New Year's resolutions have been discarded, which shows how quickly people can throw their goals aside until another year rolls around. Thus, creating a timeline for when you want to accomplish which goals can help keep you on track. While having deadlines for a certain amount, you want to lose can be helpful, don't become too rigid with your timeframe. If you can't keep up with what you thought you could do, adjust your plan instead of falling terribly behind and quitting. Allow yourself to adapt to how your body reacts to dieting so that you never lose sight of what you want while still being open-minded.

Allow your goals to change over time. What you want out of hypnosis, and your weight loss journey may change over time, which is why you should be ready to change your goals when your interests shift. Goals should give you the drive you need to complete them, but if they don't, that's a clear indicator that you need to reevaluate what is motivating you and find new motivators.

CHAPTER 24:

Change Bad Eating Habits through Hypnosis

Do you ever feel like your life spins around Food? From occasions and birthday celebrations to dinnertime with the family, Food is a significant piece of our lives each day.

However, regularly, we've been adapted to have an undesirable relationship with Food. We've figured out how to pine for garbage, and vast numbers of us long for sugar. A few, for example, use nourishment for comfort during times of pressure – they're passionate eaters. Others continually battle yearnings to enjoy. What's more, some go to Food when they're exhausted. The explanation is necessary: Our inner mind has been adapted to utilize Food as a well-being cover.

It's hard to believe, but it's true. Our inner mind – that considerable storehouse of data that controls 85-95 percent of our contemplations – needs us to have a sense of security. The battle or flight reaction is a particular subliminal barrier component; it protects us when we're in harm's way.

Those occasions when we're surrendering to the allurements of sugar, the psyche is in safeguard mode when we're protected. That is the reason we're consequently constrained to go after bites or indulge. Our subconscious has discovered that sweet snacks or that sentiment of being overfull liken to "well-being."

Conquering food habits requires something more than resolve. Indeed, you heard that right; you DO NOT require determination to overcome food habit. You need to retrain your psyche brain to help and discharge those programmed yearnings.

That is the reason hypnosis for food dependence can be so useful. Hypnosis permits us to get to the inner mind. Furthermore, when we talk legitimately to the inner mind, we can start discharging unfortunate propensities and retraining our psyche as a supporter. It's in reality significantly more straightforward than it sounds.

You might be pondering, "How does hypnosis for food compulsion work?" You can consider it like this: Hypnosis opens a direct line of correspondence with the psyche. We can talk legitimately to it and feed it positive insistences and new data to utilize. On account of Hypnosis, we can reinvent our cognizance.

Food compulsion has numerous clinical names, and individuals can have any number of undesirable associations with Food. Voraciously consuming food Disorder, for instance, happens when individuals intend to eat an over the top measure of Food consistently. A gorge eater will, in general, eat a great many calories in a short step of time, regularly carelessly, and these gorges have genuine well-being suggestions. The inclination to the canyon is frequently unreasonable—Hypnosis encourages us to oversee and get these desires leveled out.

Urgent gorging, then again, is comparable. Habitual overeaters are frequently overpowered with yearnings—for sugar, dairy, or carbs, most regularly. Furthermore, they feel an absence of authority over their desires, as indicated by the National Center for Eating Disorders. The Hypnosis instructs us to perceive yearnings and reconstructs the inner mind to be increasingly steady in assisting with defeating desires to indulge.

Hypnosis for a sugar habit, for example, can help us reframe how the inner mind sees sugar, and necessarily, that can assist us with releasing our yearnings. Despite the sort of enslavement, numerous food addicts experience similar indications:

- Eating rapidly.
- Proceeding to eat in any event, when full.
- We are eating in any event, when not feeling hungry.
- Subtly eating.
- Feeling blame or regret for gorging.

Furthermore, feeling constrained or "driven" to eat.

So what causes this undesirable relationship with Food? Overwhelmingly, the main drivers of our food addictions lie in the psyche mind. We've been molded to join positive relationships with particular kinds of Food or to gorge or gorging, for instance, and these affiliations are established somewhere down in the psyche.

How Our Thoughts Reinforce Food Addictions

Indulging, gorging, or exceptional longings aren't the issues—the issue is the negative reasoning examples that drive us to settle on undesirable eating decisions. Sadly, these affiliations are profoundly imbued. We've spent our lifetimes molding ourselves to eat horribly.

Gatherings, weddings, and preparing treats with Grandma—we've discovered that sweet bites and greasy nourishments are our companions. Many of us use them to compensate ourselves, fix weariness or uneasiness, and a few of us eat when we feel pushed.

Also, all the time, our desires are activated automatically. We experience pressure and B.A.M.! We venture into the bureau and eat without honestly thinking about why. We regularly don't think about our psyche minds—that region where research recommends 85-95% of cerebrum movement lies. What's more, this is the territory of the brain where food enslavement lives. Our subliminal considerations are programmed, and they've been strengthened by a lifetime of experience. For instance, after a horrible youth occasion, we may have discovered solace in Food, finding out that Food assisted with desensitizing sentiments of agony or disgrace.

Festive occasions can likewise be attached to our desires. Envision this: Someone may connect desserts with heating with grandmother. This way, desserts are related to adoration and well-being in their inner mind. That is why such a large number of us go to Food in enthusiastic circumstances or when we're pushed—we need to be enhanced!

The uplifting news: The psyche can be retrained. Hypnosis causes us to hold the subliminal regularly and successfully. What's more, it's been appeared to help with numerous conditions that are brought about by unfortunate reasoning examples, similar to nervousness and stress.

Hypnosis can assist us with being hyper-mindful of our longings. We figure out how to remember them. So regularly, they happen consequently, and without thought; in any case, when we figure out how to recognize them, we gain control over our yearnings.

Furthermore, we can utilize Hypnosis to get to the inner mind and furnish this fantastic archive of data with new, progressively supportive data. Consider it like pulling weeds to plant new, sound seeds. For instance, we may reframe how we consider low-quality nourishment and urge the psyche to search out and ache for more beneficial choices.

Hypnotherapy for Food Addiction

At this point, you have a thought of how Hypnosis encourages: It enables us to be aware of our longings and reteaches the psyche how to consider Food. However, how precisely accomplishes that work? Here's a look at the better purposes of Hypnosis for food dependence, and a piece of the numerous ways it can engage us to have more beneficial existences.

- **Careful Eating:** Almost all food addictions share a comparable manifestation: We regularly gorge without thought. It's become an impulse and something that we don't ponder. With Hypnosis for careful eating, we can show the psyche to be progressively mindful of our yearnings, of how full we feel, and of the genuine demonstration of eating. Hypnosis for careful eating permits us to perceive longings and physical sentiments of appetite and to be insightful about eating. We gain control over Food and our desires.
- **Breaking Habitual Thoughts:** Again and again, constant reasoning gets reactionary and negative. What's more, regularly, our longings or indulging is activated by these contemplations. You may encounter an upsetting circumstance at work. As opposed to slowly inhaling and saying there is no reason to worry, you begin to believe you're under-qualified, or the pressure goes to tension. Without disposing of these spiraling reasoning examples, we can't discharge our food addictions. Hypnosis enables us to recover control of our contemplations, and transform our subliminal into a ground-breaking partner.
- **Fixing Underlying Conditions:** Food compulsion can be propagated by any number of conditions: Depression, nervousness, an absence of self-esteem, to give some examples. Hypnosis can engage us to oversee and move past these conditions.
- **Reestablishing Confidence:** An absence of self-assurance or love can keep us from making a move. If we don't believe in ourselves, or we don't cherish ourselves, we may permit our negative behavior patterns to proceed. Hypnotherapy is a useful asset for picking up certainty and figuring out how to entertain ourselves more. This is significant for food addictions. At the point when we adore and have faith in ourselves, we're

considerably more liable to confront desires and work toward settling on a more advantageous way of life decisions.

Self-Hypnosis for Bad Eating Habits

Individuals have a couple of choices with regards to hypnotherapy: One-on-one meetings with a subliminal specialist, tuning in to hypnosis chronicles, and self-hypnosis. Self-hypnosis is one of the most advantageous because you can utilize it in the solace of your own home or at the workplace. It's additionally energetically suggested for food addictions. Look at this video to figure out how to utilize self-hypnosis from Grace. As should be obvious, the procedure is straightforward. Here are a few focuses you might need to remember:

- **Note you're Well-being:** How are you feeling? It's useful to survey how you think so that you can reconsider it toward the finish of the meeting.
- **A Guided Countdown:** You may decide to commencement from 10. This enables the psyche to go into a condition of Hypnosis.
- **Positive Affirmations:** Once you're loose, you can talk legitimately to the inner mind. Offer it certifications; positive proposals intended to recondition the brain. For instance, with food compulsion, you may rehash something like: "I am liberated from indulging. I tune in to my body to realize when to eat. I decide to eat healthy nourishments in impeccable portions. I stay away from sweet nourishments. I feel more advantageous regular. ."
- **Imagining the Change:** After you've given your subliminal positive recommendations, envision how you will follow the more advantageous way. See yourself living with a stable relationship with food. This fortifies the thought and empowers it to grab hold and support.

Repugnance Therapy and Hypnotherapy: Reframing the Mind

Sweet, salty, or greasy nourishments convey various symptoms. Overindulgence is connected to stoutness, diabetes, an absence of vitality, and even gloom. This prompts misfortunes in profitability, a brought down sex drive, and nervousness, to give some examples. In any case, yet, we're despite everything constrained to eat these nourishments.

Consider the possibility that we could assist the psyche with stopping wanting unfortunate nourishments. Imagine a scenario where when we saw a brownie or chocolate cake, the mind would not say I like to eat a ton of that.

Repugnance hypnosis is one system that prepared trance specialists to offer that can assist us with doing only that. It's not always essential, yet for food enslavement, it's regularly one of the best arrangements.

Believe it or not, we're not vast devotees of revolution treatment for most subjects (we'd much rather have our customers center around what they need, similar to a thin solid body than on a negative variant of what they don't need, similar to a cake canvassed in ants), nonetheless, with regards to food and sugar, we find that repugnance treatment can be so useful in tipping the scales for customers that we needed to incorporate it here as a potential arrangement.

CHAPTER 25:

Mistakes to Avoid

Are you ready to begin your journey to intuitive eating? The process is straight forward but takes some practice to adapt to your body and needs. Set goals for yourself: learn to read your body's signals and communication.

Avoid Skipping Meals

This is good advice for anyone. Skipping meals is sometimes inevitable, especially if your schedule doesn't allow much time to take a break. If you expect this to happen and can prepare ahead, get up early to start breakfast early. Pay attention to your level of hunger in the morning, to determine how much you want to eat. Bring a light snack to work or school, just in case there is an opportunity to satisfy your hunger, should you feel this way and need to prolong or skip lunch. Whether you eat small or large meals, ensure that you have something nutritious and tasty, just in case. Even the best-planned schedules can change at the last minute and being prepared can alleviate a lot of unnecessary stress.

Not Drinking Enough Water

Hunger can be a symptom of dehydration. If you feel hungry, drink water first. Being hydrated is one of the most important ways to stay healthy. It can also regulate your hunger signals so that when you feel like eating, it is a response to hunger and not for other reasons. If drinking water during the day doesn't appeal to you, try adding lemon, lime or cucumber. Sparkling water can be another alternative. Herbal teas are great during colder months to ensure you are hydrated. Fruit contains a lot of water and natural sugar, which can provide a boost in energy in between meals if needed. Coffee is acceptable in moderation, though alternate drinking coffee with water, as it can have a dehydrating effect.

Setting Unrealistic Goals

Many of us set goals when we diet, and often, they can be unrealistic. Magazines, advertisements and diet programs promote quick fixes and sure-fire ways to lose weight fast, but this is only good in the interim. In extreme cases, where weight loss is necessary for health reasons, a medical professional or nutritionist may provide a specific guideline for eating. Even within this plan, mindful eating can be practiced, by noticing how the food you eat impacts you and when you eat. Choosing healthy foods can be counterproductive if we eat when we're not hungry or too much when we are, therefore, not listening to our signals.

Focus on one goal at a time, if necessary, to avoid discouragement and disappointment. In other words, don't expect to lose a lot of weight, reduce your anxiety and lower your sugar levels all at once, though if you eat relatively healthy and exercise, even moderately, you'll likely see positive results within a few weeks.

The key is not to expect overnight transformations that you can post on social media for a shocking response. Even the most successful people, when it comes to losing one hundred pounds or becoming athletic, must dedicate months, even years, to achieving their goals.

When the goal is reached, maintenance is still needed and must continue. Mindfulness can instill that level of maintenance from the very beginning so that it becomes part of your everyday way of living.

Obstacles to Intuitive Eating: Emotional Response to Food and Changing Habits

We all have habits that are difficult to break or change, and it's not something that can be achieved overnight. Recognizing a negative habit is a start to making an improvement, as it shows we are aware of it. Habit-forming traits often happen as a response to something else in our life. For example, we may overeat when we feel emotionally upset or as a way to make ourselves feel better when we have a challenging experience. This can happen when someone is grieving or feeling a sense of loss. Food can often take the place of that loss in order to cope. When you are going through a difficult time, it's important not to blame yourself, especially for eating habits. Realize that it is temporary, and in time, when you are ready, you can change the way you think about eating. The key is awareness. A helpful approach is a meditation, to give yourself that space to reflect, without judgment, and set realistic goals.

Avoid Multitasking When You Eat

Meeting a deadline, chatting online or in person, and getting work done are all activities that many people try to accomplish during a meal. This happens most often during lunch break, as a "working lunch" or as a way to save time and alleviate the stress of having to complete the work after lunch, though the opposite will occur. As you try managing both tasks, you're eating habits and connecting with your body's signals will interfere. This breaks the connection between your food and you. It is during this multitasking that you may feel more anxious to rush back to work from lunch, or in a more social and conversational atmosphere, lose that sensation you experience when you enjoy your meal alone and without distraction. Even if you are pressed for time, leaving a minimum of twenty minutes to enjoy a meal is a good start. Put down the files, leave the computer screen and go for a walk in a quiet and serene place. Meals, whenever you choose to enjoy them and when you can find adequate time and space for them, should take center stage, and all other events put on pause until you are finished.

If you enjoy eating with coworkers, family, and friends, make it an enjoyable event. Keep it positive and fun. If a working lunch is what you want to do, find that enjoyment in your food when you can and chew, savor every mouthful. Keep multitasking to a minimum, if you have to keep tasks in motion during your break. Your team may notice how you slow down to eat and enjoy the taste of your food. It may be appropriate to talk about the food and appreciate what you have. This may encourage others to see how you approach intuitive eating and could motivate them as well!

CHAPTER 26:

Additional Tips to Help You Lose Weight

Now, if there's one thing many people are still dealing with in the world today, it's unnecessary weight gain, which is triggered by too much fast food. But with the aid of your side's fitness book, and a few ideas you can try out, you will significantly reduce your body's excess fat to give you the youthful look you've had in the past.

While it is a process that takes some time, if you need to get rid of your new body stance at all, you, as the victim, will demonstrate a lot of persistence as well as discipline. And what are some of the tricks with the fitness manual by your side that will make you lose weight within the shortest amount of time? The first thing you can work out is to eat a lot of fruits and vegetables and minimize fat-rich foods.

Having that in mind, you should have a routine follow-up practice that you can do, including taking a short stroll, if you find it challenging to perform rigorous workouts. This will encourage you to eat very balanced foods and do a few light fitness manual exercises from the guidebook.

The other advice is to eat healthy, organic meals, which will contain more vegetables and fruits, and drink green tea after every heart-warming meal you take. This method is very successful, specifically for those who prefer slimming down the natural way. Less calorie intake would also significantly help to decrease the bodyweight because too many calories in the body begin to slow down the body's metabolic process, thereby contributing to the weight already gained.

This is one difficult decision that many people may not be gracious enough to take, but it is the only way out of the weighty issue. Besides, if you choose to consume fewer calorie foods and perform different fitness manual exercises, then your vital body metabolism rate will bounce back into shape faster than you expected. Did you notice that drinking a lot of water will help you lose weight quickly as well?

When you're on a strict diet to lose weight, the body needs to be hydrated all the time to maintain its optimal levels and reduce the excess weight gain and water retention that might be present in the body. You're good to go, with a little fitness boost. Many tips to help you lose weight faster include eating potassium-rich foods, calcium, routine workouts using the fitness guide book or video, a healthy diet plan, and a positive attitude throughout.

Forget the anguishing stories you read about how tough it is to lose weight. Make it easier for yourself to help you lose weight by following these ten quick and easy tips. Implement one tip every day, and you'll be at your target weight before you know it: no hassle, and there is no need to turn your whole world upside down either. Don't waste any more time on medications and expensive treatments or hard-earned cash, start to use these tips today and also be lean and healthy.

1. The first trick to help you lose weight is to have healthy eating habits. In this way, you can not only obtain more food quantity, but you can also use natural low-calorie seasonings such as onions to enhance the taste. It is known for long-term well-being and weight loss as the diet burden itself is eliminated.
2. Trim the fat always off the meats that you cook. Or if it is chicken-like, cut the fat. Chop it up and add it to something like pasta, if that is too bland!

3. Get a friend accountable for your diet program. People tend to be more committed after a week or two when they know, and need to check in with others. For starters, find someone to walk with, a close friend or even a diet-boyfriend. Say your goals! Sometimes trying to do something by yourself can be a lot harder.

4. To keep track of calories, carbohydrates, proteins, etc., write down everything you consume. You would be shocked if you didn't write down your menu, how many extra items you would drink. Either plan with your dietary intake or start keeping a food log to see!

5. Using a non-stick canola cooking spray, if you need to fry stuff. It will save you plenty of calories over oil cooking. One tablespoon of cooking oil, for example, contains 120 calories! Considering that a 2.4-second PAM spray contains just 16 calories.

6. Keep the outlook optimistic, and never give up. When/if you leave, it's the only time you struggle. It may take further work or some other strategy, but it will "will" happen. Studies indicate that the majority of people struggle to try their first time. Nothing will take the place of determination! Not intellect, not talent, absolutely none! All the rest is secondary.

7. Their diet and wellness programs are 50/50 partners in the weight loss program. When one or the other is missing, you'll have less chance of success! You can work out until you pass out, but you would not see drastic improvements in your appearance if you take too many calories in. And if you don't do exercise, the body is more likely to use muscle rather than fat for energy. Aerobic exercise causes fat burns! Hunger burns up fat!

8. Reflect on the loss of fat and not just the overall weight loss. What matters is your size, and not how much you weigh. You may be surprised because the muscle is more

substantial than fat! So know calories burns with the muscle! So eat meals regularly and don't miss it. When you wait for more than four hours, your metabolism will start slowing down.

9. Know where fat appears to get the body. Women seem to accumulate fat around their thighs and glutes. Men gain it on their bellies and around their waist. This is because of the lack of circulation in those regions. Fat isn't taken as quickly into the bloodstream as other regions. That's why fat burning agents such as ephedrine work alongside a long-term weight loss plan. Help even to blood-thinning agents such as aspirin. Still, before using any replacement, make sure you read the labels, directions, and alerts!

10. Keep your weight loss program clear. If you start missing meals or skipping workouts, it slows your progress to the point of discouragement. How bad do you want that to happen? Select and stick to a good plan. Know, what you put in you gets out of it!

Most people are becoming more conscious of their weight, not just because of how it impacts the way they look but also because of the consequences of their well-being. If you're one of those looking to get a leaner body, you certainly should be entertaining the simple but successful techniques.

Turn Your Back on the World of Fast Food

Of course, ordering food from a drive-through or over the phone is more relaxed, but if your heart is set to lose significant weight, then this is the first step towards achieving such a goal. You'll have to start eating at home as an option, or if you're a busy person and can't handle such a job, you can always eat at restaurants that have a healthy menu on offer. Turning your back on fast food will also mean giving up processed foods like crispy chips and carbonated drinks.

Apply More Liquids to Your Diet

Water is a significant factor in the weight loss cycle since it is the carrier of all the nutrients from the food you consume. Keeping this in mind, make sure you drink at least 8 full glasses of water a day, as well as a few glasses of fresh fruit juice. Citrus fruits and berries make excellent shakes because they taste fantastic, and they contain a lot of antioxidants too.

Find the Right Weight-Loss Supplement—some people are vehemently opposed to using all kinds of weight loss aids, such as fat-reduction tablets, but having a little boost is nothing wrong. Nonetheless, it is imperative to choose the correct form of supplement and to steer clear of "quick-fix items" that are currently very common on the market.

Dedicate 1 Hour per Day for Exercise

Allot at least one full hour for cardio, no matter how busy you are at home or work. If you have home gym equipment, you can produce quicker results as you can work out daily. An alternative would be to run around your neighborhood block every day for a total of 30 minutes to an hour.

Set Realistic Objectives

Never expect too much of yourself, and you won't get too upset if your plans don't work out. The best method is to take it one day at a time and let your body adjust to your new diet and exercise routine.

As it's more widely known, celiac disease or Gluten allergy is increasingly becoming more prevalent in the industrialized world in which we reside. Weight gain and celiac disease aren't something that goes hand in hand with weight loss being one of the main factors in Celiac Disease. Have you been diagnosed with Gluten Intolerance lately, and struggled with adding the pounds? Let me give you a few quick tips to add to your diet to help you shed the extra pounds.

I stated above that weight gain, and celiac disease is not generally associated with one another, but that doesn't mean that many people don't have a problem. It's true that almost suddenly, about 99 percent of people will see a dramatic weight loss, and that can have a surprising effect in their daily lives.

Weight gain and suffering from celiac disease. And why do I pour on the pounds?

I'm going to try to explain that quickly and easily. It is essential to know why you could gain weight so you can step on and get rid of the extra weight in your new lifestyle. When you change your diet into Gluten-Free items, many of these don't have the number of nutrients your body wants to perform correctly, and that is an obvious issue. You can get tired, lethargic, and you can feel unwell. No movement or exercise would mean that you don't lose any calories and that you gain weight.

Some of the other causes, and the primary one for many sufferers, is the sudden change in the diet to more high-fat foods. Many people believe it's always low in fat, since a product is gluten-free, and that's not the case. Always read the labels about the products you buy in supermarkets. Many of your local supermarket's pre-packed gluten-free foods might not be as safe as you think, but that does not say that they are not suitable for you. Gluten-free diets are just like any other labeled food; just read the labels first.

CHAPTER 27:

Mindful Eating Habits

Mindfulness is a simple concept that states that you must be aware of and present in the moment. Often, our thoughts tend to wander, and we might lose track of the present moment. Maybe you are preoccupied with something that happened or are wondering about something that might happen. When you do this, you tend to lose track of the present. Mindful eating is a practice of being conscious of what and when you eat. It is about enjoying the meal you eat while showing some restraint. Mindful eating is a technique that can help you overcome emotional eating. Not just that, it will teach you to enjoy your food and start making healthy choices. As with any other skill, mindful eating also takes a while to inculcate, but once you do, you will notice a positive change in your attitude toward food. In this, you will learn about a couple of simple tips you can use to practice mindful eating in your daily life.

Reflection

Before you start eating, take a minute and reflect upon how and what you are feeling. Are you experiencing hunger? Are you feeling stressed? Are you bored or sad? What are your wants and what do you need? Try to differentiate between these two concepts. Once you are done reflecting for a moment, you can now choose what you want to eat, if you do want to eat and how you want to eat.

Sit Down

It might save some time if you eat while you are working or while traveling to work. Regardless of what it is, you must ensure that you sit down and eat your meal. Please don't eat on the go, instead set a couple of minutes aside for your mealtime. You will not be able to appreciate the food you are eating if you are trying to multitask. It can also be quite difficult to keep track of all the food you eat when you are eating on the go.

No Gadgets

If all your attention is focused on the TV, your laptop or anything else that comes with a screen, it is unlikely that you will be able to concentrate on the meal that you are eating. In fact, when your mind is distracted, you tend to indulge in mindless eating. So, limit your distractions or eliminate them if you want to practice mindful eating.

Portion your Food

Don't eat straight out of a container, a bag or a box. When you do this, it becomes rather difficult to keep track of the portions you eat, and you might overindulge without even being aware of it. Not just that, you will never learn to appreciate the food you are eating if you keep doing this.

Small Plates

We are all visual beings. So, if you see less, your urge to eat will also decrease. It is a good idea to start using small plates when you are eating. You can always go back for a second helping, but this is a simple way to regulate the quantity of food you keep wolfing down.

Be Grateful

Before you dig into your food, take a moment and be grateful for all the labor and effort that went into providing the meal you are about to eat. Acknowledge the fact that you are lucky to have the meal you do, and this will help create a positive relationship with food.

Chewing

It is advised that you must chew each bite of food at least thirty times before you swallow it. It might sound tedious, but make it a point to chew your food at least ten times before you swallow. Take this time to appreciate the flavors, textures and the taste of the food you are eating. Apart from this, when you thoroughly chew the food before swallowing, it helps with better digestion and absorption of food.

Clean Plate

You don't have to eat everything that you serve in your plate. I am not suggesting that you must waste food. If you have overfilled your plate, don't overstuff yourself. You must eat only what your body needs and not more than that. So, start with small portions and ask for more helpings. Overstuffing yourself will not do you any good, and it is equivalent to mindless eating.

Prevent Overeating

It is important to have well-balanced meals daily. You shouldn't skip any meals, but it doesn't mean that you should overeat. Eat only when you feel hungry and don't eat otherwise. Here are a couple of simple things you can do to avoid overeating. Learn to eat slowly. It isn't a new concept, but not many of us follow it. We are always in a rush these days. Take a moment and slow down. Take a sip of water after every couple of bites and chew your food thoroughly before you gulp it down.

Don't just mindlessly eat and learn to enjoy the food you eat. Concentrate on the different textures, tastes, and flavors of the food you eat. Learn to savor every bite you eat and make it an enjoyable experience. Make your first-bit count and let it satisfy your taste buds. Now is the time to let your inner gourmet chef out! Use a smaller plate while you eat, and you can easily control your portions. Stay away from foods that are rich in calories and wouldn't satiate your hunger. Fill yourself up with foods that can satisfy your hunger and make you feel full for longer. If you have a big bowl of salad, you will feel fuller than you would if you have a small bag of chips. The calorie intake might be the same for both these things, but the hunger you will feel afterward differs. The idea is to fill yourself up with healthy foods before you think about junk food. While you eat, make sure that you turn off all electronic gadgets. You tend to lose track of the food you eat while you watch TV.

CHAPTER 28:

Frequently Asked Questions

Can I Use Hypnosis to Lose Weight?

Weight loss hypnosis can help you lose excess weight if it is part of a weight-loss plan that includes diet, exercise, and counseling... Hypnosis is usually done with the help of a hypnotherapist using repeated words and spiritual images.

How Well Does Hypnosis Work For Weight Loss?

For those who want to lose weight, hypnosis may be more effective than just eating and exercising. The idea is that it can affect the mind to change habits like overeating... The researchers concluded that hypnosis might promote weight loss, but there is not enough research to convince it.

Is Hypnosis Dangerous?

Hypnosis performed by a trained therapist or medical professional is considered a safe and complementary alternative. However, hypnosis may not be appropriate for people with severe mental illness. The side effects of hypnosis are rare, but may include the following:

Can Hypnosis Change Your Personality?

No, hypnosis doesn't really work at all. But that is a fun premise. That said, hypnosis helps with stress, bad (and good) habits, sleep deprivation and quality, and pain management... In that case, no, hypnosis cannot change personality.

How Can I Tell If Someone Is Hypnotized?

The following changes do not always occur in all hypnotic subjects, but most are seen sometime during the trance experience.

- Stare
- Pupil dilation
- Change in blinking reflection
- Rapid eye movement
- The eyelids flutter
- Smoothing facial muscles
- Breathing slows down
- Reduced swallowing reflex

How Long Does It Take for Hypnosis to Work?

Depending on what the client's goal is, the client will appear on average between 4–12 sessions. Imagine for some time that you are my client and that you are sitting in my comfortable "hypnotic chair."

What Are the Negative Effects of Hypnosis?

There are several risks associated with hypnosis. The most dangerous is the possibility of creating incorrect memories (called confabulations). Other potential side effects include headache, dizziness, and anxiety. But these usually disappear immediately after the hypnosis session.

What Is the Hypnosis Success Rate?

The study found that hypnosis had long-term changes in an average of six hypnosis sessions, while psychoanalysis took 600 times. In addition, hypnosis was very effective. After 6 sessions, 93% of participants had a recovery rate of only 38% in the psychoanalysis group.

Does Hypnosis Work When I Sleep?

Hypnosis is not sleep (a meditation with a goal), but if you are tired, you can fall asleep while listening to hypnosis... Fortunately, hypnosis reaches the subconscious even if it falls asleep.

How Much Weight Can I Lose With Hypnosis?

Most studies show a slight weight loss, with an average loss of about 6 pounds (2.7 kilograms) over 18 months. However, the quality of some of these studies has been questioned and it is difficult to determine the true effectiveness of weight loss hypnosis.

Does Meditation Lose Weight?

Although there isn't a lot of research that shows that meditation can directly help you lose weight, meditation can help you better understand your thoughts and actions, including those related to food.

Can Everyone Be Hypnotized?

If we understand hypnosis as a focused state of attention, where there is not necessarily a loss of consciousness or lack of memory about what has happened in the session, the answer is yes. But if we understand this question as if the whole world can reach deep trance (sleepwalking)— understood in terms of classical hypnosis—with practically total suggestibility and loss of consciousness, the answer would be a relative

NO. Getting a light or medium trance is relatively easy. Reaching a deep trance is more complex; approximately 80% of subjects can reach a deep stage without much difficulty. The remaining 20% would be difficult due to several complicated variables of knowing or controlling (fear of losing one's conscience, prejudices or beliefs, lack of confidence in the inducer, etc.) Despite this fact, if we use hypnosis at the clinical level or doctor, in most cases a medium trance is enough to obtain results.

Who Can Hypnotize?

Hypnosis is essentially a technique. Therefore, anyone who knows it enough and learns to apply it can hypnotize. Another thing is that the inductor can then confront and solve the different situations that arise during the session. If the hypnotist does not have concrete and sufficient theoretical-practical knowledge (even if they are doctors or psychologists), it could cause serious damage to the hypnotist. Even more so if the inducer pursues unlawful ends and tries to violate the physical, psychic or moral integrity of the inducer, which has happened numerous times, manipulating the hypnotized.

Can Someone Fall Asleep Forever?

It is completely impossible for it to happen. Whether we practice self-hypnosis (about ourselves), or hetero-hypnosis, that is, about another person, we will always end up leaving the hypnotic state. If, for any reason, the hypnotist disappeared, the induced subject would progressively move from the hypnotic trance to natural sleep and would gradually wake up and clear. It sometimes happens that the person is in such a placid situation that he resists waking up. In that case, we can make a counter-suggestion such as: "If you want to stay or return to this state in the future, you must wake up now"—and will normally abandon hypnosis. Or we just let it rest until it wakes up after a time that is usually short.

Does Hypnosis Have Contraindications?

Hypnosis and all similar states and techniques produce a great benefit to the organism since it helps eliminate physical or emotional tensions, slightly reduces blood pressure, regulates the heart and respiratory rhythm, balances the cerebral hemispheres and if we talk in energetic terms, rebalances the body's bioenergy. Therefore, if we are normally healthy people, we will not be in any danger.

However, there are two absolute indications: in general, hypnosis should not be performed on people with schizophrenia or serious mental illness. Why? Because we could aggravate their symptoms, and, apart from that, they would be difficult to induce. The second case is about people with epilepsy or who have had recent crises of this type: during hypnosis, one of these crises could occur, so prudence advises not to submit them.

Does the Hypnotist Have Any Special Power?

Strongly NO. When hypnosis is used as a show, the hypnotist usually presents himself with an aura of exceptional mental powers; this is part of the suggestive environment that the inductor will use to achieve its spectacular effects. It all depends on how suggestible and impressionable we are.

Really if a person does not want it, it is very difficult to be induced, unless there is such an extreme fear or conviction that the hypnotist has such (fictitious) power that our own belief or conviction will make us fall into hypnosis even sometimes instantaneously to the slightest suggestion or touch of the inductor. To hypnotize, you do not need special skills, but a minimum of skills. For example, a shy, doubtful and insecure person would be a bad hypnotist or hypnotist.

Can Someone Be Induced to Do What They Do Not Want?

Although several authors deny this possibility, our practice only for experimental purposes shows us that YES. Everything depends on many different variables, but if the induced subject has a sufficient degree of hypnotic depth, he can accept, in whole or in part, the possibility of refusing the suggestions imposed by the hypnotist. There have been numerous cases of rape and mental manipulation under states of hypnosis—this is nothing new—that is why we should not be hypnotized by people who do not have our confidence.

Can We Hypnotize Ourselves?

Of course. Self-hypnosis is one of the most interesting aspects of this technique. For this, we can use—for example, a cassette, where we will record an induction to relax progressively, including suggestions such as: "I am getting calmer, my muscles are released, little by little I feel a pleasant and deep reverie... "In the end, we will add the suggestions that we want to implement for various purposes, such as studying more and better, quitting tobacco, being calmer, etc.

Can You Hypnotize Us Without Us Noticing?

Hypnosis is more present in our lives than we imagine. In fact, if this is only a state of attention more or less acute and focused, every day, we suffer to a greater or lesser extent one or more "hypnosis." Advertising—especially on TV aims to hypnotize us (suggest us) to buy a product... politicians use very elaborate communication and image techniques to capture our attention, even where the final impression is more important than the speech itself. But returning to classical hypnosis, there are subliminal techniques to induce a subject to hypnotic states and induce him, without the need for loss of consciousness—to certain behavior or attitude.

Is There Instant Hypnosis?

Yes. For example in hypnotic shows, when the inductor realizes that someone among his audience is very suggestible and even shows some fear when approaching him, his own fear and the fact that the hypnotist is seen wearing a special power, will make the slightest hint of it, the viewer immediately falls into hypnosis (normally it will be a light or medium trance and will have to be deepened).

The other case would be when once an induction is achieved, the subject is left implanted with a post-hypnotic order such as: "when you wake up and on the next occasions when I tell you, you will immediately fall into this same state" If the achieved state is deep enough, it is implanted in the subject's deep mind and can last even for an indefinite period.

Can You Hypnotize from a Distance?

This is one of the most Apasio Nantes research fields in the field. It is disturbing to see that on many occasions under hypnosis mental activity, its scope and scope of knowledge will exceed space and time. Our nervous system is a true network through which low voltage electricity circulates; where there is electricity, electro-magnetism can be given, so that the network of extended neurons throughout our anatomy becomes a virtual frequency transmitter that can incorporate certain information.

CHAPTER 29:

From Fat to Thin Thinking

Are you beginning to see that the path to having a slim and healthy body is an inside job? That the steps to weight mastery begin inside your mind and not outside of you in a diet?

Unlike the Weight Struggle Cycle that keeps you in the un-merry-go round-feeling of yo-yoing from good or bad, on or off, all or nothing, the steps of weight mastery form a long-term journey forward for the rest of your life.

The Weight Mastery Journey

The following list of steps is in the order with which you begin your journey.

Step 1. The Weight Struggle Cycle

At the beginning of the journey, you are typically starting in the prison of your own fat thinking, limiting beliefs and habits—stuck in the Weight Struggle Cycle. At this point, your mind is wired to keep things playing out in this frustrating all-or-nothing, good-or-bad, yo-yo weight pattern.

Step 2. Start the Journey

Now you make the powerful decision to leave your victim-based, Weight Struggler mindset behind and take control of your weight mastery. By making four mental SHIFTS (Forgive, Decide, Vision,

100% Belief) in this process, you begin breaking up the old fat thinking wiring that has kept you stuck by changing your mental focus and seeing yourself in a new light. You take yourself out of your Weight Struggler Cycle prison and start out on the road to weight mastery as an open-minded and open-hearted apprentice.

Step 3. Meet Your Inner Coach

Now that you are beginning your journey from fat to thin thinking, you need a guide, an inner voice of reason and wisdom that can inspire you and lead you through releasing your weight and achieving your ideal weight and weight mastery. This new way of communicating with yourself is focused on problem-solving, learning and adjusting, and improving old fattening behaviors. This new rational, self-respecting, strategizing, and solution-thinking way of interacting with yourself gives you consistency and long-term staying power. So that even in those moments when you want to give up and say, "I blew it, so screw it," this part of you can "show up" and help you keep going and staying consistent.

Your Inner Coach has been with you all along, but its voice has been masked by the louder voices of your Inner Critic and Rebel. This step in the Weight Mastery Journey allows you to hear that voice, connecting you to your Inner Coach to create a new inner communication system that will guide you to success.

Step 4. Practicing the Nine Skills of Weight Mastery

During the Shift Weight Mastery Process, practicing the Nine Skills builds a foundation for thin thinking. Remember, these skills are the behaviors and mental processes of people who have achieved significant weight releases and have maintained their weight for more than a year.

Consistently practicing Weight Mastery skills may sound overwhelming, but think of all the skills involved in, say, driving a car. With practice, those driving skills become automatic, and you barely think of them consciously. The same is true of the Nine Skills of Weight Mastery. They evolve from something you have to think about, specifically to becoming a part of who you are.

When you become masterful at anything in life, you use the skills involved in that activity continually to maintain them. Likewise, no matter how long a Weight Master has been maintaining a healthy, ideal weight, the Weight Master continues to use and hone the Nine Skills.

Step 5. The 30-Day Thin Thinking Practice

It takes about 21 to 30 days to create the roots of new habits and beliefs. The 30-Day Thin Thinking Practice was designed to give you the support and structure to begin shifting from fat to thin thinking. Once you begin to think of yourself as the Apprentice, with your Inner Coach as your guide, you will begin to use your Nine Skills within the 30-Day Thin Thinking Practice and begin "building your Weight Mastery Home." This is the foundational network of thin thinking wires—the new habits, beliefs, and systems that will support your weight release, help you achieve your ideal weight and maintain it. During these 30 days, you will use daily meditation and hypnosis to program these changes into your deeper mind so that they become permanent. By the end of the 30 days you will:

- Be releasing weight at a rate you decide.

- Feel free of the cravings and fake hunger of out-of-balance eating.

- Have begun breaking the Weight-Struggle Cycle.

- Be engaged in daily habits and self-supportive communication that allows you to stay consistent on your continuing journey forward.

Research shows that when you reinforce new healthy behaviors, the less prominent the neurological pathways of bad habits will become. By day 30, your new thin thinking wires will be established and getting stronger as the old, fat thinking wires weaken and fade.

Step 6. Continue Releasing Weight, Reach Your Ideal Weight, and Maintain a Healthy Weight

This step is pretty straightforward. So why has releasing weight and maintaining the loss been so hard in the past? Because when you diet, you usually focus solely on losing weight and not on establishing the mastery habits and communication skills that allow you to be successful in the long run. By embarking upon a journey to weight mastery, you are changing the lens with which you see yourself. You are no longer one who struggles but one who is consistently mastering a healthy, slim, and confident lifestyle that allows you to live life at your ideal weight and be your best you.

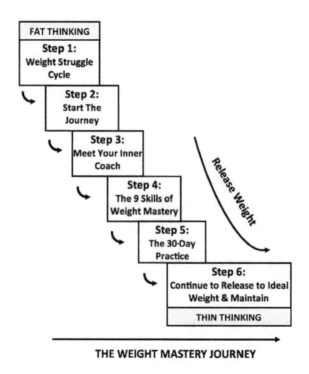

THE WEIGHT MASTERY JOURNEY

Never stopping, never "Starting Over"

So there you have the Weight Mastery Journey! You can see that it is quite different from the Weight Struggle Cycle. There is no stopping and starting over as with the Weight Struggle Cycle. The Weight Mastery Journey keeps you moving toward a slim and healthy body and confident thin thinking mind. (Chart C)

Sanity over Vanity

I like to say, "Choose sanity over vanity." What I mean is that although releasing weight is wonderful, ultimately, it is your rational, respectful, and confident relationship with food, exercise, and yourself that is the most thrilling part of weight mastery. Yes, the skinny jeans are great on the outside, but it's who you have become that is more beautiful and interesting on the inside.

I began my journey over 20 years ago when I made the decision to take back my power and said, "No more!" to diets. I saw a vision of what my life could be—slim, healthy, and free. Little did I know that this journey would open the door to a new relationship with myself. Not only was my weight going to change for the better, but everything else in my life would improve as well.

The day I stood on the scale and saw I had reached my goal of 140 pounds, I didn't celebrate. It was a busy day. My life was full. Indeed, I now had a life! I was training to be a hypnotherapist, knowing that what I wanted to do was help people take back their power and shift into weight mastery.

A few months later, I still weighed 140 pounds. This was a plateau I was enjoying being on! After years of rushing to the scale and hoping that my weight would be down, I was quite at peace with it reading the same weight day after day. Sure, the glamour and thrill of the dramatic weight losses were gone, but so was all the drama and pain.

I will be honest and say that the scale has moved up and down three to five pounds over twenty years. There have been days, weeks, and even months that didn't look so good, and my eating habits started to swing back to some of my old ways. But because of my relationship to my Inner Coach and my commitment to continuing to practice the Nine Skills, I was always able to stay on my Weight Mastery Journey. I'm 5' 9" tall, and my weight has ranged from 139 to 144 pounds for two decades.

Weight Mastery Sum Up: The Weight Mastery Journey

- Unlike the Weight Struggle Cycle that keeps you in a frustrating cycle of "on" or "off" behavior, the Weight Mastery Journey is focused on continually honing the weight, environment, and mind skills that allow you to release weight and keep it off long-term.

Making Your Shift during your 30-Day Thin Thinking Practice, you will incorporate the Nine Skills into your life and learn to depend on your Inner Coach. Over the 30 days, these new practices and healthy living habits will become second nature. You will lose weight and the old struggle will soften.

The 30-day program of daily writing exercises, along with the hypnosis and coaching resources available online, will help keep your mind in thin thinking mode as you begin releasing weight and feeling confident in your new emerging weight mastery.

"After years of struggling and feeling like a failure I can finally check this one off my list." Dina E. (Released 45 pounds, maintaining at 3 years.)

CHAPTER 30:

Overcoming Emotional Eating

Techniques for Cultivating Mindfulness

It's easy to eat well when you're prepared, well-rested, and praised for your creativity and hard work, right? But what about when you reach a deadline in the office, the mortgage payment is due, the children are ill, and you know that your trousers are getting smaller somehow? Most citizens resort to food to offer them warmth.

Food cravings also represent a symptom of emotional tension. We react by emotional eating that can function for a brief period but typically ends in us feeling much worse. Have you noticed internally when you're starving and seek to satiate that with food, it doesn't work very well? That is because nutritious food isn't an effective way to satisfy mental hunger. To combat emotional eating, we need to build better coping mechanisms to affect our emotions, feelings, and behave differently. Below are a few observations.

Using sensitivity to create a difference in any sort of hunger you feel. Would you get food cravings because the body requires calories (physical hunger), when you want to make sure you have enough nutrition (mental hunger), whether you experience internal pressure to feed (own hunger), or when you need to deal with an intense appetite (stressor)? To become mindful of your reasons for feeding, continue listening to your emotions and feelings. Listen even to what secret convictions you have regarding yourself (I am frail, I will never do this). Beware of how you sound before and after consuming some fruit. Tell yourself, "What type of feed will be suitable? Take time to pinpoint your rituals and triggers.

Upon waking up, will you head directly to the coffee pot? Speed your way to work by a bakery that offers your dream treat? Using consciousness to know whether you feed when you're sleepy, hungry, frustrated, etc. If you don't know when food is activated, consider the rapid journaling. If you're getting shocked, note down what happened before the sensation. In the end, you may see a similar thread. Our understanding of our behaviors and causes gives us the information we need to develop new strategies for coping. Most individuals claim they have absolutely no room for a safe lifestyle.

This is the adult version of "the dog was eating my homework" Not getting enough time can be just a case of failure to establish the goals. What's your priority? Dr. Edward Viljoen of Santa Rosa's Center for Spiritual Living says, "Investigate what the mental, physical, and social beliefs are so that you can be fully conscious of them. Tell yourself, are the acts of my life in line with what I think is essential, worthwhile, and true? Fashion your life for what you think. "Make in-depth goals, and have some responsibility. Particularly many women struggle with this problem because they may have a deep selfish conviction than to take care of themselves before others. I encourage you to accept the notion that self-care is not selfish. Your cup needs to be full in a safe way. Everything you're offering is in excess. Holding yourself up helps you take control of others. It lets you set your family and others around you a good example. "When you've developed a safe, fulfilling friendship with yourself, you've got something worth sharing with others." Make a list of emotional-eating alternatives.

Identify the causes, write down what you have typically done in response to them in the past, and then come up with at least three ways to adapt to the triggers in a way that promotes well-being. Examples include walking, contacting a relative, eating healthy stuff, meditating, and so on. Hold yourself on this thread. We may not be able to remember such self-nurturing options when we are anxious. Also, if you don't think they can perform, make an undertaking to test them out before you decide to eat. Set the limitations.

Make a list of which food is a "yeah," which is "maybe, at times," and which is a "no." I recommend that borders be made clear, stable, scalable, and conscious. This is particularly helpful when you experience pressure from society to consume unhealthy food. Respect your own rules, and you may see people following them too. We, individuals, tend to live up to your expectations because you don't have to dread having them. Consider thinking you do not need permission or recognition from others. Inside you, you will build a foundation of protection that another individual does not need to give and that no one else can take away. Check-in with yourself when considering a difficult decision.

Hear your ego or the best self. Play the judgment options out to the limit of your head and check in with how you feel at the moment. Be responsible for your emotions.

No matter what happens, inside of you, the response is decided. When you accuse someone else of how they believe you are being disempowered from finding solutions. Be in attendance.

It empowers you to live with the current body option and not linger in the past or predict what's going to happen in the future—using perceived failures of the past as learning experiences. Don't let the potential mold the past. Any new experience represents an opportunity to make new choices. If you're off-line, just start over again. The emotions that drive you to consume mentally have a meaning that you need to get across to you.

Listen and consider what they have to tell (not tolerate but embrace), so you won't have to repress them with milk. They would obviously let you go. Instead of listening to your thoughts, you can then react. Remember always that all the experiences are impermanent. To savor the joy of eating.

Most feeding is performed habitually without knowledge. Look out for the light, the scent, the touch, the sound, and the taste of food. Have you ever got to the end of a meal and remember that you didn't know how it tasted? Do you get more because you want to try it? Eat from the outset, attentively. Recognize the difference between "complete" and "not hungry any longer" Get over the idea of washing your plate, just consume it until you feel full. It is designed to be effective.

Tell yourself, is my lifestyle/environment enabling my aim to manifest itself? Will you have all the necessary cooking supplies to prepare healthy meals? Did you remove your household from the temptations? Should you spend time with those individuals who inspire you? What restaurants do you want to eat? Do you go out to meet a friend for a meal or a stroll in the park? Do you talk about the things you're aspiring to and interested in, or what you're worried about or what you don't like? Visualize Erfolg.

How often in our minds do we fail to watch ourselves? Or does our error replay? What if you honestly imagine yourself? Refocus your feelings.

Replace the "I can't have that" feeling with "I want something else" Focus your attention on wealth and appreciate what you do, instead of dwelling on weakness or loss. And note, starting to like new things. Define your feelings.

Will you view the "I just eat something terrible" feeling as "I'm a bad person" or "I won't be able to do this?" React to these thoughts in the way a friend would have you. Using yourself as a kind, caring expression. This could contradict those thoughts: "I made a decision that was not in my best interest. That is not to say that I am a failure or that I cannot make healthy decisions. Just now, I feel that way because I've already made a bad decision, but every moment is another great opportunity to make a different choice. So now, at this moment, I will be present and make a good decision. Feast on when you excel!

Pay attention to how comfortable you do and love the sensation as you make a good decision. To get you going, keep a journal of your achievements. You can't force trust, or bravery, or patience, but you can plant it, nurture it, and evolve with it.

Affirmations are a tool to nourish yourself. In the present tense, affirmations are positive statements designed to train one's consciousness in a constructive direction. "Repeating an assertion brings the subconscious to that state of consciousness in which it acknowledges what it wants to believe," Dr. Ernest Holmes states tips or come up with your own, Google's "personal assurance" Write them all over the home or memorize one so you can remind yourself while you're in a tough circumstance. Annual body and mind cleansing can bring immense benefits to support a healthy lifestyle. Water fasting, like in True North Health Center, will reset the taste buds, and the nutritious treats will taste more appealing. Silent mediation retreats may be emotionally and psychologically focused and motivated. Lastly, I invite you to consider the possibility of you being able to have health. Was it something you accepted? Were you clinging to that negative image of yourself? Are you able to let go of those feelings or identity? Will you owe yourself permission to remain healthy?

Important Tips

The USDA reported that, on average, Americans spent 67 minutes per day eating and drinking, even when engaged in some operation.

Practicing mindfulness gives you a complete focus on the meal. And it continues to pay attention to the food you consume when you raise the pot.

A few suggestions for feeding mindfulness are as follows:

- Consciously consider which products to purchase from the grocery store. This involves determining the worth of each object on a shopping list, thinking about each transaction, and stopping buying by impulse.
- Eat when the hunger is mild. When you are waiting for your stomach to grumble, you must aim for the most urgent incentive. To avoid gorging, feed yourself according to a timetable.
- Take a peek at the cravings. Ask whether you have real hunger or are inspired by something else to feed (e.g., pain, habit, time of day, etc.). Analyze what induces the cravings and what triggers them to fade.
- Only feed gently! This will be beneficial to use the non-dominant side because it allows you to take your time.
- Take little bits. Position your utensils on the side of your plate as you chew and bring your attention to the food's flavors.
- Express thanks. Contemplate the measures you have taken to bring the meal to your bed.

Note, the capacity to be conscious is talent. Through diligent practice, it is difficult to understand the full effects, even as a reflection on mindfulness raises gray matter over time.

CHAPTER 31:

The Mindfulness Diet

The Mindful Eating Diet

Being obvious, eating reliably alone isn't an eating regimen. No extreme purifying, no expulsion of specific fixings, no clearing of pantries, no prevailing fashions, and no quick fixes. Cautious eating can be utilized as a system to help manage increasingly cautious nourishment choices that could prompt weight reduction, even though it is important that at whatever point we pick sustenance dependent on a specific outcome, we don't eat mindfully—we eat with an unfortunate obligation that is perhaps reckless.

Essentially careful eating urges us to be available while cooking or eating, empowering us to enjoy our sustenance with no judgment truly, blame, uneasiness, or inside a remark. Regular eating routine culture makes a lot of our eating pressure, carrying with it a pile of weight, power, and false desires. Accordingly, a large number of us will, in general, consider nourishment to be a reward or punishment. That is the reason we accept we're "meriting" some nibble or bite or a spoonful of something and considering it as "a treat," as though we were a respectful pooch or infant. Individuals fixated on being flimsy may under eat and stifle hunger feelings, while people who gorge may dismiss completion feelings.

Furthermore, when people disguise considerations developed around eating regimen—getting tied up with promoting that shows weight reduction is as straightforward as 1-2-3—at that point, the weight and sentiments increment. Cautious eating expects to fix such reasoning, urging us to relinquish the customary win or bust mentality and eat as per our characteristic body weight as opposed to the bodyweight determined by magazine pictures and media-fueled weight. There is no inclusion in technique or calorie checking. We're simply endeavoring to be cognizant.

The brain is quieter when we are progressively cognizant; when the psyche is more settled, we are less inclined to be fomented or pushed or eat inwardly. We have also improved clearness with the goal that we can all the more likely observe our eating designs, and that lucidity liberates us from settling on better choices. We feel increasingly happy with the way we eat when we are quieter and clearer. We are increasingly thoughtful towards ourselves when we are more settled, more clearly, and content, thus we are less self-judgmental on those occasions when we slip or eat inwardly.

Carrying attention to the table suggests a progressively innocent, gentler eating methodology. It's not really about adjusting the nourishment we expend (even though it might be); it's tied in with modifying our contemplating sustenance.

Being aware of our thoughts and sentiments is a certain something, yet being aware of what is happening in our stomach prompts our awareness of an entire layer.

Our stomachs emit a hormone called ghrelin, which sends a sign to the "hunger center" in our minds to help our craving when we have consumed all the nourishment in our midsections and low glucose levels. On the other hand, when we are finished, a hormone called leptin is emitted by fat tissues, which demonstrates to the cerebrum that we are finished. The issue is that it takes a decent 20 minutes before that message is gotten, most specialists concur. Subsequently, during this 20-minute window, a lot of our indulging happens.

Through cautious eating, we can change by our bodies and become increasingly aware of the sensations going before this "totality acknowledgment" in the cerebrum and gage better when we are satisfied without hanging tight for 20 minutes. Truth be told, we figure out how to be a stage in front of ourselves.

We tend not to perceive such signs because a significant number of us have been instructed as youngsters to overlook their bodies: "You don't leave the table until you complete your plate!" Or "you can't go hungry!" Or "Do you need seconds for sure?" Our food habits start at a young age. So, when we converse with our very own children, we can utilize similar signs to show them how to tune in to their appetite and completion state as opposed to overlook them. Mindfulness infers not exclusively being available in its fullest sense, yet also, being interested and intrigued, willing to find how and why we accept and feel how we do—without judgment. This is not any more proper to the extent our dietary patterns are concerned.

Think about the inquiries that the vast majority don't pose to themselves: how hungry am I? What's my body requiring? How satisfied is this supper that I feel part of the way through? Am I honing or making the most of my nourishment? Do I deny myself that I like nourishment since I trust it's "awful?" Is this part to an extreme or inadequate?

We each have our frames of mind and lead designs around nourishment, regardless of whether because of hereditary qualities, conditions, or molding in the family. The consciousness of these roots offers the reason for principled eating, yet the best way to grasp our nourishment association is to invest energy with that relationship.

Care embeds a respite to help us realize how to settle on our own choices. It's as though we were hindering a chronicle from seeing our stage-by-organize process: the signs, the emotions that kick in, and the entire eating tactile impact. Just when we quit seeing this chain of events, would we be able to start to adjust our direct or sustenance thinking.

A Seven-Day Plan in Mindful Eating

Day 1

Download a snappy nourishment plan for you toward the start of your week. You might need to eat out every night or attempt another fixing each day. You can see it in your mind, however, recording it will help concentrate your arrangements and expel the worry of settling on nourishment decisions during the time at the time. Remember your arrangement while shopping or grabbing nourishment.

Day 2

Enjoy a reprieve to check in with your body and reflect Halfway through a supper today. How complete would you say you are feeling from 1–10? At that point, put it all on the line in case you're as yet ravenous! In case you're not, interruption and spare your morning or second breakfast dinner or return to it later when you're ravenous once more—the scraps are fabulous.

Day 3

Grab a chair if you can, plunk down without different errands to expend your sustenance, regardless of whether it's only a tidbit. Plunking down and eating simply confines your diversions, but above all enables you to focus on each delightful chomp. Eating without taking any kind of action else may feel abnormal from the outset. However, it empowers us to appreciate our enthusiastic connection to nourishment.

Day 4

Convenient updates are inconceivably hard to make sure to eat mindfully—especially following a protracted day of eyes on a scrumptious supper. Consider joining a string to your wrist or wearing specific arm jewelry or ring as a delicate suggestion to eat mindfully.

Day 5

Draw in your faculties with your eyes shut whenever you eat. Notice the surface, the crunch sound, and any superb flavor and smell. How are the surfaces feeling? What are you getting a charge out of about this?

Day 6

Be caring to yourself if you don't have time or vitality to approach every feast deliberately that is OK. Be delicate and excuse yourself—there is constantly another feast around the bend to be drawn nearer mindfully. Make an effort not to accept that nourishment is decent or terrible. It's everything nourishment! Nourishment has no ethical centrality; your body requires simply delectable fuel.

Day 7

Keep on practicing like contemplation, eating mindfully is a capacity that requires reliable practice. Remember the tips you've learned (or investigate the tips beneath) and practice at whatever point conceivable.

For any get-healthy plan to work, it begins with shaping an association with nourishment. When they must be aware of how they eat, why they eat, and the health benefit of what they eat. The motivation behind trance for weight reduction is to empower an individual to be aware of their eating examples and nourishments to have a fruitful adventure in weight reduction.

CHAPTER 32:

Control Your Calories

In eating right, there a couple of pointers that you can adhere to every day, and they're not going to deny you of the foods that you enjoy but deal with those foods as expensive products, so you enjoy them more.

Burning up the Calories

To keep your weight continuous, you have to maintain an equilibrium between the power you eat food calories and the energy you use up for a real job so that you can balance your weight. In warm weather, it's a great idea to take an additional 1/2 walk daily, or preferably go for swimming instead, which is a unique type of exercise. The crucial point is to enhance your level of daily tasks. A couple of mins of official workouts regular aid to tone your muscles and to improve your stance and deportment. However, unless you genuinely work fairly robust for 1/2 hour, they have no substantial result on your power balance. No slandering project is complete without the aid of exercise. It tightens up slack muscles, tones the body, and leaves you feeling healthy and dynamic. More crucial, it aids you in keeping that low level of weight you've worked so hard for.

Fats

Extreme amounts of fat in the diet can cause health issues. It is crucial to have small quantities of fat in your diet because your body requires vital fatty acids to function appropriately.

Their chemical framework identifies fats, and they can be filled, polyunsaturated or monounsaturated as well as the majority of the fat that you eat should be monounsaturated

A diet high in saturated fats can trigger your body to generate even more cholesterol, which might add to your threat of establishing cardiovascular disease and also some cancers. Saturated fats are mainly located in fatty meat, butter, full-fat milk items, cream lard as well as lots of takeaway and processed foods. They are additionally discovered in some plant food, such as hand or coconut oil. Select meat that has been trimmed of and lowered fat milk products, especially if a heart problem is common in your family. All kinds of fat are abundant sources of power. There are around 27 kilojoules of energy in each gram of fat that you consume. Your body will undoubtedly save any kind of excess calories eaten as body fat, which can cause obesity.

Sugars

Most individuals enjoy pleasant food, and also aside from sugar's effect on oral health and wellness, it is not almost as dangerous to wellness as fat. Many foods that are high in sugar are likewise high in fat, so eating soft foods can result in high-fat consumption.

Sugar is included in small amounts to make valuable processed foods, and also these items need not be excluded from your diet. High fiber morning meal cereals, as well as food such as canned baked beans, are nourishing, reduced in fat, and high in fiber and serve foods to include in a healthy and balanced diet.

Processed foods commonly have vast quantities of sugar included in them during processing. During digestion, sugars such as sucrose and lactose and other carbs, such as starch, can harm the body when it is in excess.

Salt

Salt has several purposes, and also it escalates the natural flavors, color, and structure of foods. Our body needs percentages of salt to operate because it is a crucial nutrient that the body cannot make by itself. Nevertheless, when salt is consumed in excess, it can increase your risk of developing high blood pressure. The National Health and also Medical research study Council recommends one teaspoon of salt each day. Also, if you don't include spice to your food, you might obtain this quantity of salt from eating produced food like potato pies, sausages as well as crisps.

Caffeine

Lots of people are gently addicted to caffeine. Tea, coffee, delicious chocolate, cocoa, and some soda pop beverages include caffeine.

A diet high in saturated fats can cause your body to produce more cholesterol, which might contribute to your danger of establishing heart conditions and also some cancers. Saturated fats are primarily found in fatty meat, butter, full-fat milk products, cream lard, and several take-away refined foods. There are approximately 27 kilojoules of power in each gram of fat that you eat. Your body will store any type of excess calories taken in as body fat, which can lead to weight problems.

Caffeine stimulates your mind and also the nervous system, and different physical results vary from one person to another. These effects consist of enhanced performance, high heartbeat, and urinating more.

Some researches have revealed that high levels of caffeine can somewhat elevate blood pressure, while other studies have discovered reduced blood pressure in people that eat high levels of caffeine. There is no scientific proof to recommend that caffeine-containing beverages trigger particular issues if these are consumed in small amounts.

To help, keep an appropriate level of high levels of caffeine in your diet, restrict your high levels of caffeine intake to less than 600mg daily, this would undoubtedly be 2-4 ordinary toughness mugs. Beverages that assist in keeping you sharp, such as Red Bull and V, include about 2 1/2 times the amount of caffeine discovered in regular cola beverages. If you are limiting your high levels of caffeine consumption, prevent these supposed wise beverages. There are numerous caffeine choices on the market.

Food Additives

Preservatives are included in foods for a particular objective and is not taken into consideration to be food themselves. The human-made sweetener aspartame is added to numerous beverages, yogurt, eating gum, and various other food to keep the calorie content of the product low. Some additives help to preserve or improve the top quality, color, preference, and also texture of food and prevent them from spoiling.

- GI

GI means glycemic index, which is a ranking from 0–100 that informs you whether a carbohydrate food will increase blood glucose degrees dramatically, moderately, or just a little. It offers you a step of how a carbohydrate will undoubtedly impact your blood sugar.

- Oil

Choose poly or monounsaturated spreads anywhere possible, search for salt-reduced varieties. If you want to lose weight, a reduced-fat range with just 50% fat will certainly help. If you have high cholesterol, think about a sterol spread such as sensible or Pro-active. They can aid in minimizing your cholesterol degrees if consumed in the amount suggested.

- Saturated Fats

It is best to stay away of these kinds of fats, which are found in butter, stuff, fatty meat, cheese, and also oils used in fast food. Instead, switch to monounsaturated or polyunsaturated oil. Choose from sunflower, safflower, soybean, olive, and peanut or canola oil and stay clear of saturated fats such as coconut and palm.

Reduced GI Foods consist of carbohydrates that slowly release sugar right into the bloodstream. This is optimal for those slimming down and also diabetics.

Tips to Decrease Your Fat Intake

- **Grilling instead of frying:** Use a shelf filled with a little water when barbecuing, cooking, or roasting meat. Season lean meat in a mixture of soy sauce, white wine, natural herbs, garlic, or spices. These will certainly protect against the flesh from drying while barbecuing.
- **Steaming:** It's an excellent means of cooking most veggies? The food is swiftly prepared using the vapor and also does not need any type of fat.
- **Microwave:** Microwaving oven is an excellent method for cooking. The microwave allows foods to keep their flavor as well as wetness while they prepare.
- **Stir Fry:** Make use of a frying pan or non-stick frying pan. Make use of a spray-on oil, red wine, stock, or water to fry your vegetables and after that quickly mix in your lean prepared meat.
- Baked Vegetables

Parboil veggies, spray with veggie oil, place in a dry pan, and chef in a stove on high up until crisp.

- Butter

Include reduced-fat yogurt or home or ricotta cheese to vegetables.

- Cream

Replace cream with vaporized skin milk or blend skim milk with ricotta cheese.

CHAPTER 33:

Emotional Eating Hypnosis

One simple method to perform this is to keep a food journal and a mood journal. Write down each time you know you've consumed unhealthy foods. Look back later on what feelings make you eat. You'll be able to recognize patterns or beliefs that make you overeat as time goes by. When you know what is causing your emotional eating, you will start working on how to avoid it and find ways to eat healthier.

Find Other Ways to Fuel Your Emotions

When you can't find another way to deal with your feelings without requiring food, so breaking this practice would be almost impossible. One of the reasons diets fail is that they give rational nutrition recommendations under the premise that lack of awareness is the only thing that stops you from eating properly.

That form of suggestion only works if you can control eating habits.

It's not enough to recognize your causes and grasp your process to stop emotional eating—you need to find new ways to cope with your emotions. You can call or have a hangout with a friend who makes you feel better when you're depressed or lonely, visit places you like, read an interesting book, watch a comedy show or play with the cat.

When Cravings Arrive, Pause

This might not be as simple as it sounds, because it is all you might think about when the desire for the food hits. You feel right there, and then, the need to feed. Taking at least five minutes before you give up on the craving, this gives you time to think about the wrong decision you're about to make. You can change your mind within that time, and make a better choice. Start with 2 minutes if 5 minutes is a lot for you and increasing the time as you get better with it.

Learn to Embrace Good Feelings and Negative Ones

Emotional eating comes from being unable to cope with the feelings on the brain. Find a friend or therapist who will speak to you about the problems and concerns you have. Being willing to accept negative and good emotions without having to include food would improve change.

Commit to Healthy Lifestyle Habits

Exercise, rest and adequate sleep will make it easier for you to deal with any emotional or physical problem you may experience. Create time for at least five days a week for a 30-minute workout, relax, and sleep 7 to 8 hours a day. It's also essential to surround yourself with caring people who will empower you and help you cope with your issues.

The first thing to keep emotional eating in mind is the addictive effect food has on you. You may encounter cravings that often feel uncontrollable, and you may feel as though you are addicted to food much as a smoker is addicted to smoking. The trick is to properly control your emotions and feelings and train your brain not to respond to stressful or unpleasant feelings by merely having to eat food (your preference brain drug) to calm down.

There are a few other useful methods and approaches that you can use to avoid emotional eating and lose weight, including: abandon the Diet!

Dieting ruins your metabolism, and you can eventually find yourself taking on weight. In reality, dieting will only work in the short run and will lower your fragile self-esteem.

Adjust Your Way of Thinking

Thin or lean women typically appear to think differently than overweight or obese males. People don't add emotion to food, and they don't use the menu to self-medicate themselves to make them feel better. Learn other methods to relax and de-stress. Recognize the food causes instead of feeding.

Evite or remove the food you know puts you on weight and fuels your cravings and emotional eating—these are usually fried foods, cakes, cookies, etc. But get checked out for food allergy or aversion to feeding too. Even some healthy foods may contribute to your dietary addiction and weight gain. The simple way to lose weight would be you removing something very ordinary from your diet and releasing years of unhealthy fat exercise.

This doesn't have to be boring, sweaty gym workouts. Think brain and body exercises such as yoga, Pilates, or even walking in a beautiful park will do wonders for your mind, self-esteem, and body. Relax more.

Taking some time out to spend relaxing by yourself. Many people don't know how to relax properly, so believe it's enough to sit in front of the Screen—it's not. Learn some basic techniques of meditation, which will allow you to relax completely.

Don't Equate to Anyone

When you lose weight, it is crucial not to equate your weight with the importance of those around you. If you're unhappy with your weight, comparing yourself to the skinny girls you see in magazines or on television could prolong your recovery process by adjusting your lifestyle habits with eating, exercise, and mind control; you'll find it much easier to stop emotional eating and lose the weight you want much faster and longer-term.

When you've mastered techniques for managing your eating causes, your emotional food cravings should cease.

In a person who is in control of their emotions and has more constructive ways of coping with negative feelings, emotional eating cannot thrive—it is unlikely. You can eat intuitively before you know it, and be free from raw food and excess body fat for good.

Over-food is still not given the due treatment it deserves. It is always seen as not a real issue and to be laughing at something. That view is entirely false because it is a horrific illness that needs urgent care. The positive news is that taking action to help yourself avoid emotional eating forever is easy to do. I say that because I did it myself.

Stage # 1 - Identifying the Causes

For each person, emotional eating is caused differently. Some people get the cravings when stressed out, and some when depressed or bored. You have to think a bit to figure out what your emotional causes are. When you know what they are, you will be given early notice when the desire to eat comes upon you.

Step # 2 - Eliminating Temptation

The one thing many people don't know about emotional eating is that often the craving is for one particular food. It is mostly ice-cream or candy for kids. Usually, for people, it's pizza. If you couldn't satisfy this temptation, that's not going to bother you as much. Clear out any of these temptations from your house. Throw out any nearby pizza delivery places. Once you know your tempters, get rid of them and make overeating hard for you.

Step # 3 - The Link Breaks

When the impulse hits, it's intense and instant. You are now feeling like eating. Good! You need to break this immediate bond by giving yourself some time between the desire and the eating to avoid this. Call a friend · Count to 60 · Write down what you feel · Do some exercises · Go outside for a walk · Take a shower. Whatever you can do to let the urge subside do wonder. Take these three steps, and you'll be doing them easier early and conquer emotional eating for good.

Would you like to learn the best ideas on how emotional eating stops working? It's emotional eating that satisfies your sensitive appetite. It has nothing to do with your kitchen, but in your mind lies the issue. What are the most potent methods to overcome the emotional eating temptation?

Make a list to relieve your cravings for food. In this scenario, distracting yourself does not amount to behaving mindlessly. It's not about texting while driving, or being terribly out of sight. If you divert yourself from your cravings for food, it means you're turning your focus to something else. It does have more meaning. Do something, or concentrate on some other task or event. If you feel like gorging food voraciously, consider getting a piece of paper and list five things from five types of something, like the names of five people you can ring if you feel frustrated, angry, or depressed. Perhaps you should mention five things that will help you be happy. When do you want to calm down, to what five places can you go to? What five feel-good things would you do to yourself when you're stressed up? How about five things you can do to avoid having to eat? If this list is made, show it on your kitchen or fridge shelf. The next time you're overwhelmed by your convincing food cravings, click through your list and do one of the 25 things shown here.

Prepare for Future Emotional Eating Issues

Draw a piece of paper and a pencil over the weekend and take a route about your activities in the days ahead. Your map will show the stops you intend to make and potential detours. Choose an icon that reflects emotional eating. Place the image over an occurrence or activity that could cause your cravings for food, like an early lunch with your in-laws. Prepare ahead for that case. Look for the restaurant menu online so you can order something delicious but still good.

Clear the Fears Inside Out

It helps if you take a deep breath, anytime you are nervous. Another thing you should do is to do a visual trick to detoxify yourself from the stress. Breathe in deeply and imagine a squeegee put near your head (that piece of cloth you use to clean your window or windshield). Breathe out slowly, and believe the squeegee is wiping clean your heart. With it taking away all the worries. Do this quad.

Self-Talk as If you're Royalty

Usually, self-criticism goes to emotional eating. Toxic words you say to yourself, such as "I'm such a loser" or "I can't seem to be doing anything right," force you to drive to the closest. Don't be misled even though these claims are brief. Such feelings are like acid rain, which is slowly eroding your well-being. The next time you're caught telling yourself these negative words, counteracting by moving to a third-person perspective. In moments when you think "I'm such a mess," then remind yourself that "Janice is such a mess, but Janice will do what it takes to make it work out and make herself happy." This approach will help you out of the negative self-talk loop and give you some perspective. Pull up and be positive, and you'll have the strength to avoid emotional eating.

CHAPTER 34:

Types of Food to Avoid Losing Weight

There are different types of food that you can choose if you intend to lose weight. However, not all foods are healthy for your body, and you shouldn't be consuming all types of food. Most foods are unhealthy, and they cause a lot of risks to your body. When you eat foods that you are not supposed to eat, you put your body on the risks of high blood pressure, diabetes, cancer, health problems, and stroke. So to maintain a healthy body, you need to start avoiding these foods.

So here are the foods that you need to avoid.

Fried, Broiled and Grilled Meat

The first one is fried, broiled, or grilled meat. Any food that has been prepared under high temperatures is unhealthy for consumption, and they are very palatable and dense in calories. Having excessive calories in the body is one of the risks of being obese, and you may end up struggling from a stroke because some of your blood vessels have been blocked. So consuming foods that have been grilled fried, broiled, or grilled is very detrimental to your health. So you need to avoid consuming this food. Instead, it is better to cook your food at a very high temperature. Also, you could choose to stew, Blanche it, or boil it before consuming it.

White Bread

The next one is white bread. White bread, like all the unhealthy meals, is being prepared from the low fiber. They also lack the essential nutrients that the body needs. White bread poses the risk of high blood pressure; they are a substitute for white bread and should be a bread that you prepare from home with all the ingredients.

Pizza

The next one is pizza. Pizza is prepared from which is refined and processed meat, and it has lots of calories. It is very dangerous for your health, and it is the number one junk food, you should eliminate from your diet.

Processed Foods

The next one is processed foods. Processed food has become the norm in today's society. They are readily available, and they're easy to prepare, but you have to realize that the processed foods contain high amounts of fat sugar and salt as well. So instead of eating processed foods, try to go for whole foods and vegetables.

Fast Food Meals

The next one is fast food meals. Fast food meals are very common because they are low priced, and they have no nutritional value. They fall under the class of junk food, so you should try to avoid them as much as you can.

Processed Meat

The next one is processed meat. Processed meat has been linked to diseases like cancer, diabetes colon, and heart disease. Processed meat is unhealthy, and you should avoid them in every course. Unprocessed meat is healthy, but you have to realize that any unhealthy consumption of meat is not good for the body.

Candy Bars

The next one is candy bars. Candy bars are very unfriendly. They contain lots of sugar and processed fat, especially the ones that have been made from flour. They also lack the essential nutrients that your body needs due to the ingredients used in the preparation. They are being digested very quickly and make you hungry craving for more candies.

Ice-Cream

The next one is ice cream. Ice cream is very delicious, but they do have a lot of calories and sugar in them. And it even poses more risk to your health when you eat them as a dessert. So you should avoid eating them. Instead of eating ice cream, eat healthy foods. Or you could choose to prepare an ice cream that has less sugar and eat it.

Low-Fat Yoghurt

The next one is low-fat yogurt. Yogurt will continue playing the fact that is essential to the body. However, most locally-made yogurt is low in fat and excess sugar. This is because the sugar is used to compensate for the taste of fats that have been removed from the yogurt. Also, most of this local yogurt is being pasteurized. Pasteurizing the yogurt will kill the friendly bacteria that the yogurt is normally supposed to have. So you should go for a full-fat yogurt that is the yogurt that is being made from grass-fed animals.

Cookies and Cakes

The next one is cookies and cakes. Cookies and cakes do come in a very appealing taste, and it is very dangerous to consume them in large quantities because they are being prepared from refined sugar, with flour and added fats. They also contain lots of food preservatives, and they have high-calorie content in them. So instead of consuming these cookies and cakes, you can choose to replace them with dark chocolate or yogurt.

Sugary Drinks

The next one is sugary drinks. Surgery drinks are very unhealthy to your body because they contain so many calories in them, and they will just end up putting more calories in your body than you actually need. And a large amount of sugar in your body will lead to type 2 diabetes.

CHAPTER 35:

Hypnosis to Control Food Portion

The national holidays begin with the temptations of tasty choripanes, roasts, empanadas, earthquakes, and a lot of other foods, a situation that becomes a real challenge for those who suffer from problems to control their weight and eating disorders.

A few days before the national holidays begin, there are several who are already preparing to enjoy a weekend of celebrations. This situation becomes a real challenge for those who have problems controlling their weight. Empanadas, choripanes, anticuchos and earthquakes are the temptations and real enemies of those who suffer from eating disorders or real food addiction.

However, the good news is that, like other uncontrollable desires, appetite can also be controlled through psychological therapies or hypnotherapies with high effectiveness, which would help you enjoy an 18 with no excesses.

Hypnosis points out, eating disorders or the inability to control food consumption have various causes. "Some factors that could contribute to these eating disorders are low self-esteem, lack of control of life, depression, anxiety, anger, loneliness, personal-psychological factors.

Others are more interpersonal and can help people lose control of their diet at an unconscious level, such as family problems, difficulty expressing their feelings, and hypnosis. You can go to the source of the problem, in this case of food."

Eat portions in smaller plates and have measures to eat, for example, half of the bread, half of the vegetables, of soups, either at home or in a restaurant. Fad diets usually cause rebound. Therefore, it is recommended to eat four times a day, and only when you are hungry can work through hypnosis.

Through hypnosis, you can visualize and consume food more slowly. Be clear that in the national holidays, the food does not end," advised the professional.

Regarding treatment with hypnosis to maintain a nutritional balance, the expert explained that "it consists of two stages. First, educate the patient, tell what it is and what the scope of hypnotic therapy is. Second, explain that there is a job on their part.

As for weight control, it has to do with generating the patient a cognitive modification of their brain through hypnosis that allows them to visualize differences in physical and psychological terms and also change the eating habit in terms of the amount of food eaten.

For this, we work with reinforcements, which is where the patient takes audio recorded by the Center for Clinical Hypnosis, where there are three levels and thus gradually move towards a new vision regarding what it is and what we eat."

Unlike other methods, the specialist stressed that "does not generate rebound effect, it is so powerful when people do the work they decide to do what they taught. Such as making behavioral change, hypnotic work with reinforcement at home, that it is a natural way to understand again what food is.

The rebound effect is generated in other instances. With hypnosis, a profound change is created in the person's behavior and perception of what they eat for."

On the other hand, it is difficult not to gain weight is this holiday season, since "at least on average we gain four kilos, depending on the holidays."

Anyway, he gave some tips that can help not to overdo the diet and control weight, for example, "drink with sugar change it for one without sugar, do not use dressings such as mayonnaise or others, consume roast but with salads and not with potatoes or rice, ideally green salads that have fewer calories, or one day eat empanadas and another day roasted.

The important thing is not to mix everything on the same day and avoid canned fruit if you are going to drink alcohol, try it with a light or zero drink, and decrease the caloric intake.

How to Stop Overeating

Overeating is a disorder characterized by a compulsive diet that prevents people from losing control and being unable to stop eating. Extreme episodes last 30 minutes or work intermittently throughout the day.

An excess dining room will eat without stopping or paying attention to what you eat, even if you are already bored. Overeating can make you feel sick, guilty, and out of control. If you want to know how to stop overeating, follow these steps:

Maintaining Mental Strength

Stress managing stress is the most frequent cause of overeating. Regardless of whether you are aware, the chance is to make a fuss because you are worried about other aspects of your life, such as work, personal relationships, and the health of your loved ones.

The easiest way to reduce compulsive intake is to manage life stress. This is a solution that cannot achieve with a tip bag that can help with stressful situations.

Think about: are there some factors that are stressing your life? How can these factors be minimized? For example, living with an unbearable roommate is one of the leading causes of stress in your life; it may be time to get out of that situation.

Activities such as Yoga, meditation, long walks, listening to jazz, and classical music can be enjoyed comfortably. Do what you have to do to feel that you are in control of your life. Try to go to bed at the same time every day and get enough rest. If you were well-rested, you would be better able to cope with stressful situations.

Connect Your Mind and Body Overtime

You can get more out of your feelings by writing a diary that lets you write what you have come up with, talk about your desires, and look back after an overwhelming episode.

Taking a little time to think about your actions and feelings can have a significant impact on how you approach your life.

Be honest with yourself. Write about how you feel about every aspect of life and your relationship with food.

You can surprise yourself too. You can keep a record of the food you eat unless you are obsessed with every little thing you eat. Sometimes you can escape temptation if you know that you have to write everything you eat.

Take Time to Listen to the Body and Connect the Mind and the Body

Follow the 10-minute rule before eating a snack. If you have a desire, do not grant yourself immediately, wait 10 minutes, and look back at what is happening. Ask yourself whether you are hungry or craving. If you are hungry, you have to eat something before your desire grows.

If you have a strong desire but are tired, you must find a way to deal with that feeling. For example, take a walk or do something else to distract from your desires. Ask yourself whether you are eating just because you are bored.

Are you looking in the fridge just because you are looking for something? In that case, find a way to keep yourself active by drinking a glass of water. Please have fun from time to time.

If you have the all-purpose desire to eat peanut butter, eat a spoonful of butter with a banana. This will allow you to reach the breakpoint after five days and not eat the peanut butter jar.

Maintain Healthy Habits

Eat healthy meals three times a day. This is the easiest way to avoid overeating. If you haven't eaten for half a day, you'll enjoy the fuss. The important thing is to find a way to feed the healthy food you like.

So instead of eating what you want, you feel that you are fulfilling your duty through a dull and tasteless meal, your meal should be nutritious and delicious.

The method is as follows.

Always eat in the kitchen or another designated location. Do not eat in front of a TV or computer or even when you are on the phone. There is less opportunity to enjoy without concentrating on what you eat.

This may seem to take a while, but it prevents you from feeling when your body is full. There is a gap between the moment your collection is comprehensive and the moment you feel full, so if you bite a bit more time, you will be more aware of how much you eat.

Each meal needs a beginning and an end. Do not bob for 20 minutes while you cook dinner. Also, do not eat snacks while making healthy snacks. You need to eat three types of food, but you should avoid snacking between meals, avoiding healthy options such as fruits, nuts, and vegetables.

Eat meals and snacks in small dishes using small forks and spoons. Small plates and bowls make you feel like eating more food, and small forks and spoons give you more time to digest the food.

Managing Social Meals

When eating out, it is natural to increase the tendency to release because you feel less controlled than the environment and healthy diet options. However, being outside should not be an excuse to enjoy overeating.

You must also find ways to avoid them, even if you are in a social environment or surrounded by delicious food. The method is as follows.

Snack before departure. By eating half of the fruit and soup, you can reduce your appetite when surrounded by food. If you are in an area with unlimited snacks, close your hands.

Hold a cup or a small plate of vegetables to avoid eating other foods. If you are in a restaurant, check the menu for healthier options. Try not to be influenced by your friends. Also, if you have a big problem with bread consumption, learn to say "Don't add bread" or smoke peppermint candy until you have a meal.

Avoid Temptation

Taking steps to prevent overeating when you leave home has a significant impact on how you handle your cravings. This is what you should do:

Try to spend more time on social activities that do not eat food. Take a walk or walk with friends, or meet friends at a bar that you know is not serving meals. If you are going to a family party that you know will be full of delicious food and desserts choose a low calorie or healthy option.

Try to escape from unhealthy food when you are at a party. Modify the routine as needed. Eliminate or save a little bit of unhealthy food at home. I don't want to remove all unhealthy snacks from home and go to the stores they sell at midnight.

CHAPTER 36:

Your Path to Your Perfect Weight

Figuring out how to control your points of view requires some serious energy, however, getting mindful of the sheer volume of negative improvements that barrages you every day will push you not just to teach your mind, increment your inspiration yet permit you to imagine achievement and accomplish it as well.

If you type the words "weight loss" into Google, you'll find unlimited locales on the most proficient method to get more fit, however, more regularly individuals battle with keeping weight off or not restoring the weight in addition to additional!

Tragically craze diets, patterns, and pills typically just give you transitory outcomes. They can make you a yo-yo diet, which regularly causes individuals to feel disappointed. What's more, examine shows that traditional diets frequently lead to low self-regard, uneasiness, and melancholy. These sentiments regularly fuel the choice to pick unfortunate nourishments and the cycle proceeds.

So let me offer it to you straight! I've found in my training that 'what to eat' and 'how you work out' are just little bits of the enormous riddle.

What traditional projects ignore is that you'll confront incalculable snags to effectively embracing another daily schedule, and above all, the most elevated obstruction is regularly ourselves. Traditional weight loss programs mention to us what we ought to do, which is frequently not supportable, and they once in a while center on how we can change our drawn out conduct. With regards to getting thinner, the vast majority of us have concentrated on inappropriate things. We haven't taken a shot at the most significant piece of ourselves, our minds. And afterward, we fault and judge the 'program' or mentor as opposed to peering inside.

Regularly, the narrative of our weight starts with us. It tends to be an aggregation of inner and outer encounters we've had for the duration of our lives. Antiquated intelligence instructs, "A sound mind is a solid body." Just as a house tumbles to the ground without its establishment, your body can get overweight and wiped out without a mind concentrated on well-being and bliss!

What's the Association between Meditation and Weight Loss?

Meditation is frequently tossed out the entryway and dismissed because individuals question how sitting and not consuming calories can help them get more fit. In any case, our body is a mirror impression of what's happening in our minds. If our essential spotlight is on shedding pounds, we cut ourselves off from the emotional and mental creatures we are, and that keeps us from understanding why the weight is appearing in any case.

I've found that effective customers who get more fit and keep it off are the ones who accomplish the internal work. They're prepared to face their contemplations, emotions, love for self, and how they see themselves.

The course to your ideal weight will likely be fraught with pitfalls, land mines, and saboteurs. Any worthy intention has barriers to be overcome. This is readily spotting the one's barriers, dismissing a number of them, and taking bold action to dispose of the others.

The hypnotic trance work focuses on thoughts and ideas at the mind-body level in an effort to energize the process. Familiarize yourself with thoughts, old patterns of conduct, special social events, and regular settings that could potentially sabotage your best weight. This is the primary step closer to clearing the path to your ideal weight.

Once you're able to recognize the triggers to overeating, you simply need to exercise ways to easily brush aside the ones seemingly troublesome barriers. If this appears overwhelming, don't worry. As we've said, we will guide you on your trance work, so that you might also talk exactly what you want to say on your magnificent mind-body.

Where Are You Right Now?

As you begin your course, check where you're now. New numbers from the United States Government's National Health and Nutrition Examination Survey (NHANES) affirm that overweight and weight problems are still a chief public health concern. Overweight is described as having a body mass index (BMI) of 25 or better. Obesity is having a BMI of 30 or better. Having a BMI of 40 or higher is excessive weight problems.

Keep in mind that a person who's muscular with a low frame-fat percentage can also have a better BMI because muscle weighs extra than fats.

So, if you are 5'8" and weigh 185 pounds, your BMI is 28. To see where you're right now, in comparison with different Americans, take a look at these statistics: Nearly two-thirds of U.S. Adults are overweight (BMI of 25 or better, which includes individuals who are obese).

Nearly one-0.33 of U.S. Adults is obese (BMI of 30 or higher).

Less than half of U.S. Adults have a healthy weight (BMI better than or equal to 18.5 and lower than 25).

Getting Out Of Your Way

Safeguarding your achievement and clearing the direction to begin with you. As you study in the earlier, the whole thing starts off evolved with mind and ideals approximately what you want, how you want it, and what you can accept as true with and accept. All self-defeating thoughts have to be neutralized and converted into affirmations of your success. For example, if you always say, "My belly is the biggest part of my problem," what are you telling your thoughts-frame? What is your mind-body going to make genuine for you? Here is the confirmation that neutralizes and transforms that declaration and other statements like it: "My frame is flawlessly shaped." When you encounter thoughts that don't assist your perfect weight, recall this confirmation and follow these four steps.

- You must believe it is possible for you to have the perfect weight you desire.
- You must want it and feel you deserve it.
- Accept any challenge as an opportunity to have your perfect weight.
- Let yourself expect the results you desire, and commit yourself to remove any obstacle from within or without.

Letting Go of Old Patterns of Behavior

Patterns of behavior with food, eating, and workout should end up an increasing number of likeminded with the results you want. Here are some approaches to begin shifting your perspective:

- If you adore junk meals, you need to allow yourself to go of an everyday weight-reduction plan of junk food and welcome some new, healthier meals that aid your healthy weight.

- If you have got an aversion to work out and physical pastime, you have to welcome the everyday physical activity that enlivens and strengthens your body.

The identical is authentic for the subconsciously driven styles that create cravings. You start by means of identifying incompatible cravings as limitations and mark them for removal. This tells your unconscious that it has your permission to act to your behalf. The trancework contains pointers that empower you to welcome new styles of behavior.

Clear Away All Excuses

Clear away all excuses you supply to yourself and others. They only work towards you. Here are some excuses we hear from our clients: "I don't have time to do any purchasing and cooking."

"My job is too stressful. I couldn't likely add more pressure by means of dieting." "When the children are out of the house, then I'll have time to reflect on consideration on losing weight."

"I can't lose weight. My knees harm too much."

There is no excuse that justifies an obstacle in your achievement. This includes any excuse about the charges related to weight reduction. Yes, fine meals might cost greater than fast meals, but your ideal weight is really worth each penny and each pound lighter. We have had patients inform us that weight-loss packages are too pricey or that their health insurance will not cowl the prices of a weight reduction program. No amount of money is a legitimate excuse to keep you from achieving success. The medical situations associated with excess weight will fee you extra in the lengthy run. If your investment within the problem outweighs your investment inside the solution, you will keep the hassle.

Do no longer make excuses because you sense you lack willpower. If you've got the self-control to breathe clean air or examine this eBook, you've got the willpower essential for the whole thing else you need to your life. Become sensitive to the excuses you pay attention to others using the reasons that they are saying they cannot have what they want. Pay unique attention to individuals who are overweight as they speak approximately the limitations to their weight loss. Some different excuses we've heard are: "I don't have the time or the power to make breakfast in the morning," or "It's sprinkling out; I can't take my fifteen minute walk tonight," or "The holidays start next month; I'll wait until January." Each time you hear an excuse; make a mental note for yourself: "Not for me" or "I know better." In the television collection "In Living Color," Damon Wayans performed a reluctant clown named Homey, who could go to birthday events to entertain children. When the youngsters would ask him to do the slapstick and self-deprecating activities that clowns are well-known for, he would decline, saying, "Homey don't play that." However funny this becomes, he truly had a point. He was dressed as a clown, but he never sacrificed his self-respect or integrity for anyone, even if it turned into his job. When you hear yourself or others make any excuse that could have an effect on your perfect weight, tell yourself with a smile, "I don't play that," and "I even have a better way."

Judge Righteously

Obsessions about food or weight can be boundaries to a successful healthy weight. To break those patterns, take a formidable movement to defuse, neutralize, or transform any obsessive mind, which includes "I'm always hungry," "All I reflect on consideration on is meals," or "I ought to eat." This may mean speaking to a counselor if it is an obsession that warrants medical intervention. If you feel that you cannot change an obsessive mind through yourself, you may probably gain from expert help.

If it isn't always a critical mental obsession, begin inspecting your judgmental thoughts. That is, in case you are giving meals and/or weight too much of your mental power and mind, you could exchange the judgments and thoughts which you are making. Since your intention is to acquire your best weight, you need to cancel the thoughts that let meals manipulate you and transform those mind so you control the meals. Either your obsessive thoughts, approximately meals will power you, or you may force them. Choose to judge with the "right" mind, the mind approximately food so that it will be a route to your ideal weight. A few examples: "My breakfast changed into delicious," or "The pita pocket I packed is complete of pep and power," or "I love the grapes I had for dessert." In short, if you are going to obsess approximately food, make it be just right for you with the aid of obsessing approximately your success. Make your judgments righteous: make them accurate for you.

CHAPTER 37:

Why Do We Struggle with Weight?

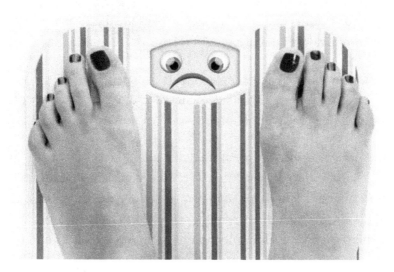

For anyone who has ever struggled with weight, life can seem like an uphill battle. In fact, it can be downright devastating to see how difficult it can be to turn things around and shed some weight.

The fact of the matter is that losing weight doesn't have to be an uphill battle. Most of this requires you to better understand why this struggle happens and what you can do to help give yourself a fighting chance.

While there may be physiological factors affecting your ability to keep unwanted pounds off, there are also a host of psychological, emotional and even spiritual causes that may be affecting your overall body's ability to help you lose weight and reach your ideal weight levels.

That is why this is about focusing on those "hidden" causes, the kinds that go beyond the obvious aspects which are widely discussed in the mainstream media and by everyday folks. We are going to be talking about how you can look inward to see how and where things may need to change so that you can begin to turn things around and make a positive impact in your life.

The Obvious Culprits

The obvious culprits that are holding you back are diet, a lack of exercise and a combination of both.

First off, your diet plays a key role in your overall health and well-being. When it comes to weight management, your diet has everything to do with your ability to stay in shape and ward of unwanted weight.

When it comes to diet, we are not talking about keto, vegan, or Atkins; we are talking about the usual foods you consume and the amounts you have of each one. This is why diet is one of the obvious culprits. If you have a diet that is high in fat, high in sodium and high in sugar, you can rest assured that your body will end up gaining weight at a rapid rate.

When you consume high amounts of sugar, carbs and fats, your body transforms them into glucose, which is then stored in the body as fat. Of course, a proportion of the glucose produced by your body is used up as energy. However, if you consume far more than you actually need, your body isn't going to get rid of it; your body is going to hold on to it and make sure that it is stored for a rainy day.

If you are asking yourself why the body does that, the answer is simple. Over thousands of years of evolution, humankind has struggled to have enough to eat. It hasn't been until about the last two hundred years that most societies have abundant amounts of food. This has enabled our generations to eat three meals a day... and a little more. Given the fact that our early ancestors would go days without eating, evolution has programmed the human body to store up as much fat as possible. If the body were programmed otherwise, it would have some sort of mechanism that would either shut off hunger and use up the fat that has been stored up or signal the body the get rid of excess fat somehow.

But, we're not there yet. Perhaps at some point in the future, the body will evolve such response. Until that happens, we need to roll with the punches and understand why we gain weight the way that we do.

Here is another important aspect to consider: sweet and salty foods, the kind that we love so dearly, trigger "happy hormones" in the brain, namely dopamine. Dopamine is a hormone that is released by the body when it "feels good." And food is one of the best ways to trigger it. This is why you somehow feel better after eating your favorite meals. It also explains the reason why we resort to food when we are not feeling well. This is called "comfort food," and it is one of the most popular coping mechanisms employed by folks around the world.

This rush of dopamine causes a person to become addicted to food. As with any addiction, there comes a time when you need to get more and more of that same substance to meet your body's requirements.

It's exactly the same with a drug addict or alcoholic. They need to consume more and more of the substance they are addicted to in order to get the same rush. In a way, the body develops a resistance to the "happy hormones" released when eating yummy food. Therefore, you need an ever-increasing amount of these hormones in order for you to get your fix.

As a corollary to diet, a lack of regular exercise can do a number on your ability to lose weight and maintain a healthy balance. What regular exercise does is increase your body's overall caloric requirement. As such, your metabolism needs to convert fat at higher rates in order to keep up with your body's energy demands.

On paper, this is a rather straightforward process. Through the process of cellular respiration, the body converts glucose (or fat back into glucose) and combines it with oxygen to produce energy. This process makes it possible for the body to transform its caloric intake into amounts of energy, which can be used to fuel the body's movements.

As the body's energetic requirements increase, that is, as your exercise regimen gets more and more intense, you will find that you will need increased amounts of both oxygen and glucose. This is one of the reasons why you feel hungrier when you ramp up your workouts.

However, an increased caloric intake isn't just about consuming more and more calories for the sake of it; you need to consume an equal amount of proteins, carbs, fats and vitamins in order to for your body to build the necessary elements that will build muscle, foster movement and provide proper oxygenation in the blood.

Moreover, nutrients are required for the body to recover. One of the byproducts of exercise is called "lactic acid." Lactic acid builds up in the muscles as they get more and more tired. Lactic acid signals the body that it is time to stop working out or risk injury if you continue. Without lactic acid, your body would have no way of knowing when your muscles have overextended their capacity.

After you have completed your workout, the body needs to get rid of the lactic acid build-up. So, if you don't have enough of the right minerals in your body, for example, potassium, your muscles will ache for days until your body is finally able to get rid of the lactic acid buildup. This example goes to show how proper nutrition is needed to help the body gets moving and also recover once it is done exercising. As a result, a lack of exercise reconfigures your body's metabolism to work at a slower pace. What that means is that you need to consume fewer calories to fuel your body's lack of exercise. So, if you end up consuming more than you actually need, your body will just put it away for a rainy day. Plain and simple.

The Sneaky Culprits

The sneaky culprits are the ones that aren't quite so overt in causing you to gain weight or have trouble shedding pounds. These culprits hide beneath the surface but are very effective when it comes to keeping you overweight. The first culprit we are going to be looking at is called "stress."

Stress is a very powerful force. From an evolutionary perspective, it exists as a means of fueling the flight-or-fight response. Stress is the human response to danger. When a person senses danger, the body begins to secrete a hormone called "cortisol." When cortisol begins running through the body, it signals the entire system to prep for a potential showdown. Depending on the situation, it might be best to hightail it out and live to fight another day.

Regardless of the outcome, the main point is to ensure survival. This evolutionary trait is what has helped preserve the human species throughout thousands of years. In modern life, though, stress plays a very different role.

In our modern way of life, stress isn't so much a response to life and death situations (though it can certainly be), rather it is the response to situations that are deemed as "conflictive" by the mind. This could be a confrontation with a co-worker, bumper to bumper traffic, or any other type of situation in which a person feels vulnerable in some way.

Over the course of our lives, we are subjected to countless interactions in which we must deal with stress. In general terms, the feelings of alertness subside when the perceived threat is gone. However, when a person is exposed to prolonged periods of stress, any number of changes can happen.

One such change is overexposure to cortisol. When there is too much cortisol in the body, the body's overall response is to hoard calories, increase the production of other hormones such as adrenaline and kick up the immune system's function.

This response by the body is akin to the panic response that the body would assume when faced with prolonged periods of hunger or fasting. As a result, the body needs to go into survival mode. Please bear in mind that the body has no clue if it is being chased by a bear, dealing with a natural disaster or just having a bad day at the office. Regardless of the circumstances, the body is faced with the need to ensure its survival. So, anything that it eats, goes straight to fat stores.

Moreover, a person's stressful situation makes them search for comfort and solace. There are various means of achieving this. Food is one of them. So is alcohol consumption. These two types of comforts lead to high consumption of calories. Again, when the body is in high gear, it will store as many calories and keep them in reserve.

This what makes you gain weight when you are really, really stressed out.

Now, suppose you go on a low-carb crash diet. Your body is already under duress from the amount of stress it is under. On top of that, you choose to take away its usual caloric intake. What do you think will be the body's response? A further deepening of its panic mode. This is the main reason why crash diets only partially work.

Another of the sneaky culprits is sleep deprivation. In short, sleep deprivation is sleeping less than the recommended 8 hours that all adults should sleep. In the case of children, the recommended amount of sleep can be anywhere from 8 to 12 hours, depending on their age.

Granted, some adults can function perfectly well with less than 8 hours' sleep. There are folks who can function perfectly well with 6 hours' sleep while there are folks who are shattered when they don't get 8 or even more hours' sleep. This is different for everyone as each individual is different in this regard.

CHAPTER 38:

What Are Body Goals?

We are currently living in an era where we are completely immersed in popular culture. Because of this, we are constantly bombarded with images of what the "ideal body" is, thus, we try to shape our bodies into what we believe is ideal. But should your body goals be the same as the goals of everyone else?

Sadly, if you focus on having the same body goals as the people you see on runways or in magazines, you might feel frustrated and dissatisfied with your body all the time. This is not the best way to live your life. Instead, the most important body goal you may try to have is learning how to embrace your body even though you're not completely happy with it. This is a lot more achievable and realistic compared to trying to have the "perfect" body but ruining yourself in the process. As part of your intuitive eating journey, your goal shouldn't just be about having the look that you desire but getting the desired feeling of looking good.

The body you have right now is the only body that you will have for the rest of your life. Therefore, when you're trying to think about your body goals, focus more on your own body, not the bodies of others. Try to learn how you can feel good about yourself, even if your body isn't considered "ideal" or "perfect." If you can learn how to love your own body and feel comfortable in your own skin, then it becomes much easier for you to tune into your body to unlock your intuitive eating potential.

Body goals are the goals you set for your own body. For instance, if you're overweight or obese and you want to improve your health, then shedding a few pounds until you reach your ideal weight is a realistic and practical body goal. But if you are already at your ideal weight and you still want to shed more pounds to have the same body as the models you see in magazines, then you might start doing things that will affect your body adversely.

To become an intuitive eater, focus more on feeling happy and good about your own body. Come up with body goals that you know you can achieve. That way, you can be kinder to yourself as you work to achieve these goals. Take some time to reflect on your thoughts and feelings about your body then try to think of the body goals that you want to achieve. The more honest you are with yourself, the more you can think of realistic and achievable goals. Make a list of these goals and once you have finalized them, you can start working on your health objectives.

What Are Health Objectives?

Once you have a list of body goals, it's now time to think about your health objectives. Health objectives are a lot like your body goals, but these also involve the steps to take to achieve them. To achieve your body goals and health objectives, you should always remember to take the right steps based on logical and ethical reasons. As an intuitive eater, you may want to focus more on your own habits, behaviors, thoughts, and choices. By doing this, you will learn how to become more intuitive, especially when it comes to your body and your health. Here are some tips to help you manage your health as an intuitive eater:

Think about your goals for proper nutrition

Ultimately, your greatest health objective should be to learn how to "eat better." This may sound simple, but it does take a lot of time and effort to achieve. If you want to eat better to improve your health and your body, try to improve your nutrition too. Take a look at your current eating habits to give you a better idea of whether you are nourishing your body with the nutrients it needs or not. If you are, keep going! If not, you may want to make better choices without forcing yourself to change things drastically. It's better to take small steps towards proper nutrition instead of trying to make huge changes that will make you feel like you're on a diet again. Remember, it's all about using your intuition.

Make sure to include proper hydration throughout the day

One of the most effective ways to ensure your health is to drink enough water each day. Drinking enough water provides your body with so many benefits. It also allows your body to adjust to your new eating habits as you move towards better health. If you're not used to drinking water, that's okay. Just try to make a conscious effort to swap out alcoholic, caffeinated or sugary drinks with this healthy beverage and you're sure to see the difference.

Eat regularly

If you want to become a healthy, intuitive eater, eating regularly is key. To eat regularly, you may want to be more conscious of what your body is feeling. If you think it will help, keep a food journal or even a nutrition app to find out your own eating patterns. After a few days or weeks of tuning into your body and using these tools, you may come to discover these patterns that are uniquely yours. By learning these patterns, you can start creating a regular routine. This is a process that takes time, so you don't have to rush it.

Start with small portions

While you don't have to strictly control your portions, it's a good idea to start with small portions whenever you eat. This allows you to eat everything on your plate without having to force yourself to finish what you have taken. If you still feel hungry after finishing the portion on your plate, then take another small portion. Keep doing this until you feel full. This is a great way to practice intuitive eating.

Focus on what you are eating

Awakening your intuition takes time and practice. When you focus on what you're eating, you can also focus on what you are feeling. Try to focus on the taste, texture, and even the smell of each bite you put into your mouth. Try to focus on what the food makes you feel. More importantly, try to focus on whether you are still hungry, or you are already full. All of these things will hone your intuition.

Set goals for the different aspects of your health

When you're thinking of your health objectives, consider your body, your mind, and your overall well-being. Therefore, you may want to include different kinds of goals and objectives, such as:

- Physical health goals like coming up with a new workout routine and practicing different breathing exercises.
- Emotional and mental health goals like establishing a relaxing morning routine and learning how to meditate.

The goals and objectives you set for yourself would depend on your own needs and on what you want to improve in your life. You can incorporate these goals into your plan for becoming an intuitive eater.

Get enough sleep each night

Never underestimate the importance of a good night's sleep. When you sleep, your body gets the chance to repair and recover from everything you have gone through each day. No matter how busy your life is, make sure that you get enough sleep each night—this should be one of your health objectives. These are some basic health objectives you can set for yourself. Some of these may apply to your own life, while others won't. As with your body goals, take some time to reflect on what you want and what you need. Then you can come up with the best objectives to improve all aspects of your health.

CHAPTER 39:

How Do I Love My Body If There Is No Reason?

You look in the mirror and you are dissatisfied. Do you wish that your shape, your nose, your legs, your hair were like somebody else's? Why do we always compare ourselves? Why aren't we reconciled with our appearance? We have heard ad nauseam that we should love ourselves, despite our mistakes or flaws. This includes things related to our personality as well as our bodies. However, there are very few people who can accept and be content with themselves. It is not about not wanting to change. It is a commendable endeavor when one wants to achieve or retain their looks or care about looking more attractive.

At the same time, most people are much more critical, stricter with themselves than justified. They are continuously dissatisfied with themselves and don't see in the mirror what others see. Some girls feel a significant discomfort looking at each other, both because they don't like looking at each other in general, and because they don't like what they see. Where do these reactions come from?

What usually happens is that you don't look at yourself; you only see yourself with respect to that ideal of beauty that you have in your head. This is where dissatisfaction creeps in. It has to do with the theory of social confrontation. We compare ourselves with those we consider better than ourselves; self-esteem is negatively affected. We all have a model in the head, a term of comparison that we have built by looking at years of magazines, advertising, and movies with perfect Hollywood princesses. The mantra must become one and only one: there is no need for me to compare myself to that model because everybody is a unique, generous specimen, rich in the indications of what I am.

Life would be much simpler and happier if we could accept ourselves as we are. A lot of negative emotions would be released, we would have less stress, and more of the things that really matter come into view. The bottom line is, if we really need to change something, we can't do it until we make peace with the current state. This is a vicious circle.

The mind works, in effect, in a strange way. If we resist something, we get more of it.

After all, if we focus our attention on what is bad, we reinforce the bad. And what we pay the most attention to as we think about something will come true.

Everything that comes from you that relates to you is just yours: your feelings, your voice, your actions, your ears, your thighs, your hopes and fears. That's why you are unique. Be happy that you are different from anyone, that you look the way you do and that it is just you. Start to feel that it's your own body, not something separate that you need to live with.

Do you want your house to be just like anyone else's? Or do you love the little things that carry memories? Don't you love the atmosphere of your messy place after playing with your kids? And the plain curtain that you know you should replace, but which your mom sewed and looks so good? Or the piece of furniture that everyone says you should throw out, but you insist on it?

That's how you should feel about your body. You should understand that you don't need to compare it with anyone else's because it's impossible to compare unique things. In addition, who determines what beautiful and ugly mean? You should not compare your body to the celebrities' perfect-looking bodies. First, because they are adjusted with Photoshop and other programs, and they are not real. Second, because you are different, as is everybody.

You're not them. You are neither the next-door girl who, after three children, looks like she did at twenty, nor your friend who you think is gorgeous. You should not only accept your body, but you should fall in love with it. Do you think like Bonnie? Do you think no one could love you because you have some extra weight? Then ask yourself the following questions. Could you fall in love with someone only if they are perfect looking? Would you really love someone because of their body? I'll go further.

Do we really love perfect looking people? I bet you prefer your imperfect companion instead of a perfect looking bodybuilder. You like the little faults of your wife, husband, kids, and friends because they belong to you too. We love imperfections better than perfections.

See? We don't measure people based on their weight. In addition, if you are happy with your body and your existence, it will also manifest in your radiance.

How Should You Love Your Body?

Sandra Díaz Ferrer, a researcher at the University of Granada, works with women who do not like their bodies and suffer from eating disorders. After years of observations, she published a study in the Journal of Behavior Therapy and Experimental Psychiatry, which reveals how looking at the mirror correctly can help in the treatment of bulimia nervosa. Her technique can be fundamental for all women dissatisfied with their image, or those who suffer from eating disorders. Imagine you have a fear of bugs that obsesses you. The psychologist might ask you to look closely at bugs until you get used to them, desensitizing yourself to the features that first terrified you. You can apply the same procedure to your body (Ferrer, 2015).

Here's an exercise that can help those who struggle to be happy about their own imperfections. You have to stand in front of a large mirror and look at yourself as if you were doing it for the first time in your life, like never before, taking time for yourself. It must be a constructive and very careful observation. No distractions, no work commitments, no notification to pull your attention. Only you and the mirror. Next time you hate your body or any part of your body, stand in front of a mirror and look at yourself. Go from top to bottom and sort out your "mistakes." You will have to start looking at yourself from head to toe, objectively observing all the details, without comparisons or judgments.

- Remember what that part of your body has done for you. When did it help, when did it protect you, when did it do something physically useful for you? Say thank you for something that was of help to you. Learn to practice gratitude.
- Appreciate what you have and love your inner self. Don't let a scale or a size define your identity and skills. It is no use to criticize yourself fiercely when looking in the mirror.

Here are some ways to cultivate enormous gratitude in everyday life. When faced with a negative situation, do not be discouraged. Ask yourself instead what you can learn for the future and for reasons to feel grateful. Promise yourself not to be negative or not to criticize yourself for three days. If you make a mistake, forgive yourself and go on your way. This exercise will help you understand that negative thoughts are just a waste of energy. Every day, list the reasons why you feel grateful. The body is a miracle and you should celebrate all the gifts it has given you. Think about the goals you have passed, your relationships and the activities you love: it was your body that allowed you to do all this. Take note of it every day. Go to the next body part and do the same.

When you have reached your toes, return to your head again, to your face, and now, going downhill, just say to all your body parts, "I love you." Even if you feel a little stupid about it, don't stop. You see, you're going to have a completely different relationship with your appearance.

And by the way, let's not forget, it's not a coincidence that it's called outer. What's inside is more important. But what's inside is visible outside. So use your inner self to love your outer, and you will be much calmer, happier, more satisfied and more confident.

Set the alarm and watch yourself for at least 40 minutes at a time. Doing so could change your life. Experts talk about the epidemic spread of body image disorder, a severe problem that leads us to see ourselves as inadequate every time we look at our bodies. According to research, 90.2% of women have an altered image of themselves and are not satisfied with their bodies, a fact that has a lot to do with how we look in the mirror. The mirror is your new weapon: from enemy to ally, but learning to use it in the right way (Ferrer, 2015).

Compliment yourself. You should consider yourself and treat yourself with the same kindness and the same admiration that you would reserve for those you love. You probably wouldn't direct the same criticisms you do to yourself, to another person. Don't hesitate to compliment yourself, don't be too hard on yourself and forgive yourself when you make a mistake. Get rid of the hatred you feel for yourself, replace it with greater understanding and appreciation. Look in the mirror and repeat: "I am attractive. I am sure of myself. I am fantastic!" Do it regularly and you'll begin to see yourself in a positive light. When you reach a goal, be proud. Look in the mirror and say, "Great job, I'm proud of myself."

Stay away from negativity. Avoid people who only talk badly about their bodies. You risk getting infected by their insecurities and dwelling on your faults. Life is too short and valuable to be consumed by hating yourself or looking for every little fault, especially when the perception you have of yourself tends to be much more critical than that of others. If a person starts to criticize their body, don't get involved in their negativity. Change the subject instead or leave. Wear comfortable clothes that reflect who you are. Everything you have in the wardrobe should enhance your body. Don't wear uncomfortable clothes just to impress others. Remember that those who accept themselves always look great. Wear clean, undamaged garments to dress the body the way you deserve. Buy matching briefs and bras, even though you are the only one to see them. You will remind your inner self that you are doing it exclusively for yourself.

Ask others what they love about you and what they consider your best qualities. This will help you develop yourself and remind you that your body has given you so much. You will probably be surprised to discover what others find beautiful about you; you have probably forgotten about them.

Surround yourself with people who love themselves. People absorb the attitudes and behaviors of the people around them. If your life is full of positive influences, you will also adopt them, and they will help you to love both your inner and outer. Look for optimistic people who work hard to achieve their goals and respect themselves.

Conclusion

A secret to women's holistic health is healthy self-esteem for women. Issues of self-esteem are women's most prevalent mental health issues. Body image is very important; it is one of the factors affecting the self-esteem of a woman. Women will build trust in their relationships, careers, personal lives, parenting skills, and the ability to live their dreams in this day and age. This will allow them to be accountable for their applecart. How much matters to a woman her looks? A woman can spend minutes to hours before the mirror just to make sure she looks her best before she heads out. A healthy self-image affects the self-esteem of a woman positively.

To define the overall sense of personal importance or self-worth of an individual, the word self-esteem is used. It is a feature of personality that includes a range of self-beliefs, such as actions, feelings, habits (habits and attitudes), values, and self-appraisal. Trust and self-satisfaction influence all aspects of one's life. This also increases your self-esteem and appreciation for yourself. Humility, modesty and humility allow your self-esteem to increase. Self-esteem is a sense of personal worth and capacity that is central to the identity of an individual. The definition of yourself has a great impact on how and what you feel about yourself. You are improving your self-esteem by loving yourself!

As a woman, believing in you is the best way to live a beautiful and happy life. Each woman has the power and potential to live her dream life, but many are not due to the low self-esteem issue.

You can enhance your self-esteem and enhance your life and live by the means described below:

- **Appreciate Your Physique:** the women you see on the pages of certain newspapers, magazines and television advertisements are often not true representations of real women. It can make you start feeling unwanted or less confident about yourself when you're always seeing size 4 people and you're a size 10. Don't think about the press! You'll see women of different sizes, styles, colors and heights walking around your community; know that being beautiful and sexy comes in various forms, including your own. Appreciate and praise yourself because God—the master builder—makes you perfectly and beautifully. Fell well with yourself.
Note: The importance you place on yourself is very important in your life.
- **Have Positive Thinking and Beliefs:** Replace negative and weak thinking with life-enriching feelings. For example, if you think you're bad because your mind is painting your reality, this will become true for you. Even if in the past you have made mistakes, forgive yourself and support yourself. Relax and talk to yourself when things don't go well. Positive thinking, apology, and doing have a positive outcome.
- **Avoid Positive Comparison:** Unhealthy comparison of yourself to another person will only make you feel bad. There are no two similar people; each woman is unique and special.

While women are referred to as the weaker sex, they have great potential to enrich lives 24/7. Self-esteem gives a woman's life strength and vigor, and with self-confidence, it can be enhanced. Do those things that make you happy and inspire you; they boost your self-esteem.

HYPNOTIC GASTRIC BAND

A Complete Guide to Achieve Weight Loss and Eat Healthy Through Gastric Band Hypnosis, Meditation, Affirmations and Motivation. Change Your Mind, Change Your Body.

Cleopatra Johnson

Table of Contents

Introduction 264
Chapter 1: What Is A Gastric Band? 268
Chapter 2: The Concept Of Hypnosis 274
Chapter 3: An Overview On Gastric Band Hypnosis 282
Chapter 4: The Power Of Visualization 288
Chapter 5: Reprogramming Your Mind 296
Chapter 6: How Gastric Band Hypnotherapy Works 300
Chapter 7: Preparing Your Body For Your Hypnotic Gastric Band 308
Chapter 8: Gastric Band Hypnosis For Food Addiction 316
Chapter 9: Techniques To Execute Gastric Band Hypnosis 320
Chapter 10: Emotional Eating 326
Chapter 11: Blasting Calories 334
Chapter 12: Meditation For Weight Loss 342
Chapter 13: A Basic Self-Hypnosis Session For Weight Loss 346
Chapter 14: Virtual Band Sample—Short Version 350
Chapter 15: Strong Hypnotic Gastric Band - The Weekly Program ... 358
Chapter 16: Positive Impacts Of Affirmations 364
Chapter 17: Motivational Affirmations 370
Chapter 18: Self-Improvement With Hypnosis 376
Chapter 19: How Hypnosis Work: Overpowered And Out Of Control 382
Chapter 20: Basics Of Meditation 388
Chapter 21: Body Image Relaxation 394
Chapter 22: Power Of Self-Confidence 398
Chapter 23: Pleasure Principle 402
Chapter 24: Eating Out On Effective Weight Loss Program 408
Chapter 25: Foods To Eat For Deeper Meditation 414
Chapter 26: The Four Golden Rules 420
Chapter 27: The Psychology About Weight Loss 428

Chapter 28: The Secret To Getting Rid Of Weight Problems 434

Chapter 29: Condition For Hypnosis To Work Out 442

Chapter 30: Your Thinner And Happier Life 446

Chapter 31: The Virtual Gastric Band Program 452

Chapter 32: Emotional Vs. Physical Hunger... 458

Chapter 33: The Disadvantages Of Emotional Eating...................................... 464

Chapter 34: Stopping Emotional Eating 468

Chapter 35: Eliminate Cravings... 472

Chapter 36: Enhance Your Motivation 478

Chapter 37: Great Techniques To Reach Your Ideal Weight 482

Chapter 38: Weight Loss Exercise 490

Chapter 39: Tips And Tricks.. 496

Chapter 40: The Final Weight Loss Puzzle 502

Chapter 41: Hypnotherapy Techniques 508

Conclusion 514

Introduction

The hypnotic gastric band system changes the size of your stomach, but it also helps you get comfortable and enjoy healthier foods. Hypno-gastric banding is a healthier, longer-term, non-evasive option. Changing your body physically cannot give you long-term results, but you can enjoy healthier alternatives by tackling the main problem of over-eating.

Your body is a genuinely astonishing machine. It produces all the energy you use. It keeps your heart thumping and your lungs breathing 24 hours every day.

It does a lot from using only the food you eat, the air you inhale, and the energy it has put away in your body. Simultaneously it fixes and keeps up itself while never halting work. When we fit your hypnotic gastric band, that fueling, fixing, and maintenance system keeps on working similarly as nature intends, however, there will be a couple of significant differences:

1. You will have less space for food in your stomach.
2. You will feel full sooner.
3. That "full" feeling will be urgent and easy to notice.
4. You are probably going to encounter changes in your food choices.
5. With the hypnotic band, there is no physical medical procedure, and therefore no physical dangers.
6. The hypnotic band is a less expensive.

As you are eating less, your body might be pickier or search out new foods to guarantee it gets all the sustenance it requires. You don't need to stress over this with your conscious mind by any means. You keep on eating exactly what you need, but you'll see that what you need to eat changes. In the early stages, those progressions might be very subtle, so it might take you a little effort to understand that you currently find various foods more appealing.

The Magic of Your Digestive System

It will be useful to have a diagram of your digestive system with the goal that you see how your hypnotic gastric band functions. A few people are interested and keen on how the body functions; others are most certainly not. Notwithstanding, whatever you deliberately think, it is significant that you read this segment with the goal that your conscious mind has all the information it needs to process my hypnotic instructions. So regardless of whether you discover this segment somewhat complex, simply continue reading because your conscious mind will comprehend and use all it needs from this clarification.

Your digestive system begins functioning when you smell your food. Your salivary glands begin to secrete saliva when the food enters your mouth; saliva begins to blend in with it to make it simpler to swallow and to start to breakdown the diet. Next, the physical movement of chewing your food sends signals to your stomach to release hydrochloric acid. When you swallow, the food goes down your throat, or in medical terms, your esophagus. At the base of your throat is a solid valve called a sphincter, which unwinds to give the food access to your stomach?

The sphincter shields your throat from the acid in your stomach. Sometimes, heartburn or overeating makes gastrointestinal reflux through that sphincter into your throat.

That builds up what we call indigestion. In your stomach, your food is blended in with acid and enzymes that break down the food into smaller particles. Proteins and fats take more time to process than sugars, so various foods take time to break down in the stomach. Vegetables do not take up to six minutes, and red meat can take a few hours to process.

You don't need to worry about this, and your body does everything naturally.

From the stomach, your food, now broken down into micro pieces, is released bit by bit into your small intestine. Then, when the food goes into your intestines, your body extracts the nutrients for sustenance. Various enzymes further break it down into particles that are sufficiently small to pass through the walls of your intestines into the bloodstream. Carbohydrates are separated into glucose, which is taken to the liver. Glucose is used to control the muscles in your body. Proteins are separated into amino acids and sent into the bloodstream circulating all through the body and used to build and repair cells and tissues.

As the food goes through your small intestine, each of the nutrients is separated into various micro-molecules. In the colon, the water and salts that helped the process are absorbed once again into your body, and the rest is excreted. Every one of these processes are controlled by a lot of hormones, or signaling chemicals, in your body. In your digestive tract, one of the most important is called Glucagon-like-peptide-1 (known as GLP-1). It is released as food enters your intestines. GLP-1 does loads of various jobs.

The two most vital jobs are:

1. It sends signals to a piece of your brain called the hypothalamus that you have had enough to eat.
2. It increases insulin secretion from the pancreas. The insulin interacts with the glucose going into your bloodstream and permits it to be stored in your muscles and liver.

Since GLP-1 does both these jobs at the same time, the feeling of fullness is connected to the process that gets energy into your muscles. This guarantees you don't feel full until your body is getting all the energy it needs. Levels of another hormone, called Peptide YY (known as PYY), also increases when you have eaten. PYY diminishes hunger and builds the capacity for nutrient absorption, so again it aids to signal you to stop eating to ensure you get what you need. Levels of a third hormone, called Ghrelin, decline after a meal. Ghrelin is one of the hormones that cause us to feel hunger.

CHAPTER 1:

What is a Gastric Band?

The gastric band (also known as a lap band) has become an increasingly popular surgical procedure for those who want to lose weight during the last decade or so. A band is fitted around the stomach and inflated in a way that significantly decreases stomach ability. This means the patient consumes less food, which leads to a fast and lasting weight loss. But surgery with the gastric band isn't without complications. With any surgery of something going wrong, there's always the inherent risk, but there are also some issues that the lap band can specifically cause. It involves a slipped band (which can result in too much or not enough stomach capacity), acid reflux, nausea, vomiting, diarrhea, regurgitation, blockages and other problems. And although the findings are unquestionably impressive, there are definitely hidden risks. But wouldn't it be awesome if there had been a way of replicating the gastric band's success without any of the risks?

Yeah, there's definitely a way in there. Recently hypnotherapists repeated the lap band treatment solely with hypnotic suggestions with great results. No scalpels, anesthetics, or wounds-pure mind-power. Hypnotherapy has become the latest craze in weight loss due to its safe and impacts the existence of the gastric band. A quick search on Google shows hundreds of happy patients who have undergone hypnotherapy in the gastric band and lost much of their excess weight. But how exactly does it work?

To understand how gastric band hypnotherapy functions, first, we need to look at hypnosis and the mental effect. Although human mental awareness is far from complete, the most welcoming theory is that the mind consists of two major components—the conscious and the subconscious. You should be most familiar with the idea of conscious thinking because this is from where the daily cycle of thought originates. Whenever you think to yourself, "I am thirsty, I should go get a drink" or something similar that is at work in your conscious mind. Your subconscious mind is much deeper and, in a way, stronger. It governs all those instinctive behaviors and responses you're not really thinking about, your routines, your impulses, and your phobias. Hypnosis operates upon the subconscious mind. The subconscious is primed by hypnosis and able to consider suggestions. Now we understand how hypnosis works; it is a little clearer how hypnotherapy works on the gastric unit. A hypnotherapist can create a hypnotic state within their client and then speak to them as if it were really occurring via the gastric band technique. There is no pain or something really happening physically at all, but it is very difficult for the subconscious mind to distinguish between illusion and reality. This is why very strong dreams can often seem all too real. If the subconscious mind assumes that the body is fitted with a gastric band, it will behave as though you are fitted with one. That means you'll feel full faster, eat slowly, and consume smaller meals. This obviously results in weight loss, which is very important. In addition to being safer than surgery, hypnotherapy by the gastric band is also much more convenient—generally ten times less costly than surgery. There are also professional hypnotherapists selling audio packs that have the very same session on CD or MP3 that are even less costly because the hypnotherapist only has to record the session once with certain clients. It will cost inferior to $100.

And if you are thinking of getting surgery with the gastric band, then the normal form of hypnotherapy might well be worth your consideration.

Hypnotherapy Gastric Band Hypnosis

If you're clinically obese—BMI over 30—there's hope with a virtual gastric band placed under hypnosis—sure, hypnotherapy may be the best all-round weight-loss choice.

I have run two successful tandem weight loss programs and so have had great experience supporting other people with their weight issues—both programs have the same philosophies at their heart. Many people on a diet are eating the items they shouldn't eat or go back to their old ways after dieting and losing weight. Some of their diets that exclude certain foods—leaving an unbalanced diet that puts a strain on their liver and kidneys—which are potentially very dangerous.

I think it's important to get people in touch with the joy of eating healthy food and persuade them of the cost-effectiveness of consuming less good quality food rather than cheaper fat sugar and salt-saturated foods—good nutrition really provides greater value for the buck and, after all, you wouldn't put paraffin in your fuel tank? You wouldn't put fuel in the car to take the metaphor further for comfort eaters if the oil light comes on, would you? Yet the oil light is a sign that something is wrong, and putting chocolate in your mouth won't fix the problems. Comfort food fixes little but gives rise to obesity.

Some of these issues are related to anxiety tension or lack of self-confidence or childhood behaviors rooted in bad eating practices as they grew up: "you have to clear your plate," for example. I say pounds more in the waste bin than pounds on the floor!

Hypnotherapy may tackle these concerns—providing approaches to cope with anxiety and depression and loss of confidence, and using methods such as regression to cope with psychological issues that could have contributed to an unhealthy relationship with food. One lady of 21 stones came to me, and after we had dealt with her bullying problems and offered her dietary advice, she immediately started to lose weight—something she should never have done!

Furthermore, the American Health Authority also blames a lot of obesity on fast food—which you can also call "junkie" food—the food has added fat sugar and salt, and the taste buds are actually addicted to this stuff—if you've ever seen "Supersize me" you know how unhealthy it can be, especially if the eating style is skewed to junk food.

The food diary is another valuable tool to remember what you eat but also when and why you consume those foods.

When obesity hits a BMI point of over 30, then for some the option is strong: if they don't lose weight, they'll have serious health problems—they'll have tried all the diets and pills and found them to fail because they haven't solved any of the underlying reasons for overeating. Often they are left with a Gastric Band's only option, the operation will cost about £3,000-£ 7,000; in some situations the operation can be risky. I just had a client who had several strokes and two of them extreme; the risks are too great for her.

Combining good nutritional advice with learning to enjoy food properly and dealing with underlying psychological problems, can result in permanent weight loss. Alternatively, putting the Virtual Gastric band under hypnosis, using something called the Hypogastric Band system, makes weight loss even more probable. The machine works with most people, and consumers have mentioned not only being able to see and observe the procedure without discomfort but also being able to feel it when it's installed. The discomfort passes quickly, and people find that they start eating smaller portions and, like my other customers who lose weight, they eat less and exercise more and start enjoying the food again.

The procedure of the gastric band is spoken about under hypnosis, and because it is keyhole surgery, it is relatively easy-wrapping a band around the higher part of the stomach. The band can be tightened or loosened, and the golf ball-sized portion of the stomach created by the band means that the hypothalamus, the appetite regulator, informs you that you are satisfied; the food passes about naturally. The hypnotic stomach band placed under hypnosis, works the same way as a real stomach band. There are also weight reduction plans that do the same but skip wearing the gastric band if you have a BMI under 30.

And if you have tried the others and it has failed, try hypnotherapy. My experience is, it's a practical option for most people.

Do Hypnosis Gastric Bands Really Work?

Lately, there's been a lot of press reports about the virtual hypnotic gastric band, but does that work? The vast quantity of websites out there would have you believe it works, and it is successful.

Such websites will just tell you what they want you to know and will not show you the absolute truth. Yeah, there have been reports in the press, but are they not just press releases sent to their publications to improve this procedure's credibility?

There won't be any newspaper publishing an article saying the hypnotic gastric band doesn't work, so who will read it? It would be as if they were writing an article stating that children do not like eating vegetables; no one would read it. But if they released an article that says a new technique was discovered that would make kids enjoy vegetables, then it would be a different story.

Since this technique was on the market, there were no scientifically validated studies demonstrating the effectiveness of the virtual hypnotic gastric unit.

This weight-loss strategy is no different from the conventional weight-loss methods that want you to believe they have the solution to your weight problem. We want you to believe their treatment will instantly turn off the mental and physiological factors that generate the weight issue right now. No treatment can do that, particularly if it doesn't tackle the real reasons why you're having a weight issue.

Having done one of those procedures is just like cutting off the head of a plant. At first, you think it's gone, and you start making progress, but those roots begin to crave the light underground. Then gradually, they start breaking the surface of the soil, at which point the old patterns of actions begin to take over again. You could then say to yourself that you deserve this chocolate bar because you were so good. Finally, those weeds start flowering and start taking up more of your lawn, at which point you give up trying to lose weight completely.

The hypnotic band may help some people temporarily lose weight, but over time people may start stretching out the limits of this procedure, as some do with the actual surgical version. The one thing about overeating mental and physiological factors is that if they aren't treated, they will come back again. This may be during one of those times a person undergoes emotional stress. The person can then use the food as a comfort either consciously or even unconsciously.

The individual then goes back to believing after this event that they have a gastric band fitted but that one little slip up has now undermined the confidence. The next time the person goes through some emotional stress, then it's even easier for them to use food for comfort because they've done it in the past already.

CHAPTER 2:

The Concept of Hypnosis

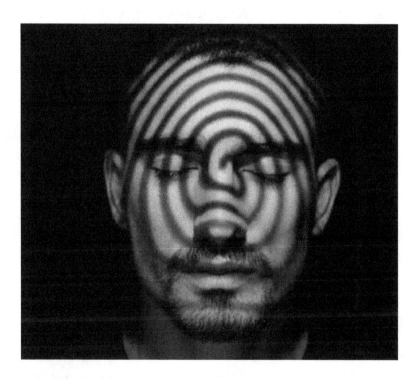

While brainwashing is a notable type of mind control that numerous individuals have about, hypnosis is additionally a significant sort that ought to be thought of. Generally, the individuals who know about hypnosis think about it from watching stage shows of members doing silly acts. While this is a sort of hypnosis, there is much more to it. This part is going to focus more on hypnosis as a type of mind control.

What Is Hypnosis?

To begin with, what is the meaning of hypnosis? As indicated by specialists, hypnosis is viewed as a condition of cognizance that includes the engaged consideration alongside the diminished fringe mindfulness that is described by the member's expanded ability to react to recommendations that are given. This implies the member will enter an alternate perspective and will be substantially more defenseless to following the recommendations that are given by the trance inducer.

It is broadly perceived that two hypothesis bunches help to depict what's going on during the hypnosis time frame. The first is the changing state hypothesis. The individuals who follow this hypothesis see that hypnosis resembles a daze or a perspective that is adjusted where the member will see that their mindfulness is, to some degree, not quite the same as what they would see in their common cognizant state. The other hypothesis is non-state speculations. The individuals who follow this hypothesis don't believe that the individuals who experience hypnosis are going into various conditions of awareness. Or maybe, the member is working with the subliminal specialist to enter a sort of inventive job authorization.

While in hypnosis, the member is thought to have more fixation and center that couples together with another capacity to focus on a particular memory or thought strongly. During this procedure, the member is likewise ready to shut out different sources that may be diverting to them. The mesmerizing subjects are thought to demonstrate an increased capacity to react to recommendations that are given to them, particularly when these proposals originate from the subliminal specialist. The procedure that is utilized to put the member into hypnosis is Knitted Hypnotic Enlistment and will include a progression of proposals and guidelines that are utilized as a kind of warm-up.

There is a wide range of musings that are raised by specialists with regards to what the meaning of hypnosis is. The wide assortment of these definitions originates from the way that there are simply such huge numbers of various conditions that accompany hypnosis, and no individual has a similar encounter when they are experiencing it.

Some various perspectives and articulations have been made about hypnosis. A few people accept that hypnosis is genuine and are suspicious that the legislature and others around them will attempt to control their minds. Others don't have faith in hypnosis at all and feel that it is only skillful deception. No doubt, the possibility of hypnosis as mind control falls someplace in the center.

There are three phases of hypnosis that are perceived by the mental network. These three phases incorporate acceptance, recommendation, and defenselessness. Every one of them is critical to the hypnosis procedure and will be talked about further underneath.

Induction

The principal phase of hypnosis is induction. Before the member experiences the full hypnosis, they will be acquainted with the hypnotic enlistment method. For a long time, this was believed to be the strategy used to place the subject into their hypnotic stupor. However, that definition has changed some in current occasions. A portion of the non-state scholars has seen this stage somewhat in an unexpected way. Rather they consider this to be as the strategy to elevate the members' desires for what will occur, characterizing the job that they will play, standing out enough to be noticed to center the correct way, and any of the different advances that are required to lead the member into the correct heading for hypnosis.

There are a few induction procedures that can be utilized during hypnosis. The most notable and compelling strategies are Braid's "eye obsession" method or "Braidism." There are many varieties of this methodology, including the Stanford Hypnotic Susceptibility Scale

(SHSS). This scale is the most utilized instrument to examine in the field of hypnosis.

To utilize the Braid enlistment procedures, you should follow several means. The first is to take any object that you can find that is brilliant, for example, a watch case, and hold it between the centers, fore, and thumb fingers on the left hand. You will need to hold this item around 8-15 crawls from the eyes of the member. Hold the item someplace over the brow, so it creates a ton of strain on the eyelids and eyes during the procedure with the goal that the member can keep up a fixed gaze on the article consistently.

The trance inducer should then disclose to the member that they should focus their eyes consistently on the article. The patient will likewise need to concentrate their mind on that specific item. They ought not to be permitted to consider different things or let their minds and eyes meander or, in all likelihood, the procedure won't be effective.

A little while later, the member's eyes will start to enlarge. With somewhat more time, the member will start to accept a wavy movement. If the member automatically shuts their eyelids when the center and forefingers of the correct hand are conveyed from the eyes to the item, at that point, they are in the stupor. If not, at that point, the member should start once more; make a point to tell the member that they are to permit their eyes to close once the fingers are conveyed in a comparable movement back towards the eyes once more. This will get the patient to go into the adjusted perspective that is knaps hypnosis.

While Braid remained by his method, he acknowledged that utilizing the acceptance procedure of hypnosis isn't constantly fundamental for each case. Analysts in current occasions have typically discovered that the acceptance strategy isn't as essential with the impacts of hypnotic recommendation as recently suspected. After some time, different other options and varieties of the first hypnotic acceptance procedure have been created, even though the Braid strategy is as yet thought about the best.

Recommendation

Present-day sleep induction utilizes a variety of proposal shapes to be fruitful, for example, representations, implications, roundabout or non-verbal recommendations, direct verbal proposals, and different metaphors and recommendations that are non-verbal. A portion of the non-verbal proposals that might be utilized during the recommendation stage would incorporate physical manipulation, voice tonality, and mental symbolism.

One of the qualifications that are made in the kinds of recommendation that can be offered to the member, incorporates those proposals that are conveyed with consent and those that progressively tyrant in the way.

Something that must be considered concerning hypnosis is the contrast between the oblivious and the cognizant mind. There are a few trance specialists who see the phase of the proposal as a method of conveying that is guided generally to the cognizant mind of the subject. Others in the field will see it the other way; they see the correspondence happening between the operator and the subconscious or oblivious mind.

They accepted that the recommendations were being tended directly to the conscious piece of the subject's mind, as opposed to the oblivious part. Braid goes further and characterizes the demonstration of trance induction as the engaged consideration upon the proposal or the predominant thought. The fear of a great many people that subliminal specialists will have the option to get into their oblivious and cause them to do and think things outside their ability to control, is inconceivable as per the individuals who follow this line of reasoning.

The idea of the mind has additionally been the determinant of the various originations about the recommendation. The individuals who accepted that the reactions given are through the oblivious mind, for example, on account of Milton Erickson, raise the instances of utilizing aberrant recommendations. Huge numbers of these aberrant proposals, for example, stories or representations, will shroud their expected importance to cover it from the cognizant mind of the subject. The subconscious recommendation is a type of hypnosis that depends on the hypothesis of the oblivious mind. If the oblivious mind was not being utilized in hypnosis, this sort of recommendation would not be conceivable. The contrasts between the two gatherings are genuinely simple to perceive; the individuals who accept that the recommendations will go fundamentally to the cognizant mind will utilize direct verbal guidelines and proposals while the individuals who accept the proposals will go essentially to the oblivious mind will utilize stories and analogies with concealed implications.

In both of these hypotheses of figured, the member should have the option to concentrate on one article or thought. This permits them to be driven toward the path that is required to go into the hypnotic state. When the recommendation stage has been finished effectively, the member will, at that point, have the option to move into the third stage, powerlessness.

Powerlessness

After some time, it has been seen that individuals will respond contrastingly to hypnosis. A few people find that they can fall into a hypnotic stupor reasonably effectively and don't need to invest a lot of energy into the procedure by any means. Others may find that they can get into the hypnotic daze, however, simply after a drawn-out timeframe and with some exertion. Still, others will find that they can't get into the hypnotic stupor, and significantly after proceeding with endeavors, won't arrive at their objectives. One thing that specialists have discovered intriguing about the weakness of various members is that this factor stays steady. If you have had the option to get into a hypnotic perspective effectively, you are probably going to be a similar path for an incredible remainder. Then again, if you have consistently experienced issues in arriving at the hypnotic state and have never been entranced, at that point, almost certainly, you never will.

There have been a few distinct models created after some time to attempt to decide the defenselessness of members to hypnosis. A portion of the more established profundity scales attempted to construe which level of a daze the member was in through the discernible signs that were accessible. These would incorporate things, for example, the unconstrained amnesia. A portion of the more present-day scales works to quantify the level of self-assessed or watched responsiveness to the particular recommendation tests that are given, for example, the immediate proposals of unbending arm nature.

As per the examination that has been finished by Deirdre Barrett, there are two kinds of subjects that are considered profoundly vulnerable to the impacts of subliminal therapy. These two gatherings incorporate dissociates and fantasizers. The fantasizers will score high on the assimilation scales, will have the option to effortlessly shut out the boosts of this present reality without the utilization of hypnosis, invest a great deal of their energy wandering off in fantasy land, had fanciful companions when they were a youngster, and experienced childhood in a situation where nonexistent play was energized.

CHAPTER 3:

An Overview on Gastric Band Hypnosis

Gastric Band Hypnotherapy is a technique used to propose that you have a gastric band connected around your stomach to the intuitive to enable you to get more fit. Gastric band medical procedure, thought about a final retreat, incorporates fitting a band around the upper segment of the stomach. This confines the amount of sustenance that you can expend physically, advancing weight reduction. It is an activity and, in this manner, involves future dangers and confusion. Hypnotherapy of the gastric band or fitting a 'virtual gastric band' doesn't include the medical procedure. Trance inducers utilize this technique to get the subliminal to think a gastric band has been fitted. The objective is to believe that you have had the physical activity on an oblivious level and that your stomach has diminished in size.

There is no medical procedure or medicine associated with the procedure, and it is thoroughly secure. In this segment, we will explore what is engaged with gastric band hypnotherapy, how it works, and on the off chance that it can work for you or not.

What is a Gastric Band?

A stomach band is a silicone flexible apparatus utilized in weight reduction medical procedure. To create a modest pack over the gadget, the band is put around the upper part of the belly. This restrains the amount of sustenance that can be put away in the stomach area, making eating enormous amounts hard.

A gastric band will likely constrain the amount of sustenance that an individual can expend physically, making them feel full in the wake of eating next to no to advance weight reduction. It is a final hotel for most people who have this medical procedure after endeavoring for other weight reduction systems. Like any medical procedure, there are perils in fitting a gastric band.

Gastric Band Trance

Gastric Band Trance can be utilized without the perils that accompany medical procedures to help people get thinner. A two-dimensional procedure is utilized by numerous trance specialists. They first hope to characterize your enthusiastic eating's underlying driver.

Utilizing trance, the specialist can urge you to recall long-overlooked nourishment related encounters that may now influence you subliminally. Before performing gastric band hypnotherapy, tending to and perceiving any unfortunate reasoning, examples concerning sustenance can be helpful.

Next, the trance specialist will play out the treatment of the virtual stomach band. The technique is proposed to recommend that you had an activity to embed a gastric band at a subliminal stage. The objective is to cause your body to respond to this proposition by making you feel quicker as though you were having a genuine medical procedure.

How It Functions

How gastric band spellbinding works using techniques for unwinding a trance specialist will get you a condition of trance. Your subliminal is progressively open to proposal in this casual state. Trance inducers are making proposals to your intuitive at this stage. With hypnotherapy of the gastric band, this suggestion is that you have joined a physical band.

The psyche is solid, so your conduct will change as needs be on the off chance that you are subliminal that acknowledges these proposals. More often than not, alongside the virtual gastric band's 'fitting,' proposals will be created about trust and conduct to help you focus on this way of life move.

Numerous specialists will likewise encourage strategies for self-mesmerizing so you can improve your activity after the session. It is likewise regularly prescribed to instruct yourself on nourishment and exercise to help physical well-being and prosperity.

The Process

Your first subliminal specialist session will likely be a unique counsel where you will talk about what you would like to get from hypnotherapy. This is an opportunity to talk about any past endeavors at weight reduction, eating rehearses, medical issues, and generally speaking nourishment frame of mind. This information will furnish the advisor with a clearer idea of what will help and whether to think about some other kinds of treatment.

The activity itself is expected to imitate the medical procedure of the gastric band to help your subliminal think it has happened. Numerous subliminal specialists will incorporate the sounds and scents of a working performance center to make the experience increasingly true. Your specialist will begin by carrying you to a condition of profound unwinding, otherwise called entrancing. You'll be aware of what's happening, and you'll generally be in order.

The specialist will address you through the system once you're sleep-inducing. They will explain bit by bit what is happening in a medical procedure, from being put under a sedative to making the primary entry point, fitting the band itself, and sewing the cut. A working auditorium's sounds and scents will improve the experience to persuade your inner mind that what is said is transpiring. As expressed before, different proposals to improve self-assurance might be incorporated during the activity. Endless supply of the system, your trance inducer may show you a few strategies for self-spellbinding to help you stay at home on the track. Some subliminal specialists will approach you to return for follow-up arrangements to screen the accomplishment of the virtual band and roll out any improvements. This happens when people additionally fit the physical band, proceeding with hypnotherapy sessions as a feature of long-term weight management, the board plan might be valuable for a few. This empowers the subliminal specialist to work with you to handle the hidden sustenance and confidence issues.

How Am I Going to Feel Afterward?

The general objective of the gastric band is to encourage a more beneficial nourishment association. If your subliminal thinks you have a gastric band fitted, your stomach will believe its lower. This, thus, makes your mind send messages that, in the wake of devouring less nourishment, you are finished. Perceiving when you are physically finished can be hard for the individuals who gorge. At times we eat only for taste (or comfort), overlooking whether we are physically ravenous or not. In developing smart dieting works on, figuring out how to perceive the physical vibes of being ravenous and being finished is helpful. In contrast to gastric band medical procedures, there are no physical symptoms in the virtual gastric band. For a few, the real medical procedure may trigger the reflux of queasiness, regurgitating, and corrosive. Since mesmerizing of the gastric band is not a physical technique, it won't trigger such side effects.

The activity ought to be a charming and loosening up understanding, with most people revealing from entrancing an impression of quiet.

Is It Going to Work for Me?

For the individuals who first attempt hypnotherapy, a well-known issue is: Is it getting down to business for me? It is anything but a simple circumstance of yes or no, lamentably; it's mostly up to you. Hypnotherapy empowers people with an assortment of issues. However, it is particularly useful in evolving propensities. Hence, helping people make great eating practices and shedding pounds is frequently viable. Like some other weight reduction plot, be that as it may, it will include your full commitment.

If you think similarly as your specialist, you're bound to get what you need from gastric band hypnotherapy. It is indispensable to be agreeable and to confide in your subliminal specialist. In this manner, it is prescribed that you require significant investment in your district to examine subliminal specialists and discover progressively about them, how they work, and what their aptitudes involve. Before the strategy, you can mastermind to meet them to ensure you are alright with them.

In case you're devoted to changing your way of life, think the methodology, and trust your subliminal specialist, the mesmerizing of the gastric band should work for you.

CHAPTER 4:

The Power of Visualization

Continual visualization directs your actions to reflect that of your mental image. This is why it is possible to acquire new skills with creative visualization. You can also use it to give yourself a new set of belief system. You only need to visualize yourself believing in the mental image you create, without allowing any resistance into your visualization.

You have to reprogram any negative and limiting beliefs if you are to achieve your goal. There are two main ways you can apply this kind of visualization in your life:

- Ensuring a healthy life and banishing bad habits
- Fostering strong relationships
- Manifesting financial abundance

Healthy Living and Banishing Bad Habits

Bad habits often start innocently; an overindulgence during a holiday season that you do not seem to break even when the holidays are over, perfectly normal social situations that slowly get you hooked to the bad behavior, peer pressure, or unhealthy lifestyles. It may be drinking, smoking, over-eating, drug abuse, or gambling.

These are all bad habits that undermine any idea you have of making your body and mind healthy. However, to have and maintain a healthy mind, you need to have a healthy and happy body.

Use Creative Visualization to Heal

The best you can do for yourself is to use creative visualization. With the help of visualization, it is easy to break off any bad habits in your life and acquire the kind of perfect and healthy life you have been dreaming of. Creative visualization can help you quit smoking, reduce drinking and eating, and return your body to better shape in no time.

Through creative visualization, you can easily develop a positive attitude to improve your health. You only need to imagine yourself in that perfect body and health you dream of, and you can easily make it into reality. According to researchers, they found out that an ill person is likely to change the situation by mentally picturing themselves combating their illness. Such action has been proven to reduce the severity of symptom in a patient and improve their quality and length of life.

However, always remember that when it comes to treating your illness with creative visualization, you must use it with tested procedures and medicines. It is good to get the best professional care and advice to be able to take care of your medical problems fast and effectively. The power of creative thinking only hastens your recovery and enhances the effectiveness of conventional medicine and professional help. It increases your defense for battling any illness you may have.

The whole process of visualizing your well-being is a partnership between you, your doctor, and your body. It is the doctor who determines what is ailing you and begins the medical treatment process to heal your condition. It is up to you to take the information you get from your doctor on where the problem is and pass it to your body. Through creative visualization, you get your body to work on the problem, and at the same time you are receiving conventional medication. This is a process that can easily help you combat any serious and minor illness you have. It involves adopting a positive outlook on your health to keep your immune system in top shape.

Use Creative Visualization to Build Strong Core Muscles

As you grow older your muscles weaken, especially if you are not active. A sedentary life makes your joints calcify and this often leads to osteoarthritis. When you are young and active, you may not think about the aches and pain of joint problems. However, when you get to your middle ages, these pains become more pronounced. What you need to do is to keep your muscles in good condition.

When using creative visualization, remember that it is impossible to build muscles simply by visualizing them. You need to get active if you want to develop your core muscles and be physically fit. Visualization helps to hasten the process and give you the motivation to keep your mind on the desired results and maintain it.

The benefits of toughening your core muscles can be realized through:

- Improved posture and less lower back pain
- Toned muscles that prevent the occurrence of back injuries
- Enhanced physical performance
- Fewer muscle aches
- Better balance made possible by having lengthened legs

According to physiotherapists and Pilates, the kind of physical and visualization exercise you engage in should emphasize to your body and unconscious mind the importance of keeping your muscles strong and fit to benefit you in all of the areas mentioned above. They believe that this technique is the key to developing core stability. This is where your abdominal wall, lower back, diaphragm, and pelvis are able to stabilize your body during movement.

How to Combine Physical Exercise with Creative Visualization

Step 1: Do abdominal bracing in a sitting position - Sit up in an alert and straight manner. While maintaining a steady breath, try pulling your navel inwards to touch your spine. It is not enough to imagine this procedure. You must carry it out.

Step 2: Channel energy to your muscles - As you hold your navel in, feel the muscles that are being employed in the process. While in this position and state of mind, visualize yourself directing energy into your muscles from within you.

Step 3: Hold the position - If you are a beginner, you can hold this position for a minimum of 30 seconds. However, the recommended time is five minutes. Always remember to keep breathing evenly.

As you continue with this exercise, you need to try to apply feelings of power, vibrant health, and motivation to your body. This makes it easy to get the inspiration to match your visualization to your physical workouts. However, this is a technique that only works for small toning cases. For an overall toning of your body muscles, you need proper exercising techniques you can combine with creative visualization. Furthermore, if you have an existing health problem, have your doctor check you up and get the relevant professional medication your body requires before you begin this exercise program.

Use Creative Visualization to Look After Your Heart

There are very many benefits you get when your heart is healthy. When you ensure your heart is in good condition, you increase your blood flow and the distribution of oxygen all through your body. This lets you enjoy:

- High energy levels and increased endurance

- Low blood pressure
- Reduced body fat and a healthier body weight
- Less stress, anxiety and depression
- Better sleep

The best way to look after your heart is to engage in aerobics. This is an exercise that causes you to breathe deeply and make you sweat for a minimum of 20 minutes. Whether it is fast walking, swimming, jogging, biking or even cross-country skiing, you should be in a position to make a conversation.

How to Combine Aerobics with Creative Visualization

Step 1: Visualize your exercise activity - In your mind, visualize taking a 20-minute jog, fast walk or any other aerobic activity. You can visualize yourself wearing the right exercising clothes and suitable running shoes.

Step 2: Visualize yourself doing the activity - Here, you need to visualize how you feel in the training wear, how the running shoes fit your feet perfectly, the country lane or suburbs in which you are running through and start the exercise. Feel the power and strength in your feet and envision your arms moving back and forth to the rhythm of your legs, feel the strength in your body and maintain your balance in a relaxed and simple position.

Step 3: Visualize yourself keeping pace for 20 minutes - In your mind's eye, you can make yourself realize that although you are getting tired, you are also energized and can well keep your pace until you are done. Imagine sweat building on your brow; you mop it away; your body feels supple and is moving easily to the finish line.

Step 4: Imagine the scenery - As you jog imagine passing trees, houses and you nod to people or wave at them. You should seem to enjoy the fact that they see you serious about your health. In your mind, breathe in and out, feel the refreshing coolness of the cool air and how refreshing it is to your lungs.

Step 5: Finish your exercise - You should continue your visualization exercise until you see yourself finish it. See yourself slowing down and returning to a normal walking pace and how your body feels fit and healthy.

While this visualization is still fresh in your mind, plan to get yourself a jogging gear to do a 20 minutes aerobic exercise. After your first jog, you will realize it is easy if you visualize the whole process and act it out as you exercise. You can do this exercise three times a week or more if you can to maintain a healthy heart. Remember to consult your doctor if you have any health issues before you start any aerobic exercises. Additionally, if you feel the exercise is painful for you or you become short of breath, you should stop.

Use Creative Visualization to Build Stamina

For you to overcome all the challenges that come with changing bad habits, you need to have both mental and physical stamina. This keeps you going and provides you the energy you need to overcome through the long haul. Your mental stamina helps you stick to your plans up to their completion. It is the physical stamina that provides you the energy you need to move your body through the whole process of your plans. When using creative visualization to build your stamina, you need breathing exercises. These exercises not only help you increase your stamina but also provide your body with the endurance you need to complete any activity you are engaged in. With the Chi breathing exercise, your goal should be to relax your shoulders and chest by breathing deeply from within your abdomen.

- Hold your hands over your lower stomach and sit in an upright position
- Breathe deeply until you cannot draw in more air then let it all out to the last gasp
- Repeat this action more than once
- Visualize yourself breathing in with your hands sucking the air down all the way to your torso and into them
- Visualize yourself exhaling with your hands pushing air back through your stomach
- Slowly take your time settling into a slow, steady and comfortable rhythm
- Imagine the deep and continuing energy each breath you take brings to you

As you breathe in and out, you should feel your abdomen expanding and contracting and the breathing moving all the way to your pelvic area. Practicing this exercise regularly is a good way to increase your endurance energy levels and build on your stamina level.

CHAPTER 5:

Reprogramming Your Mind

To reach your potential, you have to let go of some habits and some of the people you hang with. The most interesting thing about this is that many people have greatness locked up inside of them, all that they needed is to encounter someone that will unleash the beast and set them on the path of success. Many never met such people; many gave up too soon; many were even discouraged by friends. But the only way to unlocking your full potential is by discovering that you have such potential in the first place. It is after you have made this discovery that you can then move on to the next stage of development, which is to look out for ways that you can get leverage this greatness in you with life opportunities.

The main idea behind this kind of reasoning is that you have to look inward and look for ways to develop yourself. Nobody will help you if you refuse to help yourself. The earlier you realize this, the better it is. They significantly influence the level of accomplishment at each progression:

- Positive Thinking and Behavior
- Visualization
- Positive Self-Talk
- Affirmation Statements
- Dynamic Goal Setting
- Positive Action
- Assertive Behavior
- Success Strategies

These nine success strategies and behaviors are significant professional enhancers that help you to change objectives into real factors. Give close consideration to any that are new thoughts for you. They give wide-running advantages, and you can utilize them to:

- Create and support your internal drive
- Increase your certainty
- Provide mental and physical vitality
- Guide you toward objectives

Follow these means to frame the propensity for positive intuition and to help your prosperity. Intentionally spur yourself consistently. Consider yourself fruitful, and expect positive results for all that you endeavor. By practicing these inspirational desire attitude until it turns into a propensity decision making process will be impacted to a great extent by this positive vitality. The propensity will assist you with arriving at your full potential. Reflect on past victories helps, too, as this helps you to concentrate on past triumphs to help yourself to remember your capacities, and this boosts your ability to accomplish your objectives. For instance, nobody is ever brought into the world, realizing how to ride a bike or how to utilize a P.C. programming program. Through preparing, practice, and experimentation, you ace new capacities. During the experimentation periods of improvement, help yourself to remember past victories; see botches as a major aspect of the common expectation to absorb information. Proceed until you accomplish the outcome you need, and this reminds you that you have the necessary skillset to prevail since you have done it before and can also do it once more.

Certain affirmation statements are necessary for self-explanations or suggestions to help accomplish objectives. They are certain messages with a punch, "mental guard stickers," to persuade your psyche to work for you. The accompanying rules disclose how to utilize this amazing mental update strategy:

Offer the expression in the first person

- **Express yourself decidedly:** The psyche acknowledges reality in the words you give it. Utilize positive words as it were.
- **Forget about negative words:** For instance, this statement is negative: "I will be apprehensive during my meeting," while this other statement that's saying the same thing sounds positive: "I will be quiet and confident during my meeting.
- **Incorporate a positive feeling:** An expression that triggers a positive feeling reinforces a sense of determination. As a model, you could say: "My objective is important, and it energizes me."
- **Stop Negative Self-Talk:** You might rush to bother yourself since you need to be great. Be that as it may, negative self-talk is harming on the grounds that the inner mind truly accepts what you state about yourself. In case you get yourself utilizing negative self-talk, stop, and rethink. Take out the negative words. Concentrate rather on the best strategy you can take and do it.
- **Make positive correspondence a propensity:** Concentrate on the positive in objective articulations, self-talk, and all interchanges. Think about the accompanying expressions and notice how the positive words pass on certainty, duty, and energy.

Set an objective and stick to it

Characterize your objectives unmistakably by having it recorded as a hard copy. Recording your objectives/goal improves the probability of accomplishing them by 80%! Composing objectives build your feeling of duty, explains required strides in the accomplishment procedure, and encourages you to recollect significant subtleties. Make the advantages (to you and others) of accomplishing objectives clear and distinct. This is a solid spark. It gives you a clear understanding of what you need to do to accomplish your aim. Furthermore, be sure to characterize the reason for your objectives. Connect your objectives to a functional, explicit reason. To support your own inspiration, base your objectives on motivation, not simply rationale. To make this easier, you can incorporate educators, books, preparing, individuals who urge you to drive forward, gifted mentors or coaches, and printed and online research materials. Finally, build up an activity plan, set cutoff times, and act. Build up sub-objectives. Partition every primary objective into consistent, dynamic advances—set cutoff times for finishing each progression and complete strides on schedule.

CHAPTER 6:

How Gastric Band Hypnotherapy Works

Hypnotherapy for weight loss, particularly for portion control, is great because it allows you to focus on creating a healthier version of yourself safely.

When gastric band fitted surgery gets recommended to people, usually because diets, weight loss supplements, and workout routines don't seem to work for them, they may become skeptical about getting the surgery done.

Nobody wants to undergo unnecessary surgery, and you shouldn't have to either. Just because you struggle to stick to a diet, workout routine or lack motivation does not mean that an extreme procedure like surgery is the only option. In fact, thinking that it is the only option you have left is crazy.

Some hypnotherapists suggest that diets don't work at all. Well, if you're motivated and find it easy to stick to a diet plan and workout routine, then you should be fine. However, if you're suffering from obesity or overweight and don't have the necessary drive and motivation needed, then you're likely to fail. When people find the courage and determination to recognize that they need to lose weight or actually push themselves to do it, but continuously fail, that's when they tend to give up.

Gastric band hypnotherapy uses relaxation techniques, which are designed to alter your way of thinking about the weight you, need to lose, provides you a foundation to stand on and reach your goals, and also constantly reminds you of why you're indeed doing what you're doing. It is necessary to develop your way of thinking past where you're at in this current moment and evolve far beyond your expectations.

Diets are also more focused on temporary lifestyle changes rather than permanent and sustainable ones, which is why it isn't considered realistic at all. Unless you change your mind, you will always remain in a rut that involves first losing, and then possibly gaining weight back repeatedly. Some may even throw in the towel completely.

Hypnotherapy for Different Gastric Banding Types of Surgeries

There are three types of gastric banding surgeries that could be used during hypnotherapy. These include:

- Sleeve Gastrectomy
- Vertical Banded Gastroplasty
- Mixed Surgery (Restrictive and Malabsorptive)

Gastric banding surgeries are used for weight loss. Depending on what your goal is with this weight-loss method, you can choose which option works best for you. The great thing about hypnotherapy with gastric band firming surgery is that you can get similar results if you practice the session consistently.

During gastric banding surgery, the surgeon uses a laparoscopy technique that involves making small cuts in the stomach to place a silicone band around the top part of your stomach. This band is adjustable, leaving the stomach to form a pouch with an inch-wide outlet. After you've been banded in surgery, your stomach can only hold one ounce of food at a time, which prevents you from eating more than you need to in one sitting. It also prevents you from getting hungry.

Given that it is an invasive procedure, most people don't opt for it as an option to lose weight. During the procedure, you are also placed under anesthesia, which always involves some risks. Nevertheless, the procedure has resulted in up to 45% of excess weight loss, which means that it can work for anyone looking to shed weight they are struggling to lose. The procedure can also be reversed should the patient not be happy with the effects thereof. When reversed, the stomach will return to the initial size it had before the surgery. (WebMD, n.d.)

Undergoing one of these three gastric banding surgeries, there are some side-effects involved, which includes the risk of death. However, this is only found in one of every 3000 patients. Other than that, common problems post-surgery include nausea and vomiting, which can be reduced by simply having a surgeon adjust the tightness of the gastric band.

Minor surgical complications, including wound infections and risks for minor bleeding, only occur in 10% of patients. (WebMD, n.d.)

As opposed to gastric bypass surgery, gastric banding doesn't prevent your body from absorbing food whatsoever, which means that you won't have to worry about experiencing any vitamin or mineral loss in your body.

Types of gastric banding techniques used in hypnotherapy for weight loss

- **Sleeve Gastrectomy** - This procedure involves physically removing half of a patient's stomach to leave behind space, which is usually the size of a banana. When this part of the stomach is taken out, it cannot be reversed. This may seem like one of the most extreme types of gastric band surgeries, and due to its level of extremity, it also presents a lot of risks. When the reasons why the sleeve Gastrectomy is done and gets reviewed, it may not seem worth it. However, it has become one of the most popular methods used in surgery as a restrictive means of reducing a patient's appetite. It is particularly helpful to those who suffer from obesity. It has a high success rate with very few complications, according to medical practitioners. Those who have had the surgery have experienced losing up to 50% of their total weight, which is quite a lot for someone suffering from obesity. It is equally helpful to those who suffer from compulsive eating disorders, like binge eating. When you have the procedure done, your surgeon will make either a very large or a few small incisions in the abdomen. The physical recovery of this procedure may take up to six weeks. (WebMD, n.d.)

- **Vertical Banded Gastroplasty** - This gastric band procedure, also known as VBG, involves the same band used during the sleeve Gastrectomy, which is placed around the stomach. The stomach is then stapled above the band to form a small pouch, which in some sense, shrinks the stomach to produce the same effects. The procedure has been noted as a successful one to lose weight compared to many other types of weight-loss surgeries. Even though compared to the Sleeve Gastrectomy, it may seem like a less complicated surgery, but it has a higher complication rate. That is why it is considered far less common. Until today, there are only 5% of bariatric surgeons perform this particular gastric band surgery. Nevertheless, it is known for producing results and can still be used in hypnotherapy to produce similar results without the complications.

- **Mixed Surgery (Restrictive and Malabsorptive)** - This type of gastric band surgery forms a crucial part of most types of weight-loss surgeries. It is more commonly referred to as Gastric Bypass and is done first, prior to other weight-loss surgeries. It also involves stapling the stomach and creates a shape of an intestine down the line of your stomach. This is done to ensure the patient consumes less food, referred to as restrictive mixed surgery, combined with Malabsorptive surgery, meaning to absorb less food in the body.

What you need to know about hypnotic gastric band therapy

If you're wondering whether gastric band surgery is right for you, you may want to consider getting the hypnotherapy version thereof. Hypnotherapy is the perfect alternative, is 100% safe as opposed to surgery, which has many complications, and also a lot more affordable. It has a success rate of more than 90% in patients, which is why more people prefer it over gastric band surgery. Given that you can also conduct it in the comfort of your own home, you don't even have to worry about the cost involved. Overall it serves as a very convenient way to slim down, essentially shrinking your stomach.

Again, hypnosis doesn't involve any physical procedure involving surgery. It is a safe alternative that uses innovative and developed technology to help you get where you want to be. The hypnotherapy session involves visualizing a virtual gastric band being fitted around your stomach that allows you to have the same experience as you initially would during surgery, but without the discomfort, excessive costs and inconvenience.

The effect is feeling as if you are hungry for longer periods, require less food, and experiencing a feeling of being full, even if you've only eaten half of your regular-sized portion. This will also help you make healthier choices and discover that you can indeed develop a much healthier relationship with food than you currently have.

If you're wondering whether gastric band hypnotherapy will work for you, you have to ask yourself whether you have the imagination to support your session. Now, of course, everybody has an imagination, but is yours reasonable enough?

If you can close your eyes and imagine yourself looking at something in front of you that is not there, and spend time focusing on it, then you can make it through gastric band hypnotherapy successfully.

It's normal to think before you start anything, that if it isn't tailored to you specifically, it is likely to fail. However, visual gastric band hypnosis can offer you emotional healing. This supports your goals, including weight loss and health restoration. If you spend time engaging in it, you will learn that you can achieve whatever you set your intention on. You can remove your cravings subconsciously, eliminate any negative and emotional stress, as well as memories that form a part of your emotional eating pattern. Given that emotionality forms a big part of weight gain, you should know that it can be removed from your conscious mind through hypnotherapy and serve any individual willing to try it.

Gastric band hypnotherapy has a 95% success rate among patients, according to a clinical study conducted in the U.K. This study also proved that most people will be able to accept and succeed in hypnotherapy, but if they're not open to the experience, they won't find it helpful at all. People who are too closed off from new ideas, like hypnotherapy, which is often made out to be a negative practice among the uneducated, won't be able to relax properly for a hypnotherapist's words to take effect. (Engle, 2019)

After just one hypnotherapy session, you will know if it works, as it is supposed to start working after just one session. That is why hypnotherapy is not recommended for everyone. It's only suggested to anyone ready to change their feelings toward food. If you don't believe in it or that it will get you to where you want to go on your weight loss journey, it is deemed useless.

The cost of gastric band hypnotherapy sessions with a professional hypnotherapist can only be established after you've undergone an evaluation. Usually, every new patient requires up to five sessions in person. During these sessions, energy therapy techniques are also taught, which will help assist any struggle a patient may have with anxiety, anger, stress, and any other negative emotion.

CHAPTER 7:

Preparing Your Body for Your Hypnotic Gastric Band

The physical gastric band requires a surgical procedure that involves reducing the size of your stomach pocket to accommodate less volume of food and, as a result of the stretching of the walls of the stomach, send signals to the brain that you are filled and therefore need to stop eating any further.

The hypnotic gastric band also works in the same manner, although in this case, the only surgical tools you will need are your mind and your body, and the great part is you can conduct the procedure yourself. The hypnotic gastric band also conditions your mind and body to restrict excess consumption of food after very modest meals. There are three specific differences between the surgical (physical), and hypnotic gastric bands:

- In using the hypnotic band, all necessary adjustments are done by continued use of trance.

- There is absence of physical surgery and therefore, you are exposed to no risks at all.

- When compared with the surgical gastric band, the hypnotic gastric band is a lot cheaper and easier to do.

How Hypnosis Improves Communication between Stomach and Brain

How would you know when you have had enough to eat? Initially, you will begin to feel the weight and area of the food. When your stomach is full, the food presses against and extends the stomach well, and the nerve endings in the walls of the stomach respond. When these nerves are stimulated, they transfer a signal to the brain, and we get the feeling of satiety and, as the stomach fills up and food enters the digestive tract, PYY and GLP-1 is released and trigger a feeling of satiety in the brain that additionally prompts us to quit eating.

Sadly, when individuals always overeat, they become desensitized to both the nerve signals and the neuropeptide signaling system. During the initial installation trance, we use hypnotic and images to re-sensitize the brain to these signs. Your hypnotic band restores the full effect of these nervous and neuropeptide messages. With the benefits of hypnotic in view, we can recalibrate this system and increase your sensitivity to these signs, so you feel full and truly satisfied when you have eaten enough to fill that little pouch at the top of your stomach.

A hypnotic gastric band causes your body to carry on precisely as if you have carried out surgical operation. It contracts your stomach and adjusts the signals from your stomach to your brain, so you feel full rapidly. The hypnotic band uses a few uncommon attributes of hypnotic. As a matter of first importance, hypnotic permits us to talk to parts of the body and mind that are not under conscious control. Interestingly as it might appear, in a trance, we can really convince the body to carry on distinctively even though our conscious mind has no methods for coordinating that change.

The Power of the Gastric Band

A renowned and dramatic case of the power of hypnotic to influence our bodies directly is in the emergency treatment of burns. A few doctors have used hypnotic on many occasions to accelerate and improve the recuperating of extreme injuries and to help reduce the excruciating pains for his patients. If somebody is seriously burnt, there will be damage to the tissue, and the body reacts with inflammation. The patients are hypnotized to forestall the soreness. His patients heal quite rapidly and with less scarring.

There are a lot more instances of how the mind can directly and physically influence the body. We realize that chronic stress can cause stomach ulcers, and a psychological shock can turn somebody's hair to grey color overnight. In any case, what I especially like about this aspect of hypnotism is that it is an archived case of how the mind influences the body positively and medically. It will be somewhat of a miraculous event if the body can get into a hypnotic state that can cause significant physical changes in your body. Hypnotic trance without anyone else has a profound physiological effect. The most immediate effect is that subjects discover it deeply relaxing. Interestingly, the most widely recognized perception that my customers report after I have seen them—regardless of what we have been dealing with—is that their loved ones tell them they look more youthful.

Cybernetic Loop

Your brain and body are in constant correspondence in a cybernetic loop: they continually influence one another. As the mind unwinds in a trance, so too does the body. When the body unwinds, it feels good, and it sends that message to the brain, which thus feels healthier and unwinds much more. This procedure decreases stress and makes more energy accessible to the immune system of the body. It is essential to take note that the remedial effects of hypnotic don't require tricks or amnesia. For example, burns patients realize they have been burnt, so they don't need to deny the glaring evidence of how burnt parts of their bodies are. He essentially hypnotizes them and requests that they envision cool, comfortable sensations over the burnt area. That imaginative activity changes their body's response to the burns.

The enzymes that cause inflammation are not released, and accordingly, the burn doesn't advance to a more elevated level of damage, and there is reduced pain during the healing process.

By using hypnotic and imagery, a doctor can get his patients' bodies to do things that are totally outside their conscious control. Willpower won't make these sorts of changes, but the creative mind is more grounded than the will. By using hypnotic and imagery to talk to the conscious mind, we can have a physiological effect in as little as 20 minutes. In my work, I recently had another phenomenal idea of how hypnotic can accelerate the body's normal healing process. I worked with a soldier in the Special Forces who experienced extreme episodes of skin inflammation (eczema). He revealed to me that the quickest recuperation he had ever made from an eczema episode was six days. I realized that the way toward healing is a natural sequence of events carried out by various systems within the body, so I hypnotized him and, while in a trance requested that his conscious mind follow precisely the same process that it regularly uses to heal his eczema, however, to do everything quicker.

One and a half days after, the eczema was gone. With hypnotic, we can enormously enhance the effect of the mind. When we fit your hypnotic gastric band, we are using the very same strategy of hypnotic correspondence to the conscious mind. We communicate to the brain with distinctive imagery, and the brain alters your body's responses, changing your physical response to food so your stomach is constricted, and you feel truly full after only a few.

What Makes the Hypnotic Work So Well?

A few people think that it's difficult to accept that trance and imagery can have such an extreme and ground-breaking effect. Some doctors were at first distrustful and accepted that his patients more likely than not had fewer burns than was written in their medical records, because the cures he effected had all the earmarks of being close to marvelous. It took quite a long while, and numerous exceptional remedies before such work were generally understood and acknowledged.

Once in a while, the cynic and the patient are the same individuals. We need the results, but we battle to accept that it truly will work. At the conscious level, our minds are very much aware of the contrast between what we imagine and physical reality. In any case, another astounding hypnotic marvel shows that it doesn't make a difference what we accept at the conscious level since trance permits our mind to react to a reality that is independent of what we deliberately think. This phenomenon is classified as "trance logic."

Trance logic was first recognized 50 years ago by a renowned researcher of hypnotic named Dr. Martin Orne, who worked for a long time at the University of Pennsylvania. Dr. Orne directed various tests that demonstrated that in hypnotic, individuals could carry on as though two absolutely opposing facts were valid simultaneously. In one study, he hypnotized a few people so they couldn't see a seat he put directly before them. Then he requested that they walk straight ahead. The subjects all swerved around the seat.

Notwithstanding, when examined regarding the chair, they reported there was nothing there. They couldn't see the seat. Some of them even denied that they had swerved by any means. Thus, accepted they were telling the truth when said they couldn't see the seat, but at another level, their bodies realized it was there and moved to abstain from hitting it.

The test showed that hypnotic permits the mind to work at the same time on two separate levels, accepting two isolated, opposing things. It is possible to be hypnotized and have a hypnotic gastric band fitted but then to "know" with your conscious mind that you don't have surgical scars, and you don't have a physical gastric band embedded. Trance logic implies that a part of your mind can trust one thing, and another part can accept the direct opposite, and your mind and body can continue working, accepting that two unique things are valid.

So, you will be capable to consciously realize that you have not paid a huge amount of dollars for a surgical process, but then at the deepest level of unconscious command, your body accepts that you have a gastric band and will act in like manner. Subsequently, your stomach is conditioned to signal "feeling full" to your brain after only a couple of mouthfuls. So, you feel satisfied, and you get to lose more weight.

Visualization Is Easier Than You Think

The hypnotic we use to make your gastric band uses "visualization" and "influence loaded imager." Visualization is the creation of pictures in your mind. We would all be able to do it. It is an interesting part of the reasoning. For instance, think about your front door and ask yourself which side the lock is on.

To address that question, you see an image in your mind's eye. It doesn't make a difference at all how reasonable or bright the image is, it is only how your mind works, and you see as much as you have to see. Influence loaded imagery is the psychological term for genuinely significant pictures. In this process, we use pictures in the mind's eye that have emotional significance.

Although hypnotic recommendations are incredible, they are dramatically upgraded by ground-breaking images when we are communicating directly to the body. For instance, you will be unable to accelerate your heart just by telling it to beat faster. Still, if you envision remaining on a railroad line and seeing a train surging towards you, your heart accelerates pretty quickly. Your body overreacts to clear, meaningful pictures.

CHAPTER 8:

Gastric Band Hypnosis for Food Addiction

Most people enjoy food and don't even know it. Those who are discouraged by weight are ashamed of themselves. While the more people in society ignore themselves, or the real intent and tend to push for a fast fix, the more food addiction will be rife.

If I said to him/her, he or she is more than likely to look at me and say that's nuts, a slice of bread with butter that he/she is about to eat, is like a glass of scotch! Those of us who suffer from a recovery eating disorder know that's the truth.

The truth is that more people are food-suffering than is understood. The weight-loss industry is a multi-billion dollar industry because today's diets are processed sugar and starch diets, which are frozen foods, or fast foods, are easily prepared.

Today everybody is rushing from one place to the next in every hour of the day and takes less time to take care of them. Dieting does not work to change lifestyles. Slow change would have a positive impact instead of starvation and being hungry due to poverty.

The endless reminders of food on the ads, a billboard on the side of the road, a magazine advertising the scent of fresh coffee toasting are triggers. The mind is a strong device that recalls things with the five sense vision, touch, scent, taste and listening.

To improve, he or she must learn what its triggers are. Eating disorder treatment programs teach people to identify what they need to do to protect themselves from addiction. Treatment also allows patients to reschedule reactions to friends, places and events without depending on food dependency.

Eating disorder treatment programs address food addiction, both physically and psychologically. Treatment teaches you to identify and plan so that you don't have to copy food. Some people, places and stuff are not part of your life because of your affiliation.

No real relief comes from instant gratification or fast repair. What you learn in your treatment is invaluable: yes, he or she can live a life free from food dependence.

People also have food addictions and cravings while they are on a diet. There are many different therapeutic strategies to tackle all sorts of negative emotional emotions, not just emotions from craves and addictions, but also emotional eating or fear of failure in the dietary program.

For example, one technique is Neuro-Linguistic Programming, NLP. The founders of the NLP strategies initially researched what approaches the most effective psychotherapists use to build NLP. As odd as these approaches may first seem, they must be a good tool for overcoming food addictions and desires, taking into account how they are created.

Even EFT, a technique of emotional liberation, is becoming increasingly common in order to avoid unwanted emotions from desire and addiction. Although not so empirical as the context, the approach blends modern psychology with acupuncture-based concepts that the Chinese have successfully employed for thousands of years.

A new behavior pattern must be learned for both addictions and cravings, and it is also helpful to treat not only the mind, but also the body. This doesn't necessarily mean taking drugs, but rather eating whole foods, or just consuming basic foods for some time, taking vitamins and mineral supplements and recovering from unnecessary stress.

Supplements such as L-glutamine are also beneficial, as L-glutamine is known to improve food and even alcohol addictions and cravings. To conquer food shortages and cravings, regardless of their frequency, you need to know that you are coping with a learned habit.

CHAPTER 9:

Techniques to Execute Gastric Band Hypnosis

Placing

In this meditation, you will learn how to walk along a beautiful beach walk, allowing you a deeply relax. Follow me on this mental vacation as we place an emotional and mental gastric band around your stomach, which will allow you to feel a full as soon as you eat exactly as much food as you need.

So, get into a comfortable seated position, on your favorite spot, so that you are undisturbed for the rest of this session. As you relax, the gastric band will become more powerful and influential over your life. Take a big deep breath, relax, and then exhale the tension and worry as you close your eyes. Feel your body already slowing down. Take another breath and let to go with a sigh of relief. This moment is for you to practice your new lifestyle, of being full, at the perfect time. Now say to you with faith, "overeating is impossible for me."

Now breathe into the truth of these words as you breathe them out into reality. You are creating a smaller stomach. Relax and breathe and then use the power of your imagination to visualize a beautiful beach with white sand, reflecting in the sunlight. It looks like snow. You can see the turquoise waters fading to a deep blue as the ocean goes deeper.

Look down into the sand where you stand, and notice the beautiful bits of shells with all different colors and textures as you see dried seaweed scattered about something that catches your eye buried into the sand, it is your preferred color. So as you get closer, you will see that it is a small yet thick band that is as big around as your fist, and it just so happens that it is the most vivid version of your favorite color. The brightness of this hue brings you joy. The curious, round band, flashing of your most beloved color choice is called the gastric band

It is placed around the top of your stomach, cinching down the amount your stomach can hold. So, it makes your stomach feel smaller, which gives you that feeling of fullness that you've had enough to eat. This band only exists in the medical world. But, you can get the same results, using the power of your mind, by placing the band within and around your stomach in this relaxing session.

Feel your feet entering the sand and allow yourself on each step to relax more and more. Notice the powdery texture, dispersing under your feet, and allow it deeply soothe you. Feel the ocean breeze, and smell the salty air. As you walk, you will get tired. A perfect chair has appeared just for you, facing the ocean. So have a seat and recline backward with your gastric band in your hand. Familiarize yourself with its shape and size. It is like a small belt that can be tightened and loosened. This relaxing gastric band session brings you to perfect health and weight through the power of your mind. It brings about a new and improved positive attitude to life with intention, positivity, and knowing when enough is enough. Now bring your hands into the mode of prayer and notice how you feel. Notice your mind and body going back on track, firmly ready to eat the healthy amount.

Take a few calming, relaxing moments before coming back to the present moment. Take a long breath in and feel the gastric band as it's limiting your ability to overeat. Feel the band affecting the weight throughout your body. When you are ready, just gently open your eyes. And then seal this in with a grateful smile.

Tightening

Welcome to this relaxing meditation. This meditation will guide you to a pristine lake that is surrounded by mountains and help you to tighten your gastric band, making for an even smaller stomach that will fill up quickly. Get yourself into a nice seated position where you can easily fully let go, and you will not be disturbed by the surrounding world.

As you get into a powerful state of relaxation, begin to imagine that you are tightening this gastric band, and as you do so, you will find that weight-loss becomes easier and easier by the day. Now begin to breathe deeply while allowing your body to expand. Exhale all of your stress out and take another deep breath in, and as you exhale and allow, let your eyes gently closed.

Now notice how you feel. Notice how your body is settling down, and as it becomes relaxed as we go along. Let go of any current worries or obligations. Enjoying for yourself, and you begin your health and wellness journey from the first session by placing a gastric band near your stomach with the power of your mind. So, appreciate yourself for taking on this amazing opportunity.

Now say to yourself, "I will eat only as much food as I need. I need less food to feel full."

Breathe in, and allow these words to become part of every level of your awareness. Breathe out any doubt and breathe in any truth that you are capable of eating just the right amount to have the perfect shape, size, and overall wellness. Now relax, calm down, and be at complete ease. Let your body slow down just a little bit more. Activate your imagination by bringing into your mind the eye, the site of a magnificent lake that is surrounded by mountains. And the sky, which is a crisp turquoise blue dappled with the cloud. And the sun is shining all around you. The waters of this lake are crystal clear, and it's reflecting the blueness of the sky. The water is acting as a mirror for the mountain range.

Now become aware of your stomach and notice it becoming smaller from your wonderful session on the beach when you first found your gastric band. Feel how your stomach is comfortable and happy about its new size and wants to become even smaller.

As you walk toward the lake, notice the soil under your feet, becoming smooth and supportive. As you go near to the water edge, dip your toes in the cool and fresh aqua. Even though your feet are submerged, the waters of this mystical lake relax your entire body.

Notice beside you the small red canoe waiting for you. Enter into this canoe and pick up the beautiful hand-carved oar. The oar signifies the ability to be able to tighten your gastric band. Dip the oar into the water, moving to the bottom of the lake, and push off the shore. Feel as this simple movement helps to tighten your gastric band by a millimeter.

Also, visualize yourself in your kitchen now preparing your next meal. You will find that when you put the plate on your food, all of your choices are healthy. You will notice that you will only scoop a small amount of each item because you have a good ability to put the right amount of food that you need on your plate, now with your gastric band supporting you. You don't want to waste a bite of food. You should only eat the perfect amount.

See yourself eating this healthy meal, and shocked at the small food that it took for you to feel satisfied. Now, as you rise from this wonderful meditation, allow the image of the canoe and the see-through water to fade away from your mind, as well as the great mountains and along with the visual of your next meal.

Right now, bring yourself back from this experience into reality. Breathe in deeply, and become aware of your surroundings in the present moment. Wiggle around your toes and fingers a little bit and feel the fresh new energy and wisdom coming into you. And then whenever you are ready, open your eyes.

Removal

So far, you have placed this band around your stomach while walking on the relaxing beach and tightening the band while rowing your canoe on a crystal-clear lake. Right now, we will visit an ancient Japanese castle to be able to remove this band and discard it during the beautiful ceremony. Now make sure that you're in a comfortable position, in a place that you can enjoy practicing this relaxing session. This is the final step in your gastric band experience. So take a nice deep breath in and then breathe out while closing your eyes.

Relax your body. Feel it sinking into the chair or bed, soft and supportive underneath you.

Breathe in and then breathe out while noticing the gentle rise and fall of your chest as you breathe in. Now start becoming aware of your abdomen and feel how slim it is as you're, eating less food. You are becoming fuller and making hunger outdated. You know that you're supposed to eat, but eating doesn't consume your day or your mind. You only eat when you should eat and refuse to eat when you don't should eat. It's as simple as that.

Activate your creative mind again. Now imagine that you are standing in a beautiful field with tall grass, blowing in your wind. Now imagine that there's a path in front of you, and that path is made up of smooth stones. As you walk along this path, see yourself coming towards a magnificent Japanese temple that was built hundreds of years ago.

The building is well maintained with a fresh coat made of red paint as well as gold trim surrounding the windows and doors. Now make your way up to the front door and feel like the iron handle in your hand on this door is massive as you open it.

So as you step inside the temple, feel the cool air around you. Also, imagine that the interior of this structure is a work of art, crafted by sheer genius. Now notice that there is a large golden bowl in the center of the room that is set atop a marble column. Now, as you move away from this bowl, it will appear to be illuminated with a ray of sunlight, which is casting down through the window in the rooftop.

As you see, the, reflecting the light like a diamond. Now, you easily remove the gastric band and place it inside the sacred water. So you can see that it is your favorite color, yet it's a bit worn and tired from all the work that it did for your health. Now imagine as the ray of light beaming down and see it begin to dissolve the gastric band until the water is pure. Start to feel lighter than ever, and your stomach smaller, along with your figure, shrinking every day.

Feel the sensations of touch at your fingertips. Move your focus to your abdomen and to all your vital organs. Notice how your belly feels and how it is digesting. Notice your pelvis and hips, and the sensations of your weight as it's pressing it down. This should take you into a deeper state of relaxation. Your awareness should go down on each leg, over your knees, move down all the way to your feet, and touch each toe.

CHAPTER 10:

Emotional Eating

What Is Emotional Eating?

People usually eat to beat physical hunger. However, some people are relying on food as a source of comfort or to address their negative emotions. Some also use food as a reward whenever they achieve their goals or when celebrating special events like birthdays or weddings.

When you use food as a cover or a solution for extreme emotions, then you suffer from emotional eating. The feelings that trigger your eating are mostly negative, for example, stress, loneliness, sadness, or when you are grieving. However, it is not only the negative emotions that can cause emotional eating; some positive emotions such as happiness or feelings of comfort can also trigger emotional eating.

There is a difference in the way people use food to address their emotions. While some people rely on food when they are in the middle of their life situations, others may find comfort in food soon after the situation is over. They use food as a recovery tool.

A problem associated with emotional eating is that it may prevent you from utilizing other adaptive approaches to problems. You should also know that emotional eating does not solve the issues you are going through. If anything, it only serves to make you feel worse. After eating, the original emotional problem remains unsolved, and on top of it, you find yourself feeling guilty of overeating. It is, therefore, essential for you to identify the problem of emotional eating and to take timely appropriate measures to stop it.

How to Recognize Emotional Eating

The best way for you to know if you are suffering from emotional eating is to find out whether you always eat because you are hungry, or you eat impulsively. You should pay attention to your emotions and how you usually cope with them. Find out if you are utilizing food just for hunger or you are unconsciously overeating.

Once you are sure you have an emotional eating problem, take appropriate steps to stop it. This is because not all the food you eat is healthy. You will occasionally find yourself eating unhealthy food such as junk food and sweets, which could be detrimental to your health.

Common Features of Emotional Hunger

It is easy for you to mistake emotional hunger for normal physical hunger. You, therefore, need to learn how to make a distinction between the two forms of hunger. The following are some of the hints you can use to tell the difference between the two kinds of hunger:

Emotional Hunger Comes Unexpectedly

You tend to experience emotional hunger suddenly. The feelings of craving will then overwhelm you, forcing you to look for food urgently. On the other hand, feelings of physical hunger tend to grow gradually. Also, when you are physically hungry, you will not be overwhelmed suddenly by hunger, not unless you have gone for days without food.

Emotional Hunger Desires for Some Specific Food

If you are physically hungry, any food is right for you. Physical hunger is not too selective on the type of food to consume. You will feel satisfied eating healthy food like fruits and vegetables. On the other hand, emotional hunger tends to be selective on the food to consume. In most cases, emotional hunger craves unhealthy foods, such as sweets, snacks, and junk food. The craving for these foods tends to be overwhelming and urgent. You may experience strong desires for such food as pizza or cheesecake, and you have no appetite for any other type of food.

Emotional Eating Lacks Concern for Consequences

If you are involved in emotional eating, then in most cases, you find yourself eating without any concern on the consequences of overeating on your general well-being. You also eat without paying attention to the food you are consuming. You are not concerned about the quality of the food or their nutritional value. All you care about is the quantity of the food to satisfy your craving. Your goal will be to eat as much food as possible.

On the other hand, when you are eating because of physical hunger, you will be conscious of the quality and the quantity of food you are consuming. You will be concern about the health benefits of the food you are eating. You will also choose to eat a very well-balanced diet, which will prevent your body from overeating junk foods.

Emotional Hunger is Insatiable

If you are suffering from emotional eating, your hunger cannot be satisfied no matter the amount of food you have consumed. Hunger, as a craving, will refuse to get out of your mind. You will keep craving for more and more food, and soon, you will find yourself eating continuously without a break.

On the other hand, physical hunger is satisfied the moment your stomach is full. You may experience feelings of physical hunger only during specific times of the day. This could be the response of your body once you have conditioned it to receive food at times of the day.

Emotional Hunger is Located on Your Mind

Unlike physical hunger, the craving for food originates from your mind. Emotional hunger involves the obsession originating from your mind on some specific type of food. You find yourself unable to ignore or overcome this obsession. You then give in to it and reach for your favorite food. On the other hand, physical hunger originates from the stomach. You feel the hunger pang from your stomach. You can also occasionally feel growling from your belly whenever you are hungry.

Emotional Hunger Comes with Guilt and Regrets

When you are suffering from emotional eating, deep down, you know your eating does not come with any nutritional benefits. You will then have feelings of guilt or even shame. You know you are doing your health a lot of harm, and you may start regretting your actions. On the other hand, physical eating involves eating to satisfy your hunger. You will not suffer any feelings of shame or guilt for meeting your bodily needs.

Causes of Your Emotional Eating

For you to succeed in putting a stop to your emotional eating habits, you need to find out what triggers them. Find out the exact situations, feelings, or places that make you feel like eating whenever you are exposed to. Below are some of the common causes of emotional eating:

Stress

One symptom of stress is hunger. You tend to experience the feeling of hunger whenever you are stressed. When you are stressed, your body responds by producing a stress hormone known as Cortisol. When this hormone is produced in high quantities, it will trigger a craving for foods that are salty or sugary in nature as well as any fried food. These are the food which gives you a lot of instant energy and pleasure.

If you do not control stress in your life, you will always be seeking relief in unhealthy food.

Boredom

You could be eating to relieve yourself of boredom. You can also resort to eating to beat idleness. Besides, you may be using food to occupy your time because you do not have much to do. Food can also fill your void and momentarily distract you from the hidden feelings of directionless and dissatisfaction with yourself. Whenever you feel purposeless, you tend to reach out for food to make you feel better. However, the truth is that food can never be a solution to any of your negative emotions.

Childhood Habits

Emotional eating could be a result of your childhood habits. For example, if your parents used to reward your good behaviors with foods such as sweets, ice cream, or pizza, you may have carried these habits to your adulthood. You will find yourself rewarding yourself with your childhood snack whenever you accomplish a given task. You can also be unconsciously eating because of the nostalgic feelings of your childhood. This happens when you always cherish the delicacies you used to eat in your childhood. Food can also serve as a powerful reminder of your most cherished childhood memories, for example, if you were eating cookies with your dad during your outings together. Whenever you miss your dad, your first instinct is to reach out for the cookies.

Social Influences

Occasionally, you may need to go out with your friends and have a good time. During such outings, you can share a meal to relieve stress. However, such social events can lead to overeating. You can find yourself overeating at the nudge of your close friends or family who encourages you to go for an extra serving. It is easy to fall into their temptation.

Avoiding Emotions

You may use eating as a way of temporarily avoiding the emotions you are feeling, such as the feeling of anxiety, shame, resentment, or anger. Eating is a perfect way to prevent negative distractions, albeit temporarily.

Habits and Practices You Can Use to Overcome Emotional Eating to Lose Weight

Practice Healthy Lifestyle Habits

You will handle life's shortcomings better when you are physically strong, happy, and well-rested. However, if you are exhausted, any stressful situation you encounter will trigger the craving for food. In this regard, you need to make physical exercise part of your daily routine.

You also need to have enough time to sleep to feel rested. Moreover, engage yourself in social activities with others. Create time for outings with family or close friends.

Practice Mindfulness by Eating Slowly

When you eat to satisfy your feelings rather than your stomach, you tend to eat so fast and mindlessly that you fail to savor the taste or texture of your food. However, when you slow down and take a moment to savor every bite, you will be less likely to indulge in overeating. Slowing down also helps you to enjoy your food better.

Accept All Your Feelings

Emotional eating is often triggered by feelings of helplessness over your emotions. You lack the courage to handle your feelings head-on, so you seek refuge in food. However, you need to be mindful of your feelings. Learn to overcome your emotions by accepting them. Once you do this, you regain the courage to handle any feelings that triggers your emotional eating.

Take a Moment before Giving in to Your Cravings

Typically, emotional eating is sudden and mindless. It takes you by surprise, and often you may feel powerless in stopping the urge to eat. However, you can control the sudden urges to reach for food if you take a moment of 5 minutes before you give in.

This allows you a moment to reconsider your decisions and eventually get the craving out of your mind.

Find Other Alternative Solutions to Your Emotion

Actively look for other solutions to address your feelings other than eating. For example, whenever you feel lonely, instead of eating, reach out for your phone and call that person who always puts a smile on your face. Look for good alternatives to food that you can rely on to feel emotionally fulfilled. If you feel anxious, learn to do exercises.

CHAPTER 11:

Blasting Calories

We have all heard the word "calorie" and its relation to our body weight. Calories are contained in the foods we consume and are often misunderstood about how they affect us. In this topic, we seek to explain what they are, how to count them, and the best methods of blasting them to avoid weight gain.

What Are Calories, and How Do They Affect Your Weight?

A calorie is a key estimating unit. For example, we use meters when communicating separation; 'Usain Bolt went 100 meters in just 9.5 seconds.' There are two units in this expression. One is a meter (a range unit), and the other is "second" (a period unit). Essentially, calories are additional units of physical amount estimation.

Many assume that a calorie is the weight measure (since it is oftentimes connected with an individual's weight). However, that is not precise. A calorie is a vitality unit (estimation). 1 calorie is proportional to the vitality expected to build the temperature by 1 degree Celsius to 1 kilogram of water.

Two particular sorts of calories come in: small calories and huge calories. Huge calories are the word connected to sustenance items.

You've likely observed much stuff on parcels (chocolates, potato chips, and so forth.) with 'calorie scores.' Imagine the calorie score an incentive for a thing being '100 cal.' This infers when you eat it, you will pick up about as much vitality (even though the calorie worth expressed and the amount you advantage from it is never the equivalent).

All that we eat has a particular calorie tally; it is the proportion of the vitality we eat in the substance bonds.

These are mostly things we eat: starches, proteins, and fats. How about we take a gander at what number of calories 1 gram comprises of these medications:

1. Sugars: 4 calories.

2. Protein: 3 calories.

3. Fat: 9 calories.

Are my calories awful?

That is fundamentally equivalent to mentioning, "Is vitality awful for me?" Every single activity the body completes needs vitality. Everything takes vitality to stand, walk, run, sit, and even eat. In case you're doing any of these tasks, it suggests you're utilizing vitality, which mostly infers you're 'consuming' calories, explicitly the calories that entered your body when you were eating some nourishment.

To sum things up, for you, NO... calories are not terrible.

Equalization is the way to finding harmony between what number of calories you devour and what number of calories you consume or use. On the off chance that you eat fewer calories and spend more, you will become dainty, while on the opposite side, on the off chance that you gobble up heaps of calories, however, you are a habitually lazy person, you will in the long run become stout at last.

Each movement we do throughout a day will bring about certain calories being spent. Here is a little rundown of the absolute most much of the time performed exercises, just as the number of calories consumed while doing them.

Step-by-step instructions to Count Calories

You have to expend fewer calories than you consume to get thinner

This clamor is simple in principle. Be that as it may, it very well may be hard to deal with your nourishment admission in the contemporary sustenance setting. Calorie checking is one approach to address this issue and is much of the time used to get more fit. Hearing that calories don't make a difference is very common, and tallying calories is an exercise in futility. Nonetheless, calories tally with regards to your weight; this is a reality that, in science, analyses called overloading studies has been demonstrated on numerous occasions.

These examinations request that people deliberately indulge and after that, survey the impact on their weight and well-being. All overloading investigations have found that people are putting on weight when they devour a bigger number of calories than they consume.

This simple reality infers that calorie checking and limiting your utilization can be proficient in averting weight put on or weight reduction as long as you can stick to it. One examination found that health improvement plans, including calorie including brought about a normal weight reduction of around 7 lbs. (3.3 kg) more than those that didn't.

Primary concern: You put on weight by eating a larger number of calories than you consume. Calorie tallying can help you expend fewer calories and get more fit.

How many calories do you have to eat?

What number of calories you need depends on factors, for example, sex, age, weight, and measure of activity? For example, a 25-year-old male competitor will require a bigger number of calories than a non-practicing 70-year-elderly person. In case you're endeavoring to get in shape, by eating not exactly your body consumes off, you'll have to construct a calorie deficiency. Utilize this adding machine to decide what number of calories you ought to expend every day (opening in crisp tab). This number cruncher depends on the condition of Mifflin-St Jeor, an exact method to evaluate calorie prerequisites.

How to Reduce Your Caloric Intake for Weight Loss

Bit sizes have risen, and a solitary dinner may give twofold or triple what the normal individual needs in a sitting at certain cafés. "Segment mutilation" is the term used to depict enormous parts of sustenance as the standard. It might bring about weight put on and weight reduction. In general, people don't evaluate the amount they spend. Tallying calories can help you battle indulging by giving you a more grounded information of the amount you expend.

In any case, you have to record portions of sustenance appropriately for it to work. Here are a couple of well-known strategies for estimating segment sizes: Scales: Weighing your sustenance is the most exact approach to decide the amount you eat. This might be tedious, in any case, and isn't constantly down to earth.

Estimating cups: Standard estimations of amount are, to some degree, quicker and less complex to use than a scale, yet can some of the time be tedious and unbalanced.

Examinations: It's quick and easy to utilize correlations with well-known items, especially in case you're away from home. It's considerably less exact, however.

Contrasted with family unit items, here are some mainstream serving sizes that can help you gauge your serving sizes: 1 serving of rice or pasta (1/2 a cup): a PC mouse or adjusted bunch.

- 1 Meat serving (3 oz): a card deck.
- 1 Fish serving (3 oz):
- 1 Cheese serving (1.5 oz): a lipstick or thumb size.
- 1 Fresh organic product serving (1/2 cup): a tennis ball.
- 1 Green verdant vegetable serving (1 cup): baseball.
- 1 Vegetable serving (1/2 cup): a mouse PC.
- 1 Olive oil teaspoon: 1 fingertip.
- 2 Peanut margarine tablespoons: a ping pong ball.

Calorie tallying, notwithstanding when gauging and estimating partitions, isn't a careful science.

In any case, your estimations shouldn't be thoroughly spot-on. Simply guarantee that your utilization is recorded as effectively as would be prudent. You ought to be mindful to record high-fat as well as sugar things, for example, pizza, dessert, and oils. Under-recording these meals can make an enormous qualification between your genuine and recorded utilization. You can endeavor to utilize scales toward the beginning to give you a superior idea of what a segment resembles to upgrade your evaluations. This should help you to be increasingly exact, even after you quit utilizing them.

More Tips to Assist in Caloric Control

Here are 5 more calorie tallying tips:

- Get prepared: get a calorie tallying application or web device before you start, choose how to evaluate or gauge parcels, and make a feast plan.
- Read nourishment marks: Food names contain numerous accommodating calorie tallying information. Check the recommended segment size on the bundle.
- Remove the allurement: dispose of your home's low-quality nourishment. This will help you select more advantageous bites and make hitting your objectives easier.
- Aim for moderate, steady loss of weight: don't cut too little calories. Even though you will get in shape all the more rapidly, you may feel terrible and be less inclined to adhere to your arrangement.
- Fuel your activity: Diet and exercise are the best health improvement plans. Ensure you devour enough to rehearse your vitality.

Effective Methods for Blasting Calories

To impact calories requires participating in exercises that urge the body to utilize vitality. Aside from checking the calories and guaranteeing you eat the required sum, consuming them is similarly basic for weight reduction.

Here, we examine a couple of techniques that can enable you to impact our calories all the more viably.

1. **Indoor cycling:** McCall states that around 952 calories for each hour ought to be at 200 watts or higher. On the off chance that the stationary bicycle doesn't demonstrate watts: "This infers

you're doing it when your indoor cycling instructor educates you to switch the opposition up!" he proposes.

2. **Skiing:** Around 850 calories for every hour depends on your skiing knowledge. Slow, light exertion won't consume nearly the same number of calories as a lively, fiery exertion is going to consume. To challenge yourself and to consume vitality? Attempt to ski tough.

3. **Rowing:** Approximately 816 calories for every hour. The benchmark here is 200 watts; McCall claims it ought to be at a "fiery endeavor." Many paddling machines list the showcase watts. Reward: Rowing is additionally a stunning back exercise.

4. **Jumping rope:** About 802 calories for each hour This ought to be at a moderate pace—around 100 skips for each moment—says McCall. Attempt to begin with this bounce rope interim exercise.

5. **Kickboxing:** Approximately 700 calories for every hour. Also, in this class are different sorts of hand to hand fighting, for example, Muay Thai. With regards to standard boxing, when you are genuine in the ring (a.k.a. battling another individual), the biggest calorie consumption develops. Be that as it may, many boxing courses additionally incorporate cardio activities, for example, hikers and burpees, so your pulse will in the long run increment more than you would anticipate. What's more, hello, before you can get into the ring, you need to start someplace, isn't that so?

6. **Swimming:** Approximately 680 calories for each hour Freestyle works, however as McCall says, you should go for a vivacious 75 yards for each moment. For an easygoing swimmer, this is somewhat forceful. (Butterfly stroke is significantly progressively productive if you extravagant it.)

7. **Outdoor bicycling:** Approximately 680 calories for each hour biking at a fast, lively pace will raise your pulse, regardless of whether you are outside or inside. Add to some rocky landscape and mountains and gets significantly more calorie consuming.

The volume of calories devoured is straightforwardly proportionate to the measure of sustenance, just like the kind of nourishment an individual expends. The best way to lessen calories is by being cautious about what you devour and captivating in dynamic physical exercises to consume overabundance calories in your body.

CHAPTER 12:

Meditation for Weight Loss

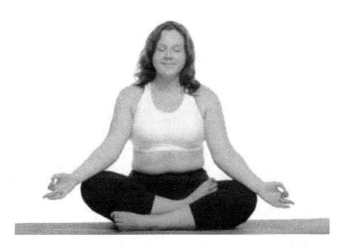

As we all know, meditation requires sitting still or even lying still. It doesn't sound like the sort of 'exercise' that'll help us lose weight, does it? How can meditation help you lose weight? Astonishing as it may be, weight loss meditation—in particular, 'meaningful meditation'—is increasingly being used by people who want to control the cravings of food and manage overeating. Often, diligent therapy may be used to reduce stress, thereby avoiding the 'comfort eating' arising out of stress. As we become more aware, we become more mindful of our cravings and can learn to pay attention to their underlying emotions, i.e., we can make a more informed decision before simply reaching for that sinful chocolate bar! When you continue feeding conscientiously every day so you will learn to like your food more over time, you'll now be more able to tell when you're full-meaning you'll continue eating fewer calories, of course. It has also been shown that consistent practice of mindful meditation lowers the stress hormone cortical. This is excellent news because high levels of cortical can cause pre-diabetes and central obesity (related to heart disease). In fact, cortical begins a process in our brains that can also lead to elevated hunger and intense cravings.

Don't Multitask

Experts say multitasking is our biggest enemy of weight control. When practicing careful weight loss meditation, it is important to concentrate on the food and the food alone. A recent study published in the 'Psychological Research' newspaper found that people who watched television at dinner were more likely to over-eat because they found the meal boring.

How Does Meditation Help You Get Weight Loss?

The truth is meditation rewires your consciousness. Feeding consciously is the opposite of feeding mindlessly. Eating more slowly helps your stomach realize when it's full—sometimes the stomach can take up to twenty minutes to signal to the brain that it's full and you shouldn't be hungry anymore. When consuming a limited amount of food, you would actually consume fewer calories all day long, resulting in a healthy and stable weight loss. There are books and CDs available which can teach you meditation techniques to reduce the urge to eat compulsively. Such training guides will help you overcome the cycle of compulsive eating so you can stick to your diet no matter what stress-causing incidents occur in your life. If it takes you a while to see results, don't be discouraged. It can take quite a bit of time to retrain your mind, so you no longer feel the temptation to overeat or eat mindlessly, particularly if it has been a lifelong problem. If you are not getting the effects you expect from directed therapy after giving it a period of time, consider consulting a counselor who is skilled in correcting compulsive behavior. Breaking the stress-based eating process is vital for your ability to stay on a diet and keep weight off after you leave the diet as you will no longer respond to stress by consuming large amounts of calories in your lifetime.

Weight Reduction Hypnosis and Self-Hypnosis

The notion of weight loss using self-hypnosis is definitely fascinating and one that would be nice to believe in. Hypnosis and self-hypnosis are now being used for various purposes, and the theory is embraced by many as much as possible. Strictly speaking, nobody is saying that by hypnosis, as if by a miracle, you can't make pounds go down. No, hypnosis is intended to reprogram your subconscious mind, so you have different behaviors. After all, your actions have much to do with your weight, as well as many other physical health aspects. It doesn't seem so hard to believe.

"Hypnosis" is a relatively new word, coined in the 19th century on the basis of a man named Franz Mesmer (from whom we got the word "mesmerism," meaning basically the same as hypnosis). It means going into a highly suggestible trance state. In more modern years, scientists have established different waves of the brain that exist during those phases. Hypnosis was initially identified with stage hypnotists and magicians, who under hypnosis, can induce people to do funny or weird stuff. However, it was also used for therapeutic purposes at the same time. It fits well with the emerging field of psychology, which stressed the subconscious mind's role in our behavior.

Using Weight Loss Hypnosis

If you were using hypnosis to lose weight, how would you go about it? Well, you might get to visit a qualified hypnotherapist. Compared to any type of traditional therapy, this would not be cheap, but it has the advantage of being fast-acting. Many hypnotherapists rely on showing you methods that you can do on your own, and you don't need to go back to them for appointments all the time. A further option is to consider one of the endless videos which will help you lose weight. These can be played at your leisure, but you are unable to play them while driving or doing anything where you need your full conscious attention. Since hypnosis's focus is on the mind, it is also up to you to discover the specific methods that function best. In other terms, you can do your research and find a healthy diet that suits your body (not all person diet works well).

The real aim of weight loss hypnosis is to enable you to do the things you need to do to lose weight without having to exert so much power of will. If your subconscious mind is more aligned with your conscious goals, there is less chance of you sabotaging yourself by cheating on your diet or dropping off your exercise program. It may sound strange or exotic to use hypnosis to lose weight, but it is really just another way to use your mind in a way that supports your goals. Perhaps not for all, but if the idea sounds appealing or at least interesting, you may want to look into some of the weight-loss possibilities of using hypnosis.

CHAPTER 13:

A Basic Self-Hypnosis Session for Weight Loss

Next, we will look at the art of manipulating your conscious and rewiring your subconscious to lose weight with the following six steps.

Step 1: Study or adjust your schedule to find time when you won't be distracted by your surroundings. This is a time set out for yourself where you are required to focus for 30 to 60 minutes to allow yourself to enter a trance state of mind where you feel completely relaxed and content without any interruptions.

Step 2: Set a weight-loss intention to reach your goals, but rather than only focusing on how much weight you want to lose, focus on all the benefits that you will reap because of it. Since a weight loss journey is also considered to be a positive and reconstructive journey, make certain you allow space for focusing on the value you place on your body. Placing value on our bodies is extremely important and helpful. It can teach us respect and motivate a greater reason behind perseverance to complete what we set out to do. Visualizing how much weight you'd like to lose in a reasonable period will set the tone for your goal before you begin. Make sure you say your goal out loud to ensure that your intention is set.

Step 3: Visualize your end-goal. What does your body look like and what size are you? How do you feel once you get closer to your goal? Also, focus on how you feel once you've reached your goal. Do you feel fulfilled and accomplished? Focus on the benefits you will reap once you've reached your goal, as well as the possibilities that will follow.

Step 4: Look the part. Close your eyes and enter a state of relaxation. Much like with meditation, your mind must be quiet and calm. Now you can engage in deep breathing for up to three minutes and choose your breathing technique, either the diaphragmatic technique or the Buteyko breathing technique. Make sure you continue to breathe until you feel calm and relaxed throughout your entire body. Now relax your body, you've entered a trance state of mind. **Step 5:** Visualize yourself reaching your goal in a trance state of mind. How good do you feel in your skin now that you've reached your goal weight? Do you miss your bad habits, and do you feel better now that you've left them behind? Do people look up to you for losing weight? Focus on the positivity surrounding the fact that you've accomplished something you possibly didn't think was possible before. Continuing with this state of mind will allow you to change your behavior and increase the desire for you to implement change into your life. **Step 6:** Return to your present state with ease, and don't rush it. You are in a relaxed state of mind and you should focus on bringing the feelings back to your reality. By doing this session daily and reminding yourself of how you feel, you will be able to adjust your mindset and increase the possibility of losing weight. You will receive new energy for taking on obstacles in your life and be able to make behavioral modifications where it is necessary.

Why Weight Loss Hypnotherapy is for You

Have you ever thought about food as your friend?

Have you ever thought about your friends and family as a priority?

If you answer both of these questions honestly, you'll come to find that food is supposed to be your friend. Thinking of it in that way, you will surely treat it with more respect. Given that we only get one body and that our bill of health deteriorates over time, we are most definitely obliged to look after ourselves. The same goes for kicking bad habits like smoking, consuming too much alcohol, possibly consuming mind-altering drugs, and even other negative factors like depriving yourself of sleep.

Hypnosis is all about bettering yourself, and if you can reach a state where you are focused on improving your health and feel willing to do so daily, you will finally change your mindset toward food, exercise, and bad habits.

Eating food that is beneficial for your health will become second nature.

Setting an attainable goal for yourself, like reaching 21-days of eating clean, will eventually lead to everything that follows thereafter if you manage to stick to self-hypnosis. Twenty-one days of consistency will allow you to create new habits and familiarities, which will keep you on track even after you've reached your weight loss goals. After a while, eating healthy won't feel like a punishment, but rather like a reward.

You Will Feel Better by Eating Better, But Also Eating Less

If you're like most people, you probably love eating and food in general, right? Just because you follow a diet and workout routine, does not mean that you can't enjoy your food. However, keeping in mind that you have three meals a day, and possibly one or two snacks, you should be mindful that your body doesn't need too much food. If our stomach is the size of your two hands clasped together in a fist, then where does the rest of the food you consume go? It gets deposited as fat storage in your body, which is exactly what you don't want. Focus on mindful eating and listen to your body. You will also find that eating less actually satisfy you more.

It shifts your attitude tremendously.

One of the biggest changes hypnosis implements is your mindset toward eating and exercising. While many individuals who engage in hypnosis do it to control their eating habits, there's a lot of change to be made to most people's sedentary lifestyles.

You are a human and you are designed to move, to hunt, to gather.

If you sit down all day and don't push your body out of its comfort zone, it will waste away and die.

CHAPTER 14:

Virtual Band Sample—Short Version

Start breathing slowly and deeply.

You are lying down and you are completely receptive to me.

You hear my voice mix with your inner voice.

My voice is now your voice.

Breathe in through your nose and out through your mouth.

Let it create a circular and continuous breathing.

Feel the air flowing in, filling the lower lungs.

The abdomen swells to the maximum inhalation, so hold your breath for three seconds. Then mentally count to five when you exhale.

Follow me:

Inhale deeply 1, 2, and 3.

Exhale slowly: 1, 2, 3, 4, and 5.

Inhale 1, 2, 3.

Exhale: 1, 2, 3, 4, 5.

Every time you exhale, you feel more and more relaxed.

Inhale 1, 2, 3.

Exhale: 1, 2, 3, 4, 5.

Every time you exhale, you feel more and more relaxed.

This will help you think much more clearly by increasing the level of oxygen reaching your brain.

You are perfectly calm and relaxed.

As you continue to breathe and relax, you are aware of the muscles in your feet and calves becoming heavy and relaxed. Let go of the tension and stiffness.

And this pleasant feeling of relaxation begins to spread to your leg muscles. You can go deeper and deeper.

Feeling peaceful and calm.

You are perfectly calm and relaxed.

You can go deeper and deeper.

Feel the sensation in your feet

Feel the force of gravity pushing them down.

Let them go.

They are heavy, relaxed.

Your calves are also heavy.

The force of gravity brings them down.

And you also begin to feel heavy and motionless legs.

Perfectly relaxed

You are calm and relaxed.

This feeling of relaxation diffuses in the body.

And every muscle in the abdomen and chest becomes calm and relaxed, free from tension and rigidity.

This sensation spreads to the muscles of the back, and the muscles become relaxed and relaxed.

Along the spine, the muscles become relaxed and relaxed. One by one. Like a mental massage from the base of the spine to the neck.

With every word I say you feel more relaxed.

Go deeper and deeper.

Enjoy this special moment where you get inside yourself and get stronger and stronger.

This feeling of relaxation spreads to the shoulders and arms.

Your right arm is heavy.

Now your left arm is also heavy.

Let go of any stiffness, and you may notice a tingling sensation on your fingertips. As your arms relax.

You feel heavy and relaxed.

You keep going deeper and deeper.

Now let go of your thoughts and feel your neck muscles relax completely, all the way to your head.

You're calm and safe, at peace with yourself, and the tension in your forehead simply begins to melt away.

The muscles of the eyebrows are relaxed.

More and more deeply.

In a few moments, I'll count from 1 to 3.

When I get to 3, your mind will be 10 times more calm and relaxed.

Let's start: 1... 2... 3...

A positive feeling spreads in you.

Today will be a special day for you.

The day of the intervention has finally arrived.

You find yourself lying on a trolley in a white surgery room.

You know that today you are going to be changed and that when you wake up you will be different.

You will be starting a new life.

You see figures in green around you.

They are slowly moving.

They are relaxed and perfectly know what they are doing.

Today they will help you change your life.

They are talking to you, asking you to relax and gently placing a mask on your face.

You almost feel a hand on your wrist briefly.

And you're vaguely aware of the noises around you and the ceiling lights.

You're happy at this moment and it's all over.

The band is fitted now, and you can visualize that band pinched around the entrance of the stomach.

That band means a lot to you.

You feel safe and secure now.

You already feel a sense of contentment and satiety.

Your new life has just begun.

You are in front of the mirror.

You can see and feel that something is profoundly different.

You can feel something different in your stomach.

There's tightness there.

Remember how you used to feel when you knew you had overeating.

Remember how it used to have that feel.

And from now on, the smallest bit of food feels huge.

Your stomach feels full all the time.

Your life is so good because you've lost weight, and you start to notice how fit and healthy you feel.

You took control of you and you are really enjoying life.

You like to feel healthy and fit because your stomach is as small as a golf ball now. One bite and you feel full.

It's a part of you now.

You're in control of your eating habits.

The surgery was perfect, and you can finally feel proud of the change.

You're really satisfied with being healthy and fit.

Your quality of life has really improved.

You have much more energy and enthusiasm.

You have much more control than many other aspects of your life...

Your self-esteem has become much stronger.

With this image of you, you feel more attractive and pleasantly regarded.

You keep feeding yourself healthy.

This is your new image.

You feel and see your body clearly.

You radiate confidence and you're proud of yourself.

You did it, you achieved your goal. This is already reality.

I'll count again from 1 to 3. When I get to number 3, you will relax 10 times more deeply, feeling focused and determined to maintain your new food balance.

Let's start: 1... 2... 3...

You are 10 times more focused.

Your mind is receptive and calm.

You feel a positive feeling spreading through your body.

You feel more determined than ever before.

Repeat after me: My stomach is the size of a golf ball.

Repeat after me: I eat the right amount of healthy, nutritious food.

Repeat after me: I like the taste of fresh, clear water.

Repeat after me: I exercise and stay fit.

Repeat after me: I eat fruit and vegetables with pleasure.

Repeat after me: I feel really full after a light, healthy meal.

These feelings take root deeply in your mind and are your reality.

Your unconscious mind continues to see this positive outcome.

You respond much better to life's difficulties.

And you continue to feel more determined.

Breathe deeply and slowly.

Living with renewed confidence and courage. Your self-esteem grows more and more.

You are satisfied with your gastric band.

It doesn't take much to make you feel full.

You think more clearly and remain calm even in the most challenging situations, calmly developing greater inner strength.

You can concentrate your mind with confidence and get what you want.

In a few moments I'll count from one to ten. With each number, you'll get more and more awake.

At number 8, you'll open your eyes, and at number 10 you'll be awake.

… 1… 2… 3… Wake up…

4… 5… Wake up…

… 6… 7… 8… Open your eyes…

9… 10…

Now you're awake and your diet is healthy and balanced.

And you can feel that band around your Stomach.

CHAPTER 15:

Strong Hypnotic Gastric Band - The Weekly Program

Practice regularly, self-hypnosis helps relieve stress, anxiety, physical pain. The first step: learn to relax your mind. Suggested by Lise Bartoli, psychologist, and hypnotherapist, these three self-hypnosis exercises will help you.

Autonomous, they can then evolve by themselves. Its program consists of several phases. Here, we'll only cover the first major step of learning to relax. But first, some tips for successful exercises.

- Choose the right time. You can test different schedules. Either early in the morning, early evening, or on weekends.

A word of advice: better avoid self-hypnosis sessions late in the evening, you might fall asleep. Plan a quiet beach. Before each exercise, make sure you are not disturbed and turn off the ringer on your phone. Even if the duration of the exercises depends on each one, allow 30 to 45 minutes of availability.

- **Choose the right place.** At home, test several places until you find the one where you feel really good to land. Once chosen, you will always put yourself in the same place when you practice a self-hypnosis session.
- **Make yourself comfortable.** Wear loose clothing and sit in a comfortable seat with your head properly seated for optimal relaxation. Avoid the lying position, which promotes sleep.

- **Memorize the course of the exercise or register.** If it's easier to relax by letting yourself be guided, record yourself reading the text of the statement. Speak in a monotone voice while articulating carefully. Leave breaks long enough to have time to respond to instructions.
- **Evolve at your own pace.** Those who are used to relaxing can do all three exercises in a row. For the others, it will be better to repeat each of them until it is fluid, then move on to the next day.

Monday - Self Hypnosis Motivation to Lose Weight

Step-by-Step to Lose Weight with Hypnosis

Losing weight with hypnosis works just like any other change with hypnosis will. However, it is important to understand the step by step process so that you know exactly what to expect during your weight loss journey with the support of hypnosis. In general, there are about seven steps that are involved with weight loss using hypnosis.

- The first step is when you decide to change
- The second step involves your sessions
- The third and fourth are your changed mindset and behaviors
- The fifth step involves your regressions
- The sixth is your management routines
- The seventh is your lasting change.

To give you a better idea of what each of these parts of your journey looks like, let us explore them in greater detail below.

In your first step toward achieving weight loss with hypnosis, you have to decide that you desire change and that you are willing to try hypnosis to change your approach to weight loss. At this point, you know you want to lose weight, and you have been shown the possibility of losing weight through hypnosis. You may find yourself feeling curious, open to trying something new, and a little bit skeptical as to whether this is actually going to work for you. You may also be feeling frustrated, overwhelmed, or even defeated by the lack of success you have seen using other weight loss methods, which may be what lead you to seek out hypnosis in the first place. At this stage, the best thing you can do is practice keeping an open and curious mind, as this is how you can set yourself up for success when it comes to your actual hypnosis sessions.

Your sessions account for stage two of the process. Technically, you are going to move from stage two through to stage five several times over before you officially move into stage six. Your sessions are the stage where you engage in hypnosis, nothing more, and nothing less. During your sessions, you need to maintain your open mind and stay focused on how hypnosis can help you. If you are struggling to stay open-minded or are still skeptical about how this might work, you can consider switching from absolute confidence that it will help to have a curiosity about how it might help instead.

Following your sessions, you are first going to experience a changed mindset. This is where you start to feel far more confident in your ability to lose weight and in your ability to keep the weight off. At first, your mindset may still be shadowed by doubt, but as you continue to use hypnosis and see your results, you will realize that you can create success with hypnosis. As these pieces of evidence start to show up in your own life, you will find your hypnosis sessions becoming even more powerful and even more successful.

In addition to a changed mindset, you are going to start to see changed behaviors.

Tuesday - Self Hypnosis to Overcome Compulsive/Emotional Eating

The "Resource Place"

Now imagine a place of relaxation that will deeply relax you.

Let your unconscious make you discover the images of a place of nature, which is for your symbol of harmony and well-being. It can be a known or imaginary place, whatever. The main thing is that you feel good in this place: whether it is a sandy beach, a corner of the countryside or a green mountain.

Look around, perceive what it is possible to feel (the sound of the waves, the blue of the sky, the smell of flowers, and the song of birds). The many sensory details developed mentally are important, because they allow you to build a place of your own, your own, a unique place of which you will feel creative.

Stay there as long as you want. You can lie down or take a walk.

Wednesday - Rest

Thursday - Self Hypnosis Motivation to Lose Weight

Interior light once plunged into the state of calm induced by the preceding exercise, continue by visualizing a soft color: blue, golden, and orange.

Imagine that the color you have chosen emanates from the earth and then goes up to you. It enters your whole body, starting with the feet. It relaxes each muscle.

The feet relax. Now bring the light up to the top of your head and enjoy this moment of relaxation. Focusing on a soft interior color leads to a number of physiological changes: lower blood pressure, slower breathing, and an even greater inner feeling of calm.

Friday - Self Hypnosis Motivation to Lose Weight

Here and now sit comfortably and choose a fixed point in front of you. It can be a painting or any other object.

While fixing this point, mentally check all the parts of your body by listing your perceptions: "I hear the rumor of the city," "I feel the warmth of the wood of the chair under my palms"... Listening to your sensations, you will gradually relax your alertness.

Fix the point until your eyelids tend to close on their own. Then continue to detail your sensations with your eyes closed. Then focus your attention on the air that you breathe, and that goes to your lungs, then guide it towards your belly. The latter inflates like a balloon and brings you more lightness. As you practice this breathing, you will feel your body becoming lighter and lighter. Savor this moment of tranquility and calm.

Saturday - Self Hypnosis for Sense of Satiety

After becoming familiar with self-hypnosis and gaining confidence, you will go into self-hypnosis, and you then ask yourself and make the most of all the bites of this much-desired food.

It starts with the eyes, you touch it with your lips, you feel it, you touch it with your tongue, you feel it in your mouth, you taste it, you breathe it, and it all happens in full consciousness, focusing on every sensation.

Then you swallow the bite, and then you open your eyes. To look again at your favorite food and wonder if you still want it. If so, then you start the self-hypnosis exercise again. All this happens slowly; in the rhythm proper to Hypnosis, and in a unique perception of the food, nothing exists anymore.

Sunday – Rest

CHAPTER 16:

Positive Impacts of Affirmations

You control the fundamental fixings that make self-hypnosis work for you. These are similar fixings that make your experience of achievement for any objective you pick. Let us take a gander at every component and how you may utilize it to perform for you.

Motivation

Motivation is the vitality of your craving, of what you need. Needing is an inclination that you can control. For the greater part of your life, you have chiefly controlled your craving or needing by restricting it or denying it. You might be truly adept at controlling your wants and needing in certain regions and powerless or natural in others. Since this is a "diet" book, you may have just set yourself up to hear that this "diet" will resemble the others that have mentioned to you what you should deny yourself or breaking point. That is, different diets have mentioned to you what not to need, and the accentuation may have been about "not needing" a few nourishments that you have developed to cherish. Welcome to another method of treating yourself; we will urge you to show signs of improvement at "needing." Denial is excluded from Rapid Weight Loss Hypnosis.

Your motivation is a key factor, one of the fundamental fixings. We need you to center your vitality of needing not toward food, yet toward the motivation that unmistakably tells your mind-body what you need it to make: flawless weight. We urge you to get great at needing your ideal weight. Here is a model. Let us state that you are in a pool, and out of nowhere, you take in a significant piece of water. At that time, you need just a single thing, a breath of air. It feels like decisive, and a breath of air is the main thing on your mind as of now. The needing is so serious and powerful that it dominates every single other idea and urges you to take the necessary steps to get that breath of air. That is the amount we need you to need the weight and self-perception that you want.

Conviction and Believing

Convictions are those musings and thoughts that are valid for you. They don't need to be deductively demonstrated for you to realize that they generally will be valid for you. Inside that, whether you know about it or not, your activities, both mindful and subconscious, depend on your convictions. Even though your convictions are as contemplations and thoughts, they shape your experience by influencing your activities throughout everyday life. If you accept that creatures make great sidekicks, you most likely have a feline or canine or parrot or a ferret or two. If you accept that espresso keeps you alert around evening time, you likely don't drink espresso before hitting the sack. The power of accepting lets you impact your body in manners that may appear to be bewildering. Fake treatment reactions, where people react to an inactive substance as though it were genuine medicine, are regular instances of how convictions are knowledgeable about the body. If an individual truly accepts that he will get well when taking specific medicine, it will happen whether the tablet contains a prescription or is inactive. Similarly, if an individual truly accepts that he can accomplish high evaluations in school, it will occur. If an individual truly accepts that he can achieve his ideal weight, it will occur.

Recollect your pretend games as a kid. Your capacity to imagine is similarly as solid now as when you were exceptionally youthful. It might be somewhat corroded, and you may require a touch of training, yet when you permit yourself to imagine and let yourself have faith in what you are imagining, you will find a powerful apparatus. You will find this is a brilliantly viable approach to convey your goals, those messages of what you need, to the entirety of the phones and tissues and organs of your body, which react by bringing that goal into reality for you. We can't state this enough: musings are things. The musings, the photos, the thoughts you put in your mind become the messages your self-hypnosis passes on to your mind-body, eventually transforming your ideal body into reality and imagining is picking what to accept and getting retained in those thoughts. Similarly, as an amplifying glass can center beams of daylight, you can center your psychological vitality to make your considerations, thoughts, and convictions genuine for your body.

Desire

You may not generally get what you need, yet you do get what you anticipate. Desires contain the vitality of convictions and become the aftereffects of what is accepted. Here is a case of how to "anticipate." When you plunked to peruse this, you didn't analyze the seat or couch to test its capacity to hold your weight. You just plunked without contemplating it. You didn't need to consider it, because a piece of you is sure, and has such a great amount of confidence in the seat, that you simply "anticipated" it to hold you. That is the way to expect the ideal body weight you want. Remembering this, be mindful of what you state to yourself as well as other people concerning your body weight desires. "I generally put on weight over the special seasons."

Mind-Body in Focus

Every one of the fundamental fixings can create powerful outcomes when centered inside the mind-body. Nonetheless, when these fixings are adjusted appropriately inside the procedure of self-hypnosis, their viability has amplified a hundredfold. Self-hypnosis is a procedure for creating your world. You may think this sounds mystical or unrealistic.

However, that is comparative with what you have encountered as yet in your life. These thoughts might be exceptionally new to you. Here is a case of the "relative" idea of new thoughts. Envision that you are given a personal jet that is flawlessly equipped with sumptuous arrangements and a very much prepared team. It is a brilliant blessing, and you get the opportunity to show this designing wonder to certain people who have seen nothing like it.

Your subconscious (mind-body) utilizes the mix of what you need (motivation), what you accept, and what you expect as a plan for activity. The outcomes are accomplished by your mind-body (subconscious), and not by deduction or breaking down. If an individual contact a virus surface that she accepts is hot, she can create a rankle or consume reaction. Then again, an individual contacting an extremely hot surface reasoning that it is cool may not deliver a consume reaction. Individuals who stroll over hot coals while envisioning that they are cool may encounter a warm physical issue (some minor singing on the bottoms of their feet). Yet, their invulnerable framework doesn't react with a consume (rankling, torment, and so on.) because their minds advise their bodies how to respond. Once more, it is the arrangement of every one of the three of the basic fixings that make this conceivable:

- Wanting to do it
- Believing it conceivable
- Expecting to be fruitful

This is the way to progress. Your body completes your convictions. Your convictions direct your activities, which like this, shape your experience.

Some portray this procedure as creating your prosperity or creating your involvement with life. In our way of life, we see this depicted inside the motivational and positive mental disposition writing. It very well may be seen in numerous zones of mysticism. You can likewise think back to the people of yore and see it depicted in the provisions of the authentic period. An individual a lot smarter than we are stated, "It will be done unto you as per your conviction." In the current period of integrative medication and brain research, we call it self-hypnosis or mind-body medication. There are currently various logical examinations that exhibit astonishing outcomes for torment control, wound mending, physical modification, and a lot of more medical advantages than we recently suspected conceivable.

Picking Your Beliefs

You can pick your convictions. You may decide to accept what you see, in the feeling of "See it to trust it" or "Truth can be stranger than fiction." This is simple to do. You experience something with your faculties, and that is a natural method of picking whether it is reasonable or not. However, you may likewise decide to trust it first and afterward observe it, which may require some training. The vast majority think that it's simpler to let the world mention to them what is valid or what to accept. The TV, media, papers, books, instructors, and specialists besiege us with what to accept. You grew up finding out about the world and yourself from numerous outside sources. This prompted a recognizable example of watching and accepting data about the world from outside yourself, and you picked which data to make a piece of your conviction framework. This included convictions about your body. For instance, when your stomach makes a thundering sound, you accept that it implies you are ravenous. Or then again, you feel queasy and trust you are wiped out. Both of these are instances of watched occasions: you watched an association once and decided to trust it.

In Rapid Weight Loss Hypnosis, we are suggesting that you turn that training around with this thought: "Trust it, and you will see it." This implies you initially pick what to accept, and afterward, your body follows up on it as evidence and makes it genuine, you would say. One of the significant messages we trust you will get from this is that your mind body hears all that you hear, all that you state, all that you think, picture, or envision in your mind, and it can't differentiate between what is genuine and what you envision. It follows up on what you need, accepts, and anticipate. In light of this, which of these announcements would assist you with encountering the ideal weight you want: "I simply take a gander at food and put on weight" or "I can eat anything, and my weight remains the equivalent"? The last mentioned. In any case, which articulation do you by and by accept to be valid for you? Once more, it will be done unto you as indicated by your conviction. We will assist you with the thoughts, language, and pictures that plan compelling hypnotic proposals, yet you have all-out command over what you decide to accept.

As you read the thoughts of this and hear the hypnotic recommendations offered during the trance work on the sound, you will settle on numerous decisions for yourself. We wholeheartedly urge you to decide to trust it so you will see it for yourself. Your subconscious (mind-body) can't differentiate and will follow up on what you select in any case. Why not select what you truly need?

The Energy of Emotions

Not all considerations and convictions show themselves into your experience. Just those that have the vitality of your sentiments (feelings), alongside your conviction and your desire that something will occur, will show themselves. Your sentiments or feelings are a type of vitality that impacts this procedure of creation.

CHAPTER 17:

Motivational Affirmations

Motivational affirmations are phrases, sentences, or even words that will enable you to stay positive, be focused, and highly motivated. You need to choose these affirmations and use them on your daily basis. They are of great help as they will help you to meditate correctly on your weight loss. You can only reduce weight when you stay focused and positive. Being true to yourself and getting motivated every time will enable you to be able to control your weight. Even though these affirmations are numerous, you need to take a look at the ones I have detailed or illustrated the most common ones in the below paragraphs. It is good to note that, these affirmations, you can use them each morning after just waking up. They will sincerely help you to jump-start your day in a much higher note. It is a challenge thrown at you that you better try this and see how your life will drastically change. Your mindset will shift, and you will only be thinking positive. You will only be staying focused on your life, and this will increase your esteem within and outside your external world. Below are some of the examples that you need to go through with much keenness.

You must embrace success. In every kind of situation or no matter the condition you are facing with, tell yourself about success. You need to talk about being successful every morning. The word "you can't" should not appear in your mind. Everyone has excuses. Some excuses emerge from fear of not trying. You need to stay focus and embrace the successful part of you. Don't get overwhelmed and overtaken by negative thinking about your success story. I challenge you to recite this affirmation every time you wake up. You will realize how important it is not only to your body but also in your external world. You need to feel unstoppable and fail to look at your excuses for not being successful. Negativity here is a BIG NO for you.

You must always be calm when faced with conflict. Conflicts are issues that always take you back to where you were. Conflict will automatically kill your daily morale leading to weak contributions of your abilities, especially within the organization and other sectors of life. You must try as quickly as possible to brush off annoyances easily. You must always agree with all sorts of disagreements so that the argument can end there. Tell yourself that you are more significant than what you are facing, and this should not drain you physically. Staying focused with a fit body and soul will make you lead a positive life.

At last, your weight will be highly controlled. You need to have that habit of doing this any time you are facing any conflict. It will only help you to stay positive and highly productive under your capacity. Reciting this affirmation every morning will be of great help. Try it as many as possible and help yourself to stay calm, relaxed, and comfortable.

You must choose to show love and gratitude every day. You need to know that life is always short, and concentrating on negativity is not good. It won't go well with you. It will only derail your success. After all these, you must radiate elements of joy to yourself and have that love of your body. Showing all kinds of gratitude will enable you to lead a happy life. It will affect not only you but also the people around you. You must embrace this no matter what happens. Staying scorned and having negative thoughts only ages you as quickly as possible and leaves you with a body shape you never wanted. Be happy always, and show love to the surrounding. You must try this and believe me, and you will have a change within the next few weeks.

You must be impressive to others. Staying positive in life is an excellent deal to yourself. Use anything under your disposal to impress those who are around you. You need to be positive in everything to be as positive as you can and never underrate yourself. No one sent a letter to be born in a certain way, so you need to accept yourself the way you are. It will enable you to stay focus and lead a real-life every day. You need to develop this habit of saying this affirmation to yourself as it is of great help. It will also help you to start your day with big morale and a notch higher.

You are free to develop your reality. Realities are things that are with us no matter what happens. Therefore, you must strive hard to create your reality. No one is supposed to create you one since you are in a better position with much knowledge about yourself. You must have a choice and choose wisely in every kind of situation you might get yourself herein. Remember, nothing should stand in between you and your happiness peak. That apex of goodness should be your cup of joy, and no one should prevent you from creating this form of reality to you. Choosing your reality every day will make you stay positive and entirely focused on life. Besides, it will be of great help as far as your body is concerned. Remember to note that your life ultimately depends on the realities within you. You can lie to people around you, but believe me, and you cannot lie to yourself. Therefore, it will be of great advice that you keep this affirmation as it will help you live and stay positive. In the end, this will automatically reflect on your body shape and image.

You need to shed off any unimportant attachment. Unimportant attachments are things that no longer have any effect on your life. These are things that will only let you down, thus derailing your life goals of achieving a mind-set full of happiness. Your future success depends heavily on this, and for you to get at that position, you will need to detach yourself from anything that might let you down. You must note that anything might also mean any person. We have people in our lives that always try very hard to put us down. These types of people are afraid of your success in life. They will try their best to pull you down, no matter how hard you try to embrace only positivity in your life. It is time to get yourself going and void them like the plague. Remember, you must live and not only live but choose a pleasant experience. It will only be possible if you manage to refuse anything or anyone that is holding you back. Since I have said this, it is now my wish that you may practice this affirmation and use it as your routine daily. Practice makes perfect, and you will only realize that when you train.

You are enough just as you are. You must release that demonic notion of having comparisons between you and others. For you to stay specific, you must have some success standards. After developing all these, set your own goals and ambitions. Your vision should relate to your mission in life. After all these, you can now judge yourself using the basis of your success. Those rules and regulations you created in your success standards should enable you to judge yourself accordingly. Just know you are just enough the way you were born. You are a complete soul, and no part of you is lacking. So never try to make a comparison with others. You should note that affirmation helps in the realization of worthiness. Within a short period, you will be able to control your body image. Also, it will be of a great deal as it helps you in achieving some of the personal goals in life, and having a sound body is one of them.

You must be in a position to fulfill your purpose. The world should know your existence, and you must be ready to show your achievement. Showing your accomplished goals will need some positive deeds that lead to a successful life. On most occasions, people who trend are our trendsetters. They trend because of having done something positive or negative. They are then known all over the world. However, in this motivational affirmation, you need to focus on positive things. You need to be a trendsetter in showing the whole world what you are capable of offering. If you have been employed somewhere to sweep, you must clean until the country president cuts short his journey to congratulate you. Achieving your best is always one decisive way to be successful and lead a happy life free from stress and distress. Remember, this affirmation reminds you that no one has that power to stop you from doing or rather fulfilling your purpose in life. Sharing this thought every morning when you wake up will eventually get you somewhere.

You must now stay focus and have this habit of telling yourself that no one can prevent you from achieving.

You must be results-oriented. In your daily life, you need to stay focus in life. Your primary focus should be on your results. It is through this that you will be able to realize your productivity.

To achieve this, you must be able to create some space for success. Get more success in your life. Avoid any derailing excuses that will only demean your reputation, thus lowering your success rate. Offer yourself these phrases every morning, and you will be in great joy for the rest of the day. You need not hold on excuses for failing to achieve something. Be yourself and have the ability to struggle until you reach that success in life. It is through this that your mind will have settled, giving you peace of mind. Peace of mind will enable you to lead a stress-free experience. It will reflect in your body image.

Be in control of your own happiness. Happiness is an aspect of life that will initiate your feelings and moods towards a positive experience. It is like a gear geared towards your prosperous life. Staying positive here will be of great importance, and for you to realize this, you must take control of your happiness. Responsibility is a virtue, and being responsible will make you bold enough to face all kinds of situations. Your joy is your key to success, and no one should tamper with it. Make happiness your priority and be responsible for it. You must let no one make you angry. Angriness will only induce you with emotional feelings that will eventually affect your life more so your body image. Having seen this, you must now be in an excellent position to embrace this affirmation. Take it as an opener to your morning and employ it entirely in your life.

CHAPTER 18:

Self-Improvement with Hypnosis

Hypnosis is rewiring your brain to add or to change your daily routine, starting from your basic instincts. This happens due to the fact that while you are in a hypnotic state, you are more susceptible to suggestions by the person who put you in this state. In the case of self-hypnosis, the person who made you enter the trance of hypnotism is yourself. Thus, the only person who can give you suggestions that can change your attitude in this method is you and you alone.

Again, you must forget the misconception that hypnosis is like sleeping because if it is, then it would be impossible to give autosuggestions to yourself. Try to think about it like being in a very vivid daydream where you are capable of controlling every aspect of the situation you are in. This give you the ability to change anything that may bother and hinder you to achieve the best possible result. If you are able to pull it off properly, then the possibility of improving yourself after the constant practice of the method will just be a few steps away.

Career

People say that motivation is the key to improve in your career. But no matter how you love your career, you must admit that there are aspects in your work that you really do not like doing. Even if it is a fact that you are good in the other tasks, there is that one duty that you dread. And every time you encounter this specific chore, you seem to be slowed down and thus lessening your productivity at work. This is where self-hypnosis comes into play.

The first thing you need to do is find that task you do not like. In some case, there might be multiple of them depending on your personality and how you feel about your job. Now, try to look at why you do not like that task and do simple research on how to make the job a lot simpler. You can then start conditioning yourself to use the simple method every time you do the job.

After you are able to condition your state of mind to do the task, each time you encounter it will become the trigger for your trance and thus giving you the ability to perform it better. You will not be able to tell the difference since you will not mind it at all. Your coworkers and superiors though, will definitely notice the change in your work style and in your productivity.

Family

It is easy to improve in a career. But to improve your relationship with your family can be a little trickier. Yet, self-hypnosis can still reprogram you to interact with your family members better by modifying how you react to the way they act. You will have the ability to adjust your way of thinking, depending on the situation. This then allows you to respond in the most positive way possible, no matter how dreadful the scenario may be.

If you are in a fight with your husband/wife, for example, the normal reaction is to flare up and face fire with fire. The problem with this approach is it usually engulfs the entire relationship, which might eventually lead up to separation. Being in a hypnotic state in this instance then can help you think clearly and change the impulse of saying words without thinking them through. Anger will still be there, of course, that is the healthy way. But anger now under self-hypnosis can be channeled and stop being a raging inferno; you can turn it into a steady bonfire that can help you and your partner find common ground for whatever issue you are facing. The same applies in dealing with siblings or children. If you are able to condition your mind to think more rationally or to get into the perspective of others, then you can have better family/friends' relationships.

Health and Physical Activities

Losing weight can be the most common reason why people will use self-hypnosis in terms of health and physical activities. But this is just one part of it. Self-hypnosis can give you a lot more to improve this aspect of your life. It works the same way while working out.

Most people tend to give up their exercise program due to the exhaustion they think they can no longer take. But through self-hypnosis, you will be able to tell yourself that the exhaustion is lessened and thus allowing you to finish the entire routine. Keep in mind though that your mind must never be conditioned to forget exhaustion, it must only not mind it until the end of the exercise. Forgetting it completely might lead you to not stopping to work out until your energy is depleted. It becomes counterproductive in this case.

Having a healthy diet can also be influenced by self-hypnosis. Conditioning your mind to avoid unhealthy food can be done. Thus, hypnosis will be triggered each time you are tempted to eat a meal you are conditioned to consider as unhealthy. You're eating habit then can change to benefit you to improve your overall health.

Mental, Emotional and Spiritual Needs

Since self-hypnosis deals directly in how you think, it is then no secret that it can greatly improve your mental, emotional and spiritual needs. A clear mind can give your brain the ability to have more rational thoughts. Rationality then leads to better decision making and easy absorption and retention of information you might need to improve your mental capacity. You must set your expectations, though; this does not work like magic that can turn you into a genius. The process takes time, depending on how far you want to go, how much you want to achieve. Thus, the effects will only be limited by how much you are able to condition your mind.

In terms of emotional needs, self-hypnosis cannot make you feel differently in certain situations. But it can condition you to take in each scenario a little lighter and make you deal with them better. Others think that getting rid of emotion can be the best course of action if you are truly able to rewire your brain. But they seem to forget that even though rational thinking is often influenced negatively by emotion, it is still necessary for you to decide on things basing on the common ethics and aesthetics of the real world. Self-hypnosis can then channel your emotion to work in a more positive way in terms of decision making and dealing with emotional hurdles and problems.

Spiritual need, on the other hand, is far easier to influence when it comes to doing self-hypnosis. As a matter of fact, most people with spiritual beliefs are able to do self-hypnosis each time they practice what they believe in. A deep prayer, for instance, is a way to self-hypnotize yourself to enter the trance to feel closer to a Divine existence. Chanting and meditation done by other religions also leads and have the same goal. Even the songs during a mass or praise and worship triggers self-hypnosis, depending if the person allows them to do so.

Still, the improvements can only be achieved if you condition yourself that you are ready to accept them. The willingness to put an effort must also be there. An effortless hypnosis will only create the illusion that you are improving and thus will not give you the satisfaction of achieving your goal in reality.

How Hypnosis Can Help Resolve Childhood Issues

Another issue that hypnosis can help are those from our past. If you have had traumatic situations from your childhood days, then you may have issues in all areas of your adult life. Unresolved issues from your past can lead to anxiety and depression in your later years. Childhood trauma is dangerous because it can alter many things in the brain, both psychologically and chemically.

The most vital thing to remember about trauma from your childhood is that given a harmless and caring environment in which the child's vital needs for physical safety, importance, emotional security, and attention are met, the damage that trauma and abuse cause can be eased and relieved. Safe and dependable relationships are also a dynamic component in healing the effects of childhood trauma in adulthood and make an atmosphere in which the brain can safely start the process of recovery.

Pure hypno-analysis is the lone most effective method of treatment available in the world today, for the resolution of phobias, anxiety, depression, fears, psychological and emotional problems/symptoms and eating disorders. It is a highly advanced form of Hypnoanalysis (referred to as analytical hypnotherapy or hypno-analysis). Hypnoanalysis, in its numerous forms, is practiced all over the world; this method of hypnotherapy can completely resolve the foundation of anxieties in the unconscious mind, leaving the individual free of their symptoms for life.

There is a deeper realism active at all times around us and inside us. This reality commands that we must come to this world to find happiness, and every so often that our inner child stands in our way. This is by no means intentional; however, it desires to reconcile wounds from the past or address damaging philosophies that were troubling to us as children.

So to disengage the issues that upset us from earlier in our lives we have to find a way to bond with our internal child, we then need to assist in rebuilding this part of us which will, in turn, help us to be rid of all that has been hindering us from moving on.

Connecting with your inner child may seem like something that may be hard or impossible to do, especially since they may be a part that has long been buried. It is a fairly easy exercise to do and can even be done right now. You will need about 20 minutes to complete this exercise. Here's what you do: find a quiet spot where you won't be disturbed and find a picture of you as a child if you think it may help.

Breathe in and loosen your clothing if you have to. Inhale deeply into your abdomen and exhale, repeat until you feel yourself getting relaxed; you may close your eyes and focus on getting less tense. Feel your forehead and head relax, let your face become relaxed and relax your shoulders. Allow your body to be limp and loose while you breathe slowly. Keep breathing slowly as you let your entire tension float away.

Now slowly count from 10–0 in your mind and try to think of a place from your childhood. The image doesn't have to be crystal clear right now, but try to focus on exactly how you remember it and keep that image in mind. Imagine yourself as a child and imagine observing younger you; think about your clothes, expression, hair, etc. In your mind, go and meet yourself, introduce yourself to you.

CHAPTER 19:

How Hypnosis Work: Overpowered and Out of Control

I'm continually contemplating nourishment and attempting to shed pounds," Mary said during her first session. "It works for some time, however then I become weary of it. Something consistently occurs and disrupts the general flow. At that point, I restore all the weight, in addition to another 10 pounds for the most part. I commit dumb errors, and I'm sluggish. I simply don't want to work out. It appears as though I harm myself. I don't have the foggiest idea of what else to do."

This sort of reasoning is normal for individuals who battle to shed pounds and keep it off - the negative self-talk, believing they're self-attacking, or there is a major issue with them—and who can accuse them? By and large, they've pursued each arrangement, done all that they "thought" they should do—despite everything it didn't work.

What they don't understand is that there are parts of science and how the brain really functions at play here, and by getting familiar with how the psyche really functions, the things that used to be keeping them down would now be able to assist them with being effective.

Prepared to Eat Wrong

We are prepared since early on to treat nourishment with a specific goal in mind. When we're little youngsters, we're frequently advised to "finish all the nourishment on your plate," or "would prefer you not to grow up huge and solid?" Huge numbers of these benevolent proclamations made by grown-ups are really neutralizing our science—supposing that you see how kids eat, you'll see they'd frequently prefer to play over eat. They're increasingly keen on investigating their general surroundings, playing with their toys and different children than eating, on the off chance that they're not really ravenous.

At that point as we get more established, we're instructed that "breakfast is the most significant meal of the day," and much of the time we're not permitted to venture out from home without eating a "decent breakfast." Lunch is at a particular time each day, so we need to eat at that point or not in any way. This frequently proceeds into adulthood where at work, we make some specific memories edge to have lunch, are as yet having breakfast toward the beginning of the day, regardless of whether we're really eager or not.

We're encouraged that nourishment is there to assist us with feeling better, "eat something and you'll feel good." We go out for dessert when we win the softball match-up, and go out for pizza when our rabbit kicks the bucket. Without our rabbit kicks the bucket. Without acknowledging it, our social reactions to nourishment are instructing us to sincerely eat.

The issue with these components that are a piece of our general public is that it's not quite we as people are structured. We have something many refer to as a craving. Our craving is the body's regular method to disclose to us when it's a great opportunity to eat, or when it's an ideal opportunity to quit eating. What's more, we're prepared out of utilizing our craving at a youthful age by being compelled to eat at explicit occasions, or eat explicit measures of nourishment when we're not ravenous. Contrast that with other basic substantial capacities—like realizing when to go to the restroom, for instance. Ask yourself—how would you realize when it's a great opportunity to go to the restroom? Do you plan it? Do you plan it, and consider it throughout the day? Most likely not.

Probably the most ideal ways we can gain power back with regards to eating, is to give the activity of realizing when it's a great opportunity to eat and what amount back to the body, and away from the reasoning procedure. This is tied in with returning to the genuine power that we're brought into the world with - our bodies' own intelligence incorporated with a significant part of our body called our craving, and start eating when our body reveals to us it's a great opportunity to eat and stop when we're fulfilled or full. It's called Mindful Eating, and it's conceivable to begin utilizing our hunger again to assist us with accomplishing the weight reduction we want. Regardless of whether you don't think you have a hunger - you may astonish yourself. Numerous customers have revealed some fear when it came to utilizing their craving to help manage their nourishment consumption, since they state they don't really have a hunger and aren't sure in the event that they realize when they're fulfilled or full. What's more, it might be valid—meds and ailment are two things that can affect our feeling of craving. Be that as it may, I generally ask them to simply attempt it—hold up until they're eager to eat and see what occurs. What's more, for each situation, customers are astonished to learn they do in reality have a craving, and it can help direct their nourishment utilization. Careful Eating implies you utilize your hunger to eat when you're eager and stop when you're full, eating well nourishment in sound parcels.

The Brain Cares How You Feel

The other component keeping individuals caught in weight gain is the mind's characteristic propensity to get some distance from torment and toward delight. There's a lot of logical foundation on how this functions, yet to streamline it, there are two contending portions of our mind that are continually attempting to help keep us sheltered and upbeat.

One is the limbic framework. It's a more established, progressively crude piece of our mind. The essential focal point of this piece of the mind is to protect us. It reacts to feelings and inspiration, is answerable for long haul memory, and it doesn't prefer to feel agitated or uncertain in light of the fact that those sentiments are dangerous.

Be that as it may, we as a whole realize we live in a universe of vulnerability, so the limbic framework is regularly miserable. When something transpires that we don't care for - for instance, we're exhausted, or tragic, or upset, this piece of the mind feels awkward, and the characteristic propensity is for this piece of the cerebrum to get us to improve. This is the place numerous individuals stumble into difficulty, since when feeling exhausted or focused on, nourishment will frequently fill in as a generally excellent distractor to offer some relief. The cerebrum is glad - quickly, on the grounds that nourishment gives prompt delight. The issue is that it's likewise fleeting, so with the goal for you to really feel much improved, you'll need to continue eating. This is the manner by which a whole sack of treats vanishes and how we eat more than we need, which thusly can make us put on weight.

The other piece of the mind at work here is the prefrontal cortex. This piece of the mind is the fresher, official capacity part of the cerebrum liable for long haul arranging. This is the piece of the mind that realizes it's bad to eat a whole pack of treats and wouldn't like to eat the whole sack either.

So the issue is that with these two contending portions of our mind at play, we regularly feel clashed—with part of us needing to eat the treats to feel better now, and part of us realizing we'll think twice about it later. Furthermore, the genuine test comes in light of the fact that the nourishment really improves. All in all, the limbic piece of the mind is really relieved by the nourishment. So truly the nourishment attempts to assist us with feeling much improved—however, it's just an impermanent arrangement—we feel better just while we're really eating. Over the long haul eating for enthusiastic reasons transforms into an unfortunate propensity and causes weight gain.

The explanation this is imperative to comprehend is that there is a superior way. The limbic framework doesn't really require nourishment—it simply needs to feel much improved, and there are numerous different things that will make this piece of the mind feel good. The issue is that nourishment works so well in the transient that numerous individuals depend upon it only—so when the opportunity arrives, and we are not feeling better, we just have one reaction. What's more, that is to eat something. At that point, we feel wild.

The initial phase in any change procedure is mindfulness. What's more, for a considerable lot of my customers just understanding this is the means by which the mind works—the explanation you go after nourishment when you feel exhausted, focused, miserable, and blameworthy is that there's a piece of your cerebrum that simply needs you to feel good—simply realizing that the procedure is mostly the cerebrum normal reaction, that can assist us with settling on a superior decision since we understand there's nothing amiss with us.

For Mary, she understood that in the event that she just took a full breath, and ventured outside, she could regularly evade the automatic reaction to passionate triggers in her day-by-day life. This gave her a quick feeling of control, regardless of whether it was just a piece of the time from the outset. In any case, gradually, after some time, the mind starts to overhaul itself. Presently, rather than simply having a solitary alternative to feel much improved nourishment, there are various choices: a walk, tea, call a companion, tune in to music. Furthermore, with those numerous decisions comes a significant part of making change: the delay. A minute to stop, reflect, and really pick the manner in which you react to a circumstance so you can get the outcomes you need.

CHAPTER 20:

Basics of Meditation

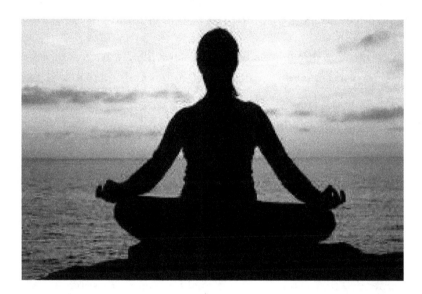

Meditation is the art of quieting the mind. It is the art of awakening our consciousness. Meditation helps us shift from a consciousness bound by a small ego to a deeper sense of self. We will achieve peace of mind, relaxation, and a positive attitude about ourselves and the world if we meditate properly. When we have a healthy mind and an increased self-esteem, the rest of our being will benefit too. We will find better health when we reduce our tension, and we can be comfortable no matter what life throws at us.

Meditation practice is mostly used as a part of meditation and other metaphysical disciplines. Some of the benefits are that you do not need any special equipment or location to do meditation.

The basic concepts of meditation are similar, there are several ways in which it can be performed. The most important, and sometimes the hardest part is to relax your mind and avoid following any distracting wandering thoughts.

It is the negative thoughts which are polluting the mind. You will find harmony and relaxation in a hectic day, by learning to keep them out. Training to keep your mind quiet helps you to concentrate on deeper, more positive thoughts that motivate you to enjoy life more.

When you trudge down life's fatiguing alleys, life always resembles a rat race. Workplace tension, frustration at home and intense soul fatigue add up to build a peculiar state. Sometimes the busy workers thought they had handled their lives better if the day had 36 or more hours in it. Yet, there are several risks that arise from persistent stress and anxiety. Indeed, almost all modern illnesses are somehow connected to the stressful lifestyle. Meditating is the best way to counter the fatigue and tiredness. Now meditation will only produce great replenishing results if you do it in the right way. Too many people know meditation's common benefits, but very few know how to meditate. If this is the first time that you intend to engage in any meditation exercises, it is recommended that you meet with a qualified trainer or someone who is experienced in such techniques. Here are a few basics of meditation for beginners to support.

How to Prepare

You need to make some arrangements before meditating. At first, try to secure in the early morning at some time. The explanation for this is that a person is usually in his best mood and health in the morning. You should perform this exercise with an empty stomach. And if you prefer meditation evening, make sure you did not take any food at least three hours before the session. Taking a cool shower before meditating is always healthy. This will help you to concentrate better.

The Right Ambience

You need a great ambience for proper meditation, which is serene and calm. Choose a place to get yourself some solitude. Mild, calming fragrance would be of great help in this. Space light should be dim, and the session should not be disturbed by noise.

Right Posture

Posture is also an essential factor influencing the action. With a sitting position or lying position, you can do it all. Yet the beginners also fall asleep while they are lying on the floor or mattress doing this. Hence beginning with a sitting posture is advisable. The typical method of meditating is to sit cross beamed on a mat or a flat mattress in a posture called Lotus. But if you have knee pain or other discomforts, consider sitting on a chair that holds the back and neck straight.

Breathing Exercises and Tips

Few special breathing techniques that are mandatory at the time of the sessions. Deep breathing is one of the most common meditation techniques, where both the process of inhalation and exhalation is long and slow. You should try to focus on thinking about one specific thing. Besides these, there are other strategies that you can get from any book or other tools on "How to Meditate."

Meditation is the best way to calm your mind and rejuvenate the damage to your soul as well. Practice it daily and track the results over a short period.

Below are a few tips to help you learn to practice the art of meditation.

Bring some comfortable clothing on first. Close-fitting trousers and tight clothes are likely to be something of a nuisance. Find something to wear that lets you relax without having to worry about being pinched or pulled. You can then play some good and calming instrumental music. If you listen to music with lyrics when you are meditating, you are likely to start singing along in your ear, which will not help you concentrate.

To help them concentrate, some people think it helps to have a candle or other item to look at. Many tend to close their eyes to help avoid anything that might disrupt their mental comfort.

Sit in a snug spot. Putting a pillow under your bottom could help you sit up straight and balanced. When you think you can stay awake during your meditation period, you can always lie in bed or on the couch. What is crucial is that the place helps you to relax as you concentrate. The position or location may also be helpful. Select a place that is free from disturbance inside your home. A place where temperature and appearance are both relaxed and friendly. There are those who decorate a specific part of a room only for meditation purposes. Switch your mobile phone off the Screen and the ringer. You may want to set the timer on your phone, so you will know when it is time to stop without having to check every minute to see how long it has been. If this is a new activity for you, simply schedule it for 5 minutes and start developing your meditation skills. As you develop your ability to concentrate and quiet your mind, you can extend your meditation practice.

Now That You Are Ready, What Are You Going to Do?

There are two rising meditation methods. One focuses on the air, during mindfulness instruction that is also a technique taught. You just focus on the air as you inhale through your nose and softly exhale through your mouth. Reflect on the wind feeling when it gets into the body. See it as it moves through your lungs, giving life to your mind and then see it as it leaves your body.

Any time an outside thought comes into your mind, accept it but do not act on it, just return your attention to your breath for the time that you set it.

The other common approach is to imagine a healing beam of light that hits your eyes, bringing to your mind and body a wave of relaxation and peace. Let it search gently across your body, starting at your head and slowly going all the way to the tips of your toes. When you feel any stress or discomfort, just imagine the soothing beam that dissolves discomfort and stress in your body.

There is really no downside to meditation practice. No physical exertion or special equipment is required. If you have any mobility problems, just sit in a chair providing you with the support you need to feel secure and relaxed.

Meditation has been shown to relieve tension and to be helpful in many ways, such as changing a person's outlook on life. It is easy to do, and yet difficult because at the same time, you are learning to relax and control your thoughts. Take 5 minutes a day and do a week or two of meditation practice. You can do it for free, and the benefits you get will significantly improve your life!

CHAPTER 21:

Body Image Relaxation

Body image meditation helps reduce stress by making you aware of how your body feels instead of paying attention to stressful thoughts. When you feel stressed out, your body also feels those effects, and it starts to show signs of stress through pain in your back, stomach or tensed shoulders. You may even experience neck ache, particularly if you have been concentrating on things that were difficult and that strained you in some way. You may just have aching bones because you are cold or because you feel worn out in general, but a body image can help you to feel much better. By practicing body image meditation, you distract your mind from the stressful thoughts by paying attention to those parts of the body that feel stressed. As a result, you become mindful of your body and forgetful of the thoughts that bring you stress. Thus, you feel relaxed and your stress levels greatly reduce. Here is a step-by-step guide on how you can perform this meditation technique.

How to Perform Body Image Meditation

The first step is to find a quiet place to perform this meditation technique, which is similar to the other techniques that I have mentioned earlier. Once you are in a quiet place with no distractions, then follow the steps mentioned below:

- Lie on your back on the floor in a position that makes you feel comfortable. Make sure that your posture doesn't make you uncomfortable. If lying on the floor hurts, then you can lie on a mattress or bed instead; there is no hard and fast rule that you have to lie on the floor.

The aim here for you is to feel comfortable. You can slide a pillow under your back if you feel uneasy or you can lie on your side: right or left—whichever makes you feel relaxed. The preferred position is on your back using only one pillow to support your head so that your airways are clear.

- As soon as you settle, take a deep breath to calm your racing mind. Sometimes, it may take you longer than just one deep breath, depending on how your day went. If that's the case, keep breathing deeply until you feel a sense of calmness in your mind. A great way to calm your racing mind is to focus on the breath as you take it. In fact, if it helps you, use the counting that you used before—8 for the inhale through the nostrils and 10 for the exhale. You can even see if you are breathing deeply enough by placing a hand on your upper abdomen and feeling it going up when you breathe in and down when you exhale.

- Once your mind is calm, bring your attention to your body. Feel every sensation in it. Start with the tingling feeling in your toes and feet. Once you feel it, slowly shift your attention from your feet to other parts of your body.

Feel the tension in each part as you move up from your toes to your head.

Feel the tension in the muscles of your legs and the sensations in your belly or the tension in your shoulders and back, depending on where you feel the most stress and pain. Feel the strain in your head, and your eyelids hurt as you open and close them.

Note: In the process of examining every sensation in your body, your mind will try to distract you by bringing in different thoughts. If that happens, bring your focus back to your body and start again from the toes and slowly move up to the head and try again to feel the tension on each part. If it helps you at all, I find that being conscious of that area of the body, followed by tensing the area and then purposely relaxing it helps a lot. As you relax that part of the body, feel the weight as the body relaxes.

- Do this exercise for 15–20 minutes at the start and then slowly increase the time as you get good at it. Remember that your mind is your #1 enemy, as it keeps distracting you from bringing in countless thoughts that only end up causing stress and anxiety. However, you have to fight it (which is a continuous struggle); with time and patience, everything can be achieved.

- Body image meditation is hard as compared to the other techniques that I have mentioned before but, if done properly, it is a great technique, as it can greatly help you to relieve stress and anxiety almost instantly. It also helps to lower your blood pressure and bring your heartbeat down, so do remember to get up slowly from the exercise and relax for a moment before going into your everyday activities again.

So far, you have learnt three of the most effective meditation techniques to reduce stress and anxiety. To get better results, it is important to enhance their effectiveness.

CHAPTER 22:

Power of Self-Confidence

Self-love is probably the best thing you can accomplish for yourself. Being infatuated with yourself furnishes you with fearlessness, self-esteem and it will, by and large, help you feel progressively positive. You may likewise find that it is simpler for you to experience passionate feelings for once you have found out how to cherish yourself first. On the off chance that you can find out how to adore yourself, you will be a lot more joyful and will find out how to best deal with yourself, paying little respect to the circumstance you are in.

Self-Confidence

Self-confidence is just the demonstration of putting a standard in oneself. Believing in yourself is one of the most significant ethics to develop so as to make your mind powerful. Fearlessness likewise realizes more bliss. Regularly, when you are sure about your capacities, you are more joyful because of your triumphs. When you are resting easy thinking about your abilities, the more stimulated and inspired you are to make a move and accomplish your objectives.

Meditation for Self-Confidence

Sit easily and close your eyes. Count from 1 to 5, concentrating on your breath as you breathe as it were of quiet and unwinding through your nose and breathe out totally through your mouth. Experience yourself as progressively loose and quiet, prepared to extend your experience of certainty and prosperity right now. Proceeding to concentrate on your breath, breathing one might say of quiet, unwinding, and breathing out totally.

In the event that you see any strain or snugness in your body, inhale into that piece of your body, and as you breathe out, experience yourself as progressively loose, quieter. On the off chance that contemplations enter your psyche, just notice them, and as you breathe out to let them go, proceeding to concentrate on your breath, taking in a more profound feeling of quiet and unwinding and breathing out totally. Keep on concentrating on our breath as you enable yourself to completely loosen up your psyche and body, feeling a feeling of certainty and reestablishment filling your being. Experience yourself as loose, alert and sure, completely upheld by the seat underneath you. Permitting harmony, satisfaction and certainty to full your being at this present minute as you currently open yourself to extending your experience of harmony and happiness. And now, as you experience yourself as completely present at this time, gradually and easily enable your eyes to open, feeling wide conscious, alert, better than anyone might have expected—completely present at this very moment.

Self-Love

Self-love is not just a condition of feeling better. It is a condition of gratefulness for oneself that develops from activities that help our physical, mental and profound development. Self-love is dynamic; it develops through activities that develop us. When we act in manners that grow self-love in us, we start to acknowledge much better our shortcomings just as our strengths. Self-love is imperative to living great. It impacts who you pick for a mate, the picture you anticipate at work, and how you adapt to the issues throughout your life. There are such a significant number of methods for rehearsing self-love; it might be by taking a short outing, gifting yourself, beginning a diary or anything that may come as "riches" for you.

Meditation for Self-Love

To start with, make yourself comfortable. Lie on your back with a support under your knees and a collapsed cover behind your head, or sit easily, maybe on reinforcement or a couple collapsed covers. For extra help, do not hesitate to sit against a divider or in a seat.

In the event that you are resting, feel the association between the back of your body and the tangle. On the off chance that you are situated, protract up through your spine, widen through your collarbones, and let your hands lay on your thighs.

When you are settled, close your eyes or mollify your look and tune into your breath. Notice your breath, without attempting to transform it. What's more, see additionally on the off chance that you feel tense or loose, without attempting to change that either.

Breathe in through your nose and afterward breathe out through your mouth. Keep on taking profound, full breaths in through your nose and out through your mouth. As you inhale, become mindful of the condition of your body and the nature of your brain. Where is your body holding pressure? Do you feel shut off or shut down inwardly? Where is your brain? Is your brain calm or loaded up with fretfulness, antagonism, and uncertainty?

Give your breath a chance to turn out to be progressively smooth and easy and start to take in and out through your nose. Feel the progression of air moving into your lungs and after that pull out into the world. With each breathes out, envision you are discharging any negative considerations that might wait in your brain.

Keep on concentrating on your breath. On each breath in, think, "I am commendable," and on each breathe out, "I am sufficient." Let each breath in attract self-esteem and each breathes out discharge what is never again serving you. Take a couple of minutes to inhale and discuss this mantra inside. Notice how you feel as you express these words to yourself.

On the off chance that your mind meanders anytime, realize that it is all right. It is the idea of the brain to meander. Essentially take your consideration back to the breath. Notice how your musings travel in complete disorder, regardless of whether positive or negative and just enable them to pass on by like mists gliding in the sky.

Presently imagine yourself remaining before a mirror and investigate your very own eyes. What do you see? Agony and pity? Love and delight? Lack of bias? Despite what shows up in the meditation, let yourself know: "I adore you," "You are lovely," and "You are deserving of bliss." Know that what you find in the mirror at this time might be not the same as what you see whenever you look.

Envision since you could inhale into your heart and imagine love spilling out of your hands and into your heart. Allow this to love warm and saturate you from your heart focus, filling the remainder of your body. Feel a feeling of solace and quiet going up through your chest into your neck and head, out into your shoulders, arms, and hands, and afterward down into your ribs, tummy, pelvis, legs, and feet. Enable a vibe of warmth to fill you from head to toe. Inhale here and realize that affection is constantly accessible for you when you need it.

When you are prepared, take a couple of all the more profound, careful breaths and, after that, delicately open your eyes. Sit for a couple of minutes to recognize the one of a kind encounter you had during this meditation.

CHAPTER 23:

Pleasure Principle

Nutrition is closely connected to our sensory perceptions, and therefore to our memories. We remember how it looks, how we feel eating it, how it tastes. The tastes and textures of the food linger on the palate, from sweet to salty, crispy to crunchy, and take the mouth and mind to a happier spot. It can be the smooth ice cream flavor that drives you—or the bittersweet chocolate abundance, the easy tart pop of fresh berries, or the crispy, chewy roast chicken goodness, or all of that, and more. Food tastes fine. This would be.

The enjoyment of taste, along with desire, is one of our essential eating motivations—a "spring," in terms of health-psychology. And still, flavor recognition is a double-edged knife. Many people who struggle with weight and eating habits see their taste buds as their downfall. "If I could only miss the taste of the onion rings, I think everything else will fall into place," said Lydia, 30, during one of our sessions, causing the rest of the room to laugh. "I am not crying!" It can sound counterintuitive, but learning to adapt to the taste of food will help prevent overeating and direct you to healthier choices. For example, distracted eating habits—eating really fast or watching TV, driving, or multitasking—short-circuit not only our hunger and fullness signals, as you discovered before but also our flavoring experience. So if you scarf down a Snickers bar from the grocery store on the way home, or eat a bowl of pasta and sauce in front of the TV, you barely notice what you're eating.

The subconscious always looks for gratification when this happens. What are you doing, then? Have some more. What's missing is a total eating experience, guided by the senses. The missing ingredient is not more food but focus. We miss the feeling though, at the same time paying attention to other items. The answer, right? Remember to be mindful of every element of the food itself. You will get flavor to work in your favor by learning to enhance your taste experiences. It offers you yet another tool in your toolkit for mindfulness.

Wired for Flavor

Satiety—the relaxed feeling that we have had enough food—causes us to avoid eating. We spoke about one sort of satiety, fullness. You have learned that one of the ways we know we've had enough food is through physical sensation—the way our bodies, particularly our stomachs, feel when we're eating or afterwards—and you've been practicing slowing down and tuning in to those sensations. One form of satiety is called "taste satiety," a phrase used by Jean Kristeller to promote comprehension of the idea of sensory-specific satiety. The satiety of the taste is not the mouth, but the tongue.

Eating food with a specific flavor—sweet, salty, sour, or bitter—builds peaks, and then starts to lose the enjoyment we get from it. The peak before decline is satiety of taste—the feeling we've had enough of a specific flavor. You know the sensation: the fourth cheesecake slice, when it goes from celestial to neutral. Once the transition happens, the neuronal activity changes within the brain. Studies show that taste satiety in our hypothalamus, which regulates our appetite, and our prefrontal cortex, which regulates most aspects of our behavior, influences brain function. A variety of factors affect taste satiety, including the size of the bites we consume, how physically hungry we are, how quickly we consume, whether we eat whole or processed food, and the flavor mix in each meal. When it works normally, our mechanisms of taste satiety tell us that we have "had enough" of a specific flavor, but you need to slow down and pay attention to get the message.

Taste satiety is intended to promote interest in nutritional quality, eating a variety of foods. When you start eating hungry, you can usually hit taste satiety long before you experience fullness signals; when you eat a good, nutritious meal, taste satiety will help you consume some of the items on your plate. (It's more difficult to consume processed foods specifically engineered to overcome taste satiety, as we'll discuss below.) Knowing how satiety taste works is also a key to "pleasure eating"—those moments when you want something sweet after dinner or you're missing the salty, creamy taste of your favorite cheese.

The Physics of Flavor

Clients are always shocked by how easily when they slow down and pay attention to the flavor, they achieve taste satisfaction. With a single kiss, most achieve taste satiety, and after that, the flavor decreases. Understanding that from one piece of chocolate, you can get as much satisfaction as from ten is powerful knowledge, particularly when dealing with cravings.

Can you not stop taking a few bites with complete attention? For decades, scientists have been researching taste satiety, so there's a strong body of research on variables and techniques that influence how happy you are with a given meal or snack. Although regular eating is rarely as attentive as in the above exercise, you can use taste satiety as a method for healthy eating by bearing in mind the following things: pace: the pace at which you eat will influence how happy you are going to be. In one test, which compared the experience of people consuming ice cream slowly (taking thirty minutes) versus quickly (in five minutes), consuming slowly led to significantly higher levels of a satiety hormone called peptide YY, or PYYY, for several hours after eating the ice cream. That suggests eating gradually keeps you happy longer—which can help reduce your total intake of food. Through our own clinical study and experience, we have found that you have to slow down the eating cycle and concentrate intensely to find differences in the taste.

Bite size: A cookie has the same calorie count, whether you eat it in three bites or ten. Yet how fulfilled you would feel from that cookie—and how much you end up eating—can differ dramatically, depending not just on your eating speed but also on the size of your bites. Which exactly is the explanation? Research shows that faster satiety is achieved, and less total food is consumed by taking smaller bites. Even if the caloric content is the same, more bites give you more sensory pleasure, so you get satiety of the taste faster.

Simple versus complex flavors: Studies and our clinical experience suggest that people with one flavor achieve satiety faster than with multiple flavors. Another groundbreaking research found that when people were given "pure sweet," like sugar water, on the third or fourth drink, they hit their taste satiety peak—much faster than you would expect. However, after many bites of a "pure" flavor like sweet or salty, some people do not tend to hit taste satiety, as described in "Taste Satiety and Weight Gain," below.

It takes longer to achieve taste satiety when complex flavors are involved, as they often are. Consider the salty-sweet blend of a Thai stir-fry, the combination of peanut butter and chocolate that has made Reese popular, or the dessert salted caramel phenomenon. When the flavors play in your mouth, your taste buds can start hitting sweet satiety but then get hit with salt, then back into sweetness, and so on. It's the difference between hearing a piece of music in its entirety (satisfying) and listening to three (confusing) overlapping tracks. The contrast is exquisite but often prevents the satiety of taste.

Whole vs. Processed: Research shows that foods that are highly processed take a long time to register in terms of taste satiety compared with whole foods. In other words, it takes a long time to feel relaxed even if you're eating slowly while you're eating flavored tortilla chips, frozen pizza with lots of toppings or a candy bar. It's not a disaster.

Food producers are well versed in taste satiety science and using it to their benefit, manipulating flavor and texture both to compensate for manufacturing processes that degrade flavor, such as dehydration and freezing, and to produce what is known as "hyper palatability." Manufactured foods—snacks, sweets, meals, condiments, and beverages—are sometimes designed to provide complex flavor combinations. And as you discovered earlier, you keep feeding when you're not full.

In other ways, too processed foods compromise our understanding of satiety. Food makers brought the sweet and salty tastes to a whole new stage, dosing processed foods with large quantities of artificial sweeteners and salt. If you regularly consume excessive amounts of sweet and salty food, that's what you expect if you consume, and your taste buds lose their sensitivity and need higher levels of flavor to reach the same satisfaction level.

There is proof that some of the sweeteners used in processed products, both calorie-laden types and low- or no-calorie sweeteners, do not register in our satiety center as natural sugars do, at a chemical stage. While glucose (natural sugar) is transferred through the brain and provides signs of satiety, high-fructose corn syrup, while caloric, does not reach brain tissue and thus does not signal satiety. In one recent research, the levels of PYYY and other satiety-related peptides did not alter when people were given the no-calorie artificial sweetener sucralose.

Processed foods are filled with sodium and artificial flavors, not only to produce a convincing taste, but also to disguise the bitter or bland aromas of chemical preservatives and other artificial ingredients. Participants do an exercise in our mindful-eating classes in which they suck the spice coating off a Dorito. They usually say there is no flavor in the chip underneath.

Processed foods do not need to ruin your taste experience forever, though. You can recalibrate your taste satiety back to a natural, balanced sweet and salty experience by moving to a full-food diet that provides more satiety per calorie than highly refined and processed foods. Because whole foods require more chewing than processed foods usually do, they appear to spend more time in your mouth. This increased "oral-sensory stimulation" may result in increased release of hormones in the gut satiety.

It will take time and patience to recalibrate your taste satiety, depending on how long you have eaten processed food and how much of it you consume. Working with hundreds of consumers over the years, we've found it takes at least two weeks to get comfortable consuming a diet that doesn't contain added sugar (and longer for a lower-fat diet). However, when you do, the natural sweetness of foods like fruit gets a lot more powerful.

Strong vs. Liquid: Approximately 18 percent of our calories come from beverages, many of which are high-calorie sodas, juices, sports drinks, and other canned drinks. Such "food calories" are a major culprit in the epidemic of obesity and a prime target for anyone who attempts to control weight. Nonetheless, a recent study by Johns Hopkins found that reducing calories from drinks contributes to greater weight loss compared with reducing calories from food. Here's what to bear in mind: while drinks can quench your thirst, they're not very successful at either satisfying hunger or satiety. If you eat liquids, natural processes of taste-satiety don't kick in the way they do with solid food.

CHAPTER 24:

Eating Out on Effective Weight Loss Program

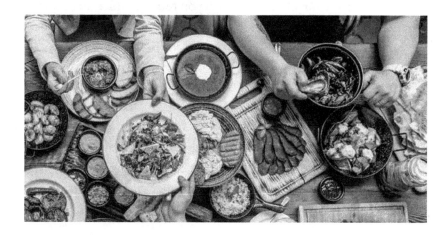

It is natural to worry about eating out, no matter what sort of diet plan you're on. There are moments when you're going to want to go out to eat to celebrate or hang out with friends, but you're concerned about finding entries that will fit inside your diet plan and still have all the tastes you want.

A successful weight loss plan is designed to help you eat based on your day-to-day daily activities. And that involves making the day that you go out to eat in order to enjoy life or do something a little special. So long as you are mindful of the food you eat when you go out, you can enjoy yourself when you go to your favorite restaurants. You're always going to have to be careful about your point values and be careful about going over or eating food that's too far from your limits and you're going to be all right.

Specific Rules for Eating Out

Every time you eat on a diet plan, you need to make sure you follow some basic guidelines that will make eating anything you enjoy easier, without having to go over your budget. Some of the guidelines you should follow to make sure you keep your diet promises:

Set a budget for food - you can set the budget for what you're supposed to do when you're going to the restaurant. How many points do you reserve for yourself, and how do you remain under this cap when you get there? When you want to know where you are going to eat in advance, you can look up some of the options before you even go.

Set the parameters early - set down the rules you are going to follow before you even go to the restaurant. Will you let yourself have an appetizer or a snack, or will you just stick to the main entrance? Was it possible to eat in the salad bar? Which sides do you allow yourself to be in? Using these instructions from the outset will help you stay on track and make this phase of decision-making simpler when you arrive at the restaurant.

Make special requests - most restaurants are used to special requests, so don't be afraid to ask questions. As long as you're not going too wild, most chefs would be able to make some changes for you. For instance, you can ask that the sauce be put on the side of your meal instead of on the main entrance. Instead of frying it, you can ask to grill the meat or go with mixed greens as the side instead of the fries or another side, which isn't as healthy.

Go for portion control - if you're really looking at the portion sizes available in restaurants, you will find these can be at least twice as large as a regular meal. So if you do anything mega-size or add on, you make the portion sizes even more insane. There are a few things you can do to make sure you keep an eye on your parts. One is taking half of the meal and putting it to go for later. This helps in preventing overeating when at dinner. You may select a salad, and then break the entrance into your group with someone else. You may also set up your own meal together, doing side dishes rather than the main meal together.

Learn the different terms - there are a lot of different terms that come up in the world of cooking, and each of them will mean different things for the points you use up when eating out. Grilled, steamed, and baked, for example, are usually healthier options, as long as there aren't many extra sauces added to the meal, while fried can be one of the worst.

Downsize - never get up while eating out from the smallest size. Each size you go up will add hundreds of calories to your diet, and several more. Pick a smaller burger with several toppings, instead of a double or larger one with no toppings. If you can find a kids option instead of the big adult alternative, then go with it. Select smaller hands, or miss them entirely, if you can.

Look at the extras - the extras are always going to cut in your scores. When you add chips, cookies, something sweet or other things that aren't steamed vegetables, you'll consume more calories than you might imagine. Skip the bacon and cheese as well as the dressings as they add tons of calories, look out for double or larger sandwiches and even be vigilant of what things add to extra bread.

Be cautious with the toppings - salad bars are available in many restaurants, so filling up a bit on a salad and then having a smaller entrance to save points is a brilliant idea. Yet a lot of the salad bars come with a variety of toppings. When you add a lot of these toppings, particularly with the dressings, to the salad, you cut into some of the points that you should eat instead. Be sure that the toppings on your salads, burgers and other items are held to a minimum and go with something like lemon juice to top it off rather than a sauce.

Watch the drinks - specialty beverages are extremely high in calories, sugars, and other unhealthy stuff for health. You don't want to squander all your points on the drinks you choose. It's better to go with something that doesn't have alcohol in it at all and nothing that might be called a dessert as these would be the ones with the lowest calorie count. Water is a good option, and if you do want the taste of soda without all the bad stuff, you can get even sparkling water. Green tea, or sugar free tea, is also a great choice.

Stop thinking you've got to clean the plate - many of us slip into the pit of thinking we ought to finish the whole meal because we paid for it. Just think about how many calories you ordered in that big meal. Typically it's way more than we need and the extra calories, and a range of unnecessary nutrients on the body can do. The easiest way to learn is to eat just as much as you like. Feed gradually because the brain knows it is a good place to start when it is full. Another idea is to bag half of the meal before it even hits you so you won't be tempted to eat more than you need to.

Eating out while you are on a diet can be a challenge. You want to go out and visit some of your favorite restaurants, but you are afraid you won't be able to stick with all the hard work you do. Yet, a successful weight loss plan recognizes that you want to go out and spend time with family and friends.

The Rules of Working Out

That said, when you get going on a new exercise regimen, there are a few things you can keep in mind. These will help you get started and make sure you get the right kind of workout to suit your needs.

Firstly, the type of exercise you select will make a huge difference. To target your whole body, you need to be able to pick out a wide range of workouts. Cardio is the first form, and you should spend three to four days a week getting some of this into your routine, as it increases your heart rate and makes sure your heart gets some of the treatment it needs.

Plus, the weight loss is really great because you can burn a lot of calories in the process.

That doesn't mean certain forms of workouts aren't important. Weight lifting can also be done a couple of days a week because it also strengthens those muscles. Your metabolism will burn much faster during the day while doing normal activities when the muscles are toned up. So while you may not burn as many calories as you do with cardio during the actual workout part, weight lifting can be amazing for the metabolism benefits.

And on stretching you can't forget. Take some time off your days, and do some stretching, like yoga or some other technique. This can help give the muscles a good time to relax after having worked so hard during the week, make them stronger and leaner and prevent injury.

Now, when it comes to how long you're supposed to work out, that will vary. When you want to lose weight, it's recommended you work out at least three days a week for 45 to 60 minutes. However, some people prefer to work out at whatever minutes for five or six days, so it's easier to fit into their schedule. When you are just beginning your fitness routine and it's been a while since you've worked out, beginning slow is best. Ten minutes is better than nothing, and from there, you can build up. Never say you don't have time to work out; you can fit three or four ten-minute sessions into the day, and you've completed a full workout once you've done it.

Make sure the workouts you select have a lot of variety. Mix the stretching, cardio, and weight-lifting days together. Test out a host of different things, including some you've never done before. Mixing it up helps to focus on various muscle groups that helps with weight loss and can make your workout easier to enjoy.

CHAPTER 25:

Foods to Eat for Deeper Meditation

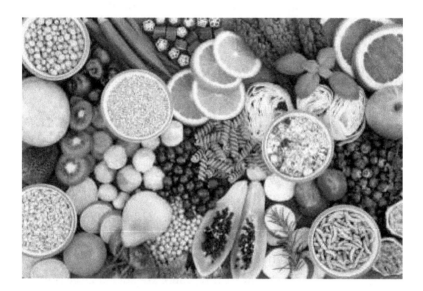

Meditation can be extreme. Take out every single stray idea? Concentrate just on your breath? Sit still for (at least) 10 minutes one after another? In any case, we are finding out increasingly more that rehearsing everyday meditation has such a large number of astonishing advantages, from helping us become progressively empathetic to empowering us to be increasingly quiet, adoring, happy, excusing and liberal. Fortunately, there are a few nourishments that we can begin to consolidate into our eating regimens, which can enable us to pick up that laser center we are hoping to encounter when we plunk down to think.

Green Tea

Numerous old societies related tea with long life and well-being. Actually, starting in China, it has been utilized as medication for a great many years. Green Tea has not exclusively been filling our mugs for quite a while yet has played a job as a key fixing in numerous a sweet. It has been the subject in various restorative and logical investigations to decide if it is since quite a while ago, toted medical advantages really convey any legitimacy. Furthermore, they do. Green tea lifts mental aptitude and standardizes glucose, so tasting on a cup before you plunk down to ruminate can be a valuable practice.

Tomatoes

Tomatoes have a lot of vitamin C, which is generally viewed as valuable in bringing down your pressure. As per an investigation led in Japan, members who ate tomatoes in excess of six times each week had an essentially lower danger of framing discouragement. Specialists are as yet attempting to make sense of whether lycopene, the synthetic segment that makes tomatoes dark red, legitimately influences the psychological prosperity. What's more, there are such a large number of approaches to appreciate them.

Nuts

Brimming with cell reinforcement Vitamin E and zinc, nuts, for example, almonds, pistachios, and pecans, are useful for boosting the insusceptible framework. They likewise contain a lot of B-Vitamins, which help you oversee pressure and despondency. Scientists have demonstrated that nuts improve the capacity of our cerebrums to tackle issues, one more significant piece of meditation.

Vegetables and Whole Fruits

Eating an eating regimen wealthy in entire foods grown from the ground is probably the best thing you can accomplish for your body. The equivalent is similarly valid for the brain. Root vegetables, including sweet potatoes, squash, and carrots, are pressed with a wide range of nutrients and minerals. However, the beta-carotene in these specific vegetables has been appeared to help your invulnerable framework to help keep you sound and keep your mind sharp. They are additionally crammed with fiber, which means they are delayed in their processing, and you will feel fuller more.

The most significant part of your meditation diet is that you start to consider nourishment to be vitality. Prior to eating, think about whether this nourishment contains the indispensable life power that you need. A few nourishments are loaded with vitality, and others will, in general, dull the psyche. As you ponder, you will become progressively delicate to what makes you feel better, and what cuts you down.

The more we can consider nourishment to be vitality, the more we will settle on savvy decisions in our eating routine. In any case, it is hard when we have spent our lives eating for eating. Attempt to see that all that you eat affects your body, psyche, and soul.

Affirmations to Heal Your Food Relationship

Our association with nourishment is personally associated with how sincerely protected, adored and sustained we feel. An expansion in craving may result from enthusiastic torment, the need to fill that excruciating, void spot with something. The something you are truly searching for is love, yet in an apparent nonappearance of adoration, you manage with nourishment. An absence of craving can demonstrate a longing to withdraw from life, sustaining the hurt inside us again, showing a requirement for affection. Our association with nourishment can be perplexing. Incredible feelings of happiness and blame get into the blend.

By dispensing with your negative convictions about nourishment and your body that are never again serving you, you make space for a plenitude of positive affirmations that will serve you in tuning in to, trusting and respecting your body's individual needs.

Here is a rundown of affirmations you can include in your everyday schedule:

- I am the main individual who characterizes what well-being intends to me.

- I discharge myself from eating regimen mindset contemplations that are never again serving me.

- I respect the space between where I am now and where I need to be with my association with nutrition.

- I respect and trust my body and its needs by eating food sources that are pleasurable, fulfilling and supporting to me, and I give myself consent to appreciate all nourishments.

- I realize that I can confide in my body to give me the prompts and flag that will prompt adjusted smart dieting as a rule.

- Nourishment is not my adversary. I express gratitude toward it for supporting me and giving me vitality.

- My weight does not characterize my value.

- I value the extraordinary and remarkable qualities of my body.

- I discharge blame and negative sentiments I have about eating.

- I have everything inside of me that I have to feel totally free around nourishment.

- It is alright for me to tune in and trust my body.

- I pick self-care over restraint.

- I can be solid and cheerful at any size.

- I need to feel better and feeling great accompanies tuning in to my body and regarding its needs.

- I feel great consistently. Consistently, I advise myself that I can settle on the decision to feel better.

- Sustaining myself brings me delight, and I am deserving of the time spent on recuperating my association with nourishment and my body.

CHAPTER 26:

The Four Golden Rules

Even however you may have instant success with the hypnotic gastric band, it's significant that you use the Four Golden Rules that are the foundation of my system. They help to support the progressions you are making. You may ask why you need the golden rules since you have a hypnotic gastric band; however, in certainty, those rules are at the core of all the healthy eating of all naturally slim individuals. Naturally, healthy individuals eat when they are hungry, they eat what they need, they focus on their food and appreciate it, and they quit eating when they are full.

As it were, healthy, thin individuals follow the Four Golden Rules naturally. It is a natural, healthy approach to eat. The splendid thing about your hypnotic gastric band is that it makes the physical changes that make it natural for you to follow the Golden Rules as well. How about we remind ourselves of them now.

Golden Rule One - When You Are Hungry, Eat!

When a few people hear me state this, they believe it's crazy. They say, "That is the issue, I can't quit eating, now, he's proposing that I eat." What I am saying is that when you are really physically hungry, get yourself a healthy meal, and eat. If you starve yourself, your body goes into "survival mode," and you slow your digestion. So, when you are genuinely hungry, and you eat, your body knows there will consistently be sufficient food, so it doesn't slow the digestion, and you have enough fuel in your "body's engine" to do the things you have to do. It's critical to make the distinction between genuine physical hunger and emotional craving. Real hunger starts gradually. It is clear and steady, and you feel it in your gut. It isn't activated by nervousness or by an emotional ache that goes ahead out of nowhere when you feel upset. It's anything but a response to fear, embarrassment, or outrage. It's anything but a plan to distract you when you are exhausted.

Real hunger is a straightforward physical feeling in your stomach. Sometimes, we confuse emotional distress for hunger. We suppose if we eat, we will feel much improved. Be that as it may, food doesn't fix emotions; it just covers them over incidentally. There are numerous, much better approaches to manage feelings than eating. If you speculate you need food because really you feel awful, you can use Havening to feel much better and afterward check in with your body and find whether you are actually physically hungry.

Recognizing Real Hunger

Proper physical appetite is a particular physical feeling, and with your hypnotic gastric band, you will think that it's simpler than at any other time to remember it. It will, likewise, be simpler to perceive when you are truly full. Be that as it may, for complete clearness and to ensure that you are precisely situated at both unconscious and conscious levels, I will request that you do a little psychological test that will help you in a split second and effectively perceive the signs for when you are really hungry and when you are full. If you have ever endured your way through a diet, you will have contorted your reaction to your body's natural signals. This activity will push your mind to recalibrate your stomach's natural sensitivity to craving and satiety.

> 1. Think about when you were super hungry—so hungry you felt swoon and even a crust of stale bread would have tasted delectable. Recall that.

2. Now, think about when you were totally stuffed—when you'd ate and eaten so much food that you were in pains, even nauseous. Remember that.

3. Do this a multiple time with the goal that you emphasize the contrast between being starving and stuffed

4. Alright, now unwind. Those two feelings are the extremes. You never need to feel both of those terrible emotions again. You never must be that hungry, and you never need to feel that full.

I have created a scale where one signifies being so hungry you are about to blackout and ten signifies being so full you believe you will explode. It will assist you with recognizing effectively where your body is whenever.

The Hunger Scale

1. Physically blackout
2. Voracious
3. Genuinely hungry
4. Marginally hungry
5. Neutral
1. Six. Wonderfully satisfied
6. Full
7. Stuffed
8. Enlarged
9. Nauseous

Starting now and into the foreseeable future, NEVER go below three or over seven until kingdom thy come!

As you see, it gets simpler to live in the middle segment of the scale, your association with food, and your body will improve. You will feel more in charge, and like anything you practice for a couple of days, it will before long become natural. With your hypnotic gastric band, every one of these stages will be as clear as light. When you are somewhere in the range of 3 and 4, the time has come to eat. When you are somewhere in the range of Six and 7, the time has come to quit eating. With your hypnotic gastric band, you can't eat as much as in the past, so when you feel full, quit eating. Try not to attempt to eat more since it will sting to attempt to squash more food into your stomach.

Golden Rule Two - Eat What You Want, Not What You Think You Should

When you make food prohibited, it turns into everything you can think about. That is the reason for your gastric band, and with my system, there are no illegal foods. It's game over. You wind up having it and beating yourself. That method for eating resembles battling with your body. It resembles driving a vehicle by stalling the accelerator and pulling on the hand brake. It is a misuse of fuel, and it trashes the vehicle. This disorder is intensified by dieting. Dieting mutilates your body's natural systems. All diets include constraining and denying the body. So, the body's reaction is to hunger for high-energy crisis foods to make up the deficiency as fast as could be expected under the circumstances. That is the reason individuals on diets all fantasy about high-fat, high-sugar foods like cakes and chips and French fries and frozen yogurt.

The more they diet, the more they need those foods. There is nothing amiss with any of them, coincidentally—but as you move away from dieting towards balanced nutrition, you might be shocked to see that what you need to eat starts to change. As you become progressively touchy, food that you never focused on begins to speak to you. You will likewise see that you start to support new food, in any event, when it sets aside more effort to cook or get ready. This happens because your body is never again attempting to save you from starvation. It isn't searching for a crisis energy fix. Presently it is allowed to move towards more noteworthy well-being. As you lose weight, it searches out the protein, nutrients, and minerals it needs to fix and explain your skin and fabricate your muscles.

The extraordinary thing pretty much every one of these progressions is that you don't need to consider them by any stretch of the imagination. Your body's natural signaling system will control you. The more you focus on your body, the more you will understand that appetite isn't only a basic requirement for energy. You will start to see you are hungry for a particular food, for example, fish, or serving of mixed greens, or cake. You will see you lean toward one vegetable to another, etc. To summarize, dieters eat what a book discloses to them they ought to eat. Healthy individuals eat what their body truly needs.

Golden Rule Three - Whenever You Eat, Do It Consciously

This is potentially the most powerful suggestion I can give you, and what I am going to let you know is currently bolstered by various scientific research around the globe. When I state eat intentionally, I mean two things:

1. Focus on what you are eating, and that's it. Give your food your total attention. Concentrate on the food and NOTHING else!
2. Slow you're eating speed directly down. Slow down to about a fourth of your past speed and bite every mouthful multiple times. When individuals eat quickly, they flood their brains with happy chemicals (neurotransmitters), and they can't hear the signs from their stomach that say, "You are full." So, they end up crazy and gorging. It's significant that as you bite every mouthful of food, you put your blade and fork down and bite your food 20—yes, 20—times!

If you can't do this, I don't think I can support you, and I don't want to believe anybody can. It's a little favor you can do for yourself that comes with an enormous reward.

Concentrate on Your Food

You can eat anything you desire, at whatever point you need, so long as you give it your total, full concentration. That never implies, at any point, eat, and do something different simultaneously. When you eat, sit at a table, eat your food from a plate, using a blade and fork, and chew your food multiple times. This may appear to be a little ridiculous to you now. However, it is completely indispensable to retrain yourself to focus on each mouthful you are eating absolutely.

This will guarantee that you truly make the most of your food. Appreciate the taste and texture of your food, and truly notice it as you swallow it and feel how it fills your stomach. By focusing on eating, you will think that it's basic and simple to notice the satiety signal that you get from your hypnotic gastric band, and you will quit eating and be fulfilled sometime before you would have expected to because you will feel how rapidly your stomach tops off.

This is the one thing I need you to do to ensure you can encounter the advantage of your hypnotic gastric band and get more fit. Conscious eating is the manner by which individuals forget about their body's natural weight control system in any case. By eating deliberately, you regard your food, and you regard yourself. Research has demonstrated indisputably that individuals consistently eat more when they sit in front of the TV. Concentrate on your food solely. That implies no TV, but also no perusing while you eat. Try not to surf the Internet or answer messages or reply to your friends. Try not to drink liquor when you eat, because it dulls your attention and diverts you from the real food. Try not to snatch snacks while driving or tuning in to music or playing a game or using your telephone.

That may sound demanding; however, it is likewise incredibly useful since it implies that you should just ever eat food that you totally appreciate.

CHAPTER 27:

The Psychology about Weight Loss

Weight Loss Is Hard

As you already know, weight loss is hard. It's intimidating, and often doesn't feel good. You put yourself through hell at the gym, and you start to dread having to get up and go through the same awful things that you think are necessary for losing weight. Losing weight becomes a burden rather than a satisfying process, and with this mindset, even if you manage to lose weight, you won't feel good about yourself in the way that you should when it's all over because you'll be swaddled by negative feelings.

During weight loss, your body will often fight against you and urge you to eat more even though that is against your diet plan. Hormonally and emotionally, you'll want to go back to eating how you used to. Hypnosis can help stave off the urges, but it helps to understand what you're up against because this information highlights that dieting takes a lot more than willpower to be successful. You need to gather all your weight loss tools, and you need to use them to undermine the hardships of weight loss, or else you'll never find the success that you want and deserve. Weight loss isn't impossible, but it can seem pretty grim, especially in the beginning when you're still getting your footing.

The statistics are not on your side. Very few people actually lose weight. Just over forty percent of men and fifty-six percent of women in the world tried to lose weight as of 2019. A whopping sixty percent of high school girls have tried to lose weight. Many people are trying to lose weight in the world at any given time, but an estimated eighty to ninety-five percent of people regain weight after losing it. Often, this regain is attributed to unmaintainable weight loss regimes that are often advertised. Weight loss can be straightforward, but keeping your weight down in the long term can be arduous. The contestants of "The Biggest Loser" show this. While some contestants of the notorious weight-loss show have been able to maintain their weight, most returned to their original weight within six years.

People often focus only on the weight loss element of physical transformation, but thinking about just weight loss itself isn't going to lead to actual results. If people refuse to acknowledge the psychological impacts of weight loss, our weight loss statistics will never improve. There's so much misinformation out there about weight loss, information that tells people they need to starve themselves and subscribe to extreme diets. People are being set up by failure by diets that promise fast results but give no emotional support or strategies for maintenance. Eating well for a while isn't going to cut the cravings. You have to change your mindset if you want to change your life.

They aren't making genuine, lasting changes to their lives. Even so, to succeed at weight loss, you need to take measures that other people don't. Hypnosis is one such step, and understanding why you might be reluctant to give your all to lifestyle changes is another important step you need to take. So many people are afraid of changes, which is why fear is one of the biggest mental blockers that you have to defeat before you can lose weight.

Don't Let Fears Hold You Back

Fears can be so damaging to your progress. It's almost impossible to commit yourself in the way you need to if you are so fixated on your fears instead of what you can do to succeed. Hypnosis is best done with willingness and openness, so don't let your fears hold you back and impede your ability to do what you've always wanted to do. Before you even start hypnosis, you need to analyze and understand what fears you have so that you can prepare for the major obstacles that will threaten your progress. Fears are valid; they stem from your brain wanting to protect you from danger, but you need to avoid overblowing them in your mind.

The fear of failure is one of the biggest fears that can disrupt your ability to give your all for losing weight. This fear can lead to you quit when you've only just gotten started. Nearly one-third of all adults in the United States have a fear of failure, and this fear can seep into every part of a person's life. It can make you feel insecure and unable to accomplish anything. This fear can make it hard to change anything too, and it can feel impossible to overcome the worry that you're just going to fail anyway. This fear can be draining because it makes you unhealthily obsessed with the things that could go wrong. Instead of thinking that you might succeed, you convince yourself that there's no chance that you will succeed. Then, you become a self-fulfilling prophecy and really do fail.

The fear of failure can easily lead to self-sabotage. When you fear failure, you'll avoid doing the things that could bring you success and choose the safety of stagnancy. You're not any happier by doing this, but psychologically, it feels safer. The truth is, though, that when you let your fears run your life, you're not better off because, in that scenario, you will never thrive. At least when taking a chance, you have the chance of triumph. When you have a fear of failure, you may subconsciously take measures to thwart your advancement. You will mess up, and then just quit because you feel like your progress has already been ruined.

You don't need to live with the fear of failure anymore. You can address this fear by knowing that you don't have to be perfect. You're human, and sometimes you're not going to do things in the best way. Hindsight allows you to see things that you didn't see before, and it can make you feel like a fool, but know that your mistakes don't mean you're a failure as a person. They are normal, and they are okay.

Look at your failures constructively. Don't even call them failures anymore because, more than anything, they are opportunities to grow. People often look at failure as something shameful, but when you have misfortune, it doesn't mean that you are incompetent or somehow bad. Use mistakes as a chance to grow. When you face failure, don't use that moment to give up or run away. Find ways you can improve. If you overeat one day, don't let yourself think that your whole diet is ruined because a good diet isn't shattered by one day of overindulgence. You need to understand that getting back on track is the biggest success you can have on this journey. For all the successes you have, you will have errors, but with a good outlook, those errors won't destroy you. They will build you up and help you learn through experience.

Imagine the worst that could happen if you put in a genuine effort. It's scary to think of the worst-case scenarios, but most of the time, the worst that you're thinking in your head is absurd and unlikely to happen. By letting yourself think of the worst that can happen, you can reduce the anxiety that you have regarding failure because the acknowledgment of what worries you is liberating. By identifying what is truly bothering you, you take away the power of that fear and can prepare yourself for any disappointment or negative feelings that you may face on your weight loss journey.

Take the pressure off yourself. Putting yourself under pressure isn't going to help you. It's just going to stress you out. Try not to put strict time parameters on your weight loss. Don't tell yourself, "I need to be ten pounds lighter by the holidays," because the pressure is going to get in your head and make it harder to stick to your diet. It's okay to want to accomplish certain goals by certain times, but if those goals don't happen at the exact time you want them too, you must avoid being hard on yourself. Sometimes, things happen, and you can no longer meet the expectations you had for yourself. That's fine, and you can adjust your expectations accordingly.

Find aspirations outside of weight loss that makes you happy so that you have other things to keep you going when you have mishaps. Your whole life shouldn't be single-mindedly focused on weight loss. If it is, you're probably miserable. You have to have other goals to strive for that have nothing to do with your weight. Find hobbies and activities that add excitement and happiness to your life because these will not only help you relax, but they will take your mind off food. It's hard to lose weight when you're thinking about food all the time, so let yourself think about other things. Be conscious about your dietary decisions, but don't allow weight to be the only thing that drives you.

The fear of not being enough, or the fear of being an imposter are also fearing that many people deal with. Many people think that no matter what they do, they will never be good enough for all the good things that they have. These self-esteem issues make it hard to find the incentive and momentum to lose weight. The fear of not being enough often also feeds into imposter syndrome. Imposter syndrome is the fear people have in certain areas of their lives, especially work, that they are imposters who seem to be competent at what they are doing to other people but are just pretending to have the necessary skills. They feel like imposters, faking their expertise to the people who they know, and they are terrified of being revealed as not worthy of what they have. People with imposter syndrome are perfectly competent, but they feel as though everyone else will see them someday as being ineffectual, which can result in these people avoiding attention and trying not to make any major changes.

To make yourself feel worthy, you can do a myriad of things, but the most important thing is to find enjoyment in who you are. See beyond what your body looks like or how well you do your job. Tell yourself that you are worth it. Affirmations are a smart way to convince yourself that something is true. Your brain believes all the things that you tell it

432

most; thus, by repeating positive things about yourself, you will build worth and start to value yourself as a person more.

Be unafraid to be yourself. Don't keep the things you love and want a secret. Feel free to share what you love, even if other people won't necessarily relate to those things. Sharing your passions is an ideal way to bond with the people around you, and when you share your passions, you're reiterating that you are worth it by allowing the things you love to be validated.

CHAPTER 28:

The Secret to Getting Rid of Weight Problems

What is the secret to getting rid of weight problems? I am going to tell you. The trick is breaking the old subconscious blocks, generating new patterns of thought and harmonizing the conscious and subconscious mind. Hypnosis will help you conquer the subconscious bloc obstacles.

You'll feel better. They're going to feel in control. You'll feel sure to be able to control your weight with encouragement and determination to keep up with your weight loss goals. Hypnosis has none of the negative or harmful side effects of diet pills or surgery. If you choose a successful diet and exercise plan and then reprogram your mind to make it no longer challenging but simple, pleasant, and efficient to follow your food and fitness programmer, you will certainly succeed.

Have fun exercising and eating healthy, so you can stop causing self-induced tension, stress, and discouragement. You will start doing the things that will help you in your aim of being safe and losing weight, obviously. You need to get rid of the unhealthy habits of thought that make you overweight. These thought patterns, which are stored in your subconscious mind, must be replaced with healthier thoughts and healthy behaviors so that you can instinctively do what you are expected to do without ever thinking twice about it.

Does that sound tricky? In reality, it's much less complicated than you would imagine. All you need is 10 to 20 minutes a day for a total of 21 days (the amount of time it takes to build a habit).

You can now have what it takes to speedily program your mind to lose weight. You see, hypnosis is one of today's world's most overlooked and powerful methods for self-change.

When you say "hypnosis," most people think of magic shows in Vegas or stupid acts on stage. Those on stage were chosen especially because of their susceptibility to suggestion. They wouldn't do anything that they normally wouldn't do on stage. For the publicity they receive, they really "do not mind" behaving stupidly on stage. If they don't perform, they know they're going to be taken off the stage and back to the seat. There could not be anything further from the facts. In theory, hypnosis is a very comfortable state of mind in which you become more receptive to suggestions. During the day, you usually go through hypnosis many times.

If the use of hypnosis for treating illness has been accepted by major medical societies, imagine how amazingly successful and beneficial it is when coping with thought patterns that stand in the way of the healthy body you deserve. The use of hypnosis has been used for more than half a century to treat illness. In addition, in 1955, the British Medical Association approved the hypnotherapy use. Its use was approved in 1958 by the American Medical Association.

In a 9-week trial-weight management group study (one using hypnosis and one not using it), the hypnosis group has continued to get results in the two-year follow-up, while the non-hypnosis group did not show any further results (Journal of Consulting & Clinical Psychology, 1985). The groups using hypnosis lost an average of 16 pounds in a sample of 60 participants, while the other group lost an average of just 0.5 pounds (Journal of Consulting & Clinical Psychology, 1986). Multiple studies showed that the addition of hypnosis increased the weight loss by an average of 97% during treatment and, more importantly, the efficacy increased by more than 146% after treatment. Hypnosis is known to perform much better over time (Journal of Consulting & Clinical Psychology, 1996). "The best way to break bad habits is by hypnosis," even Newsweek Magazine said.

Whether you want to use audio tapes or CD's for hypnosis, evaluate the script used to determine if the suggestions make sense to you. Make sure there are no negative suggestions.

The subconscious will not hear "no" or "don't," so the suggestion's emphasis would be: "I do not consume fattening foods." This will give you your objective in the opposite direction. Just use constructive feedback. "I just eat fresh foods that make me feel solid, safe, and happy" is much better.

How you perceive the suggestions is significant. If someone said, "That door should be closed," you get up and close the door or just think, maybe it should be closed and somebody else should close it. When you get up and close the door, it means you've "inferred" you're supposed to close your door. Some people don't like being asked what to do (direct suggestions). You may be making your own audio more effective. You might play a soothing audio, and then read or write your suggestions.

When you get up in the morning and before going to bed in the evening is the best time for your mind to accept these positive suggestions. You need a quiet room where nothing bothers you. When you're getting a lot of action in your house, you may need to find a room where you can shut the door and get undisturbed. It only lasts from 10 to 20 minutes.

Hypnosis is not a one-time fix for most people, the results are cumulative. The more post-hypnotic suggestions are applied to the hypnosis, the more permanent the results become. So, few people are likely to get hypnotized once to avoid smoking or lose weight. We usually create a new habit if they do, to replace the one they just quit. Most people who quit smoking begin overeating. We were replacing only one undesirable habit with another. Unless the root(s) of the problem is found, there would be no need to add another habit.

Having a specialist skilled in hypnosis and the weight-loss struggles could prove useful. Working with a specialist will help you understand the earlier programming and remove it.

Especially with weight loss, use the relaxation and self-hypnosis every morning and evening to be effective, changing and perfecting your suggestions while you lose weight. Upon reaching the weight you are comfortable with, you might want to add other goals along with strengthening your healthy eating and exercising habits.

You will need to start with full relaxation at first, but after a week or so, you will be able to go very quickly into the altered relaxed state by counting down from 10 to 1. Always end your session with a suggestion that makes you feel good, better than ever, relaxed and either alert, clear-headed, refreshed, and full of morning energy or relaxed and able to soundly sleep when you go to bed at night.

Keep a pen and paper close by to write down any insights that come to mind while listening to your suggestions or reading them. You can recall things that you were told as a child that now influence your behavior. For me, I started to remember a lot of things I was told when I was a child that I never thought had bothered me until I was much older. I just didn't connect those things that I remembered with my behavior. I became really mad when I recalled. I realized the life I missed by believing in what these people had said or taught me as a child and reinforced through the years by other people and events.

Weight Loss Affirmations: Are They Enough and How to Practice Them

Weight loss claims are one of the many daily affirmations people are practicing to improve themselves, but are they just enough to make a change, and how do you practice them effectively? This article discusses what to include with your positive weight-loss affirmations as well as ways to make them work.

First of all, when practicing affirmations of weight loss or any other affirmations of self-esteem, it's important to remember that you're "working from the inside out." What that means is that in order to make any change in your life, whether it's focused on your physical body or your finances, you want to change your mindset and inner mind (your subconscious) before any outer change appears.

While many people already know about this concept, it is not always practiced in such a way that positive claims for weight loss or other affirmations of self-esteem work as well as they might. You must really "believe" that you are thin in order to "be thin," and that is where most people "fall off the wagon" and avoid making their regular affirmations because the outer shift is not quick enough.

So, when you start, you decide to allow yourself enough time to make the inner change without any "expectation" of seeing any external changes.

Next, you will want to include other positive affirmations on a daily basis such as affirmations of self-love, spiritual affirmations, and assertions of faith and confidence. Why? For what? Because when you're trying to make progress, especially when it's about your own definition of yourself, you just want to "pour on love" to yourself and install as much "confidence" in the process as possible, and in yourself.

In fact, increasing your self-love and the ability to trust the process is critical for any self-affirmations to work on your list of affirmations because when you can increase your self-love, you have raised your "vibration" to the level of love that manifests things quicker. Often, you are more likely to view yourself better because you have greater self-confidence, and before you know it, you have lost weight effortlessly.

It is also important to trust the mechanism, because the vibration of confidence is absolutely necessary to attract what you want, which in this case is to be slim. And, by the way, it's vital that you don't use words like "don't" or "weight" when practicing weight loss affirmations, because they focus your mind on "what you "don't want."

"I don't want to overeat," for example, focuses on "overeating." On the other hand, affirmations of weight loss that contain terms like slim, attractive, fit, and safe are better options as they "rely" on being thin, attractive, fit, and healthy.

Creative Visualization

Once you find the right weight loss affirmations that make you feel great, get an image of the "perfect for your body" and place it somewhere around your bed so when you wake up in the morning you instantly see your target subsequent you. Then close your eyes and really "feel" when your body looks like that, and say your positive affirmations for weight loss and self-love affirmations.

The main thing to note at the beginning is that you want the inner change to happen first and affirmations are a great starting move, but self-hypnosis may be a better option to change your inner mind. However, self-hypnosis for weight loss is very common simply because it first works to change your inner mind which paves the way for outer change to follow.

Once you give yourself the time to make the inner change of seeing yourself thinner without any expectations of seeing the outer change actually becoming thinner, and you get the hang of visualizing your affirmations of weight loss that include affirmations of self-love and the ones of faith and trust, you'll be surprised how quickly you'll see the outer change happen.

CHAPTER 29:

Condition for Hypnosis to Work Out

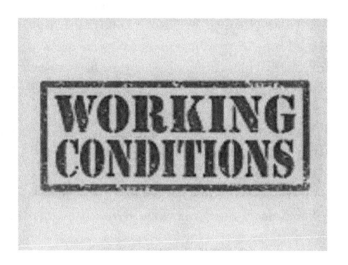

Although hypnosis itself cannot be accurately predicted, clinical experience and laboratory experiments at institutions such as Harvard and Stanford suggest that those who are most susceptible to hypnosis tend to share specific characteristics. As already mentioned, virtually everyone can benefit from hypnosis. However, studies have shown that if you have most of these characteristics, you may be easier to hypnotize than others. Here are some of the criteria for hypnosis:

Motivation

The motivation is at the top of the list. If you don't want to be hypnotized, you won't. If you are strong enough to change something, the chance is to be able to hypnotize yourself. But such motives must come from within. You need to want to improve yourself, not because other people think you should, but because it's what you need at the moment.

Optimism

Top people tend not to be skeptics if you take a continuum of hypnosis from low to high. This doesn't mean you can't hypnotize yourself if you're skeptical now. However, by the end of this topic, your skepticism will be alleviated somewhat so that you can experience hypnosis more easily. It turns out that most hypnotic people are likely to have a hopeful and optimistic view of life. To them, the bottle is not half empty but half full.

Defending

The people most susceptible to hypnosis are usually lawyers. This is an extension of buoyancy, trust, and hope reflected in their optimism. Whether it's something new in medicine, politics, art, or something that interests them, they are keen to spread the word. An opposite is a person who is very cognitive and very scientific in her evaluation. This individual demand evidence wants to read half a dozen books and scrutinizes the subject before committing himself. This attitude of the brain is not wrong. It merely means that such reality-oriented individuals must stay longer in hypnosis to get results.

Concentration

An important feature of hypnosis is increased concentration. Hypnosis deepens your concentration, but you need it to achieve this condition. The more distracting a person is, the more he responds to hypnotizing himself or is hypnotized by others. He also has to use this method more often to make a profit. Meanwhile, most people at least sometimes have a deep focus. Go to the room when they are reading and call their name.

You can't get the answer. Those people can't hear your voice because they are too concentrated. We find no significant evidence difference between vigorous situation and self-hypnosis itself.

Acceptability

Many people are afraid to be hypnotized so as not to be absorbed in the will of others. This may be called Svengali syndrome. A mysterious stranger with a black cloak and flint's eyes seizes the soul of a naked girl while bending her will to adapt to an embarrassing wish. People who are prone to hypnosis have normal or good intelligence and a core of beliefs and firm attitudes that are fundamental to life. An example of such a person is someone with a well-trained religious education that embraces new ideas. He is hard to be fooled. He is sensitive to wise suggestions. Of course, the receptivity level differs from person to person. The receptivity for new ideas is one of the determinants of how easily you can get hypnosis. On a scale of 0-5 (0 is a person impervious to hypnosis), the majority of the population falls in the middle, for example, in the range 2 to 3. However, rest assured that your level of susceptibility to hypnosis is not included in the five-point scale. At the age of two or three, hypnosis should be repeated more often. However, being at the top of the scale has both disadvantages and benefits.

Imagination

Scientists at the Hypnosis Institute at Stanford University School of Psychology studied the hypnotic differences between individuals for nearly two decades. This is a project supported by the National Mental Health Institute and the Air Force Office of Scientific Laboratory. An organization that does not tend to fund trivial efforts. Dr. Josephine R. Hilgard, a clinical professor of psychiatry at Stanford University, reported that people who have been imaginatively active as a child could have hypnosis. The theory states that the imagination and ability to participate in adventures that emerged early in life remained alive and functional through continued use. Among university students, reading, drama, creativity, childhood imagination, religion, sensory, and thirst for adventure were activities identified as hypnosis. Hypnosis is deeply involved in one or more imaginary areas (reading novels, listening to music, experiencing the aesthetic of nature, adventuring the body and mind) can do.

Dr. Hilgard found that the student in major of humanities is most susceptible to hypnosis, the majors of social sciences are comparatively less, and students of natural sciences and engineering are not much hypnotized. The experience and research of other employees in this area tend to corroborate Stanford University results. According to Dr. Lewis R. Wolberg, a 40-year authority in the field: people with the ability to enjoy sensory stimulations and can adapt themselves to different roles have more tendency to be hypnotic than others.

Dr. Hilgard's lab was the most vulnerable to those who had fictitious friends in childhood and could read, adventure, and be immersed in nature. Suspicious, withdrawn, and hostile people have discovered that they tend to resist hypnosis. "Few people appreciate all of the above criteria. You don't even have to show improvement in all areas. You can make up for what's missing in another category. Defined these criteria, Hypnosis still needs a great deal of research, and the academic and medical community has accepted it as a subject worthy of serious investigation. A lot of eye-widening results are drawn from the study.

CHAPTER 30:

Your Thinner and Happier Life

Benefits of Eating Healthy and Detoxifying

Most times, we don't eat because we are hungry, we eat because food is available. The same way you make random decisions to purchase items you don't actually need in a supermarket in the same way that you purchase food. Most times, when you get a job that offers you some financial freedom, you begin to go to that expensive restaurant you have always dreamt of going because you can now afford it.

Now that you can afford the food there, you start to visit the restaurant frequently and purchase food that you do not really need. You are just buying the food because you have the money to do so, and the food is readily available. Many of the bad decisions that make us eat food that we do not need to eat can be avoided if we start to focus our thoughts on getting what is necessary.

The process of getting that what is necessary requires you as an individual to be able to acquire some personal discipline. Before you purchase any food, you need to ask yourself if buying the food is really necessary. Ask yourself if the food that you are eating will add any value to your overall health. After asking yourself that question, you will know the right thing to do based on the response to the questions. It is an easy process to do, and it will help to save you from eating those carbs that only add unnecessary weight to your body.

Maintain a Healthy Body

Once we consume food, our bodies respond to what we have consumed. The response could be negative or positive. Different foods generate different feelings. You may not believe what some of these feelings are, except you focus your minds on realizing them. The power of meditation is that it allows you to be able to focus, concentrate on a certain thing that requires your attention. This is an easy task to accomplish, and you only should evaluate how your body reacts to the foods that you are consuming. Once you eat some foods, you will notice that you feel energized, while some foods will make you feel tired.

Once you overeat, you will experience some sudden feelings of tiredness. You will begin to feel as if your body is too heavy, and so all you want to do is take a nap or a rest. Now when this happens, you should realize that it is a sign that whatever you ate was unnecessary, and hence the body will not use the food. As a result, most of what you ate will become something that your body needs to eliminate. Thus, you will start to add extra weight, because the excess food in your body becomes excess fat in your body. On the other hand, if once you eat, it immediately makes you feel energized; it means your body was receptive to the food that you eat.

It means that your body was able to convert much of the food into energy, and each of those components present in the food will be well utilized by your body. This is beneficial for the well-being of your body, and it can help you when losing weight and prevent you from adding unnecessary weight.

Maintain the Bodyweight

Your eyes are shut. Envision coasting your desires ceaselessly. Envision what's pleasant for you to eat a day. Envision spellbinding helping you get in shape as the news seems to be. Psychotherapist Jean Fain from the Harvard Medical School gives ten trancelike recommendations to endeavor.

When I tell people how I make a lot of my life—as a psychotherapist who entrances thin individuals—they ask: Does that work? Typically, my reaction lights up their eyes with something among energy and unbelief.

A great many people don't comprehend that adding daze to your weight reduction endeavors can enable you to lose more weight and look after it. Spellbinding originates before the tallying of carb and calories by a few decades. However, this well-established technique for centering consideration presently can't seem to be completely held onto as an effective methodology for weight reduction.

As of not long ago, the real claims of prestigious trance inducers have been bolstered by insufficient logical proof, and an excess of pie-in-the-sky responsibilities from their issue kin, stage trance specialists, have not made a difference.

Indeed, even after a powerful reanalysis of 18 sleep-inducing studies in the mid-1990s demonstrated that psychotherapy clients who appropriately self-trance lost twice as much weight as compared to the individuals who didn't (and held it off in one research two years after the part of the bargain) unless if you or somebody you know has joyfully been constrained by entrancing to buy a crisp, littler closet, it might be hard to believe that this psyche over-body procedure can enable you to take a few to get back some composure on eating.

- **Seeing is thinking absolutely.** So, investigate yourself. To gain proficiency with a portion of the priceless exercises that trance must instruct about weight reduction, you don't need to be spellbound. There are ten smaller than expected ideas that are pursued contain a portion of the eating regimen modifying recommendations that my gathering and individual hypnotherapy weight the executive's clients get.

- **The power is inside.** Trance specialists believe that you have all you should to be effective. You truly needn't bother with an alternate accident diet or the ongoing suppressant of hunger. Thinning, as you do when you ride a bike, is tied in with confiding in your innate abilities. You may not recall how terrifying it was the point at which you previously endeavored to ride a bike. However, you kept on rehearsing until you had the option to ride, consequently, with no idea or exertion. Getting more fit may appear past you moreover. However, it's just about finding your balance.

- **You see your conviction.** Individuals will, in general, do what they accept they can achieve. That is even valid for mesmerizing. Those fooled into deduction they could be entranced (for example, as the trance inducer proposed they would see red, he turned the switch on a disguised red bulb) demonstrated improved mesmerizing reaction. It is essential to hope to be made a difference. Give me a chance to propose you anticipate that your arrangement should work on weight reduction.

- **Highlight the positive.** Recommendations, for example, "Doughnuts will sicken you," negative or aversive, work for some time, however on the off chance that you need lasting change, you need to think emphatically. Specialists Herbert Spiegel and David Spiegel, a dad child hypnotherapy group, considered the most well-known valuable trancelike proposition. "I need my body to live in. I owe regard and security to my body." I elevate clients to create their very own energetic mantras. A 50-year-old mother who shed 50 pounds more rehashes day by day: "Superfluous nourishment is a weight on my body. I will shed what I needn't bother with."

- **It's going to come if you envision it.** Like competitors who are getting ready for the challenge, you are set up for a successful truth by picturing triumph. Envisioning a smart dieting day will enable you to envision the means expected to turn into a decent eater. Is it too difficult to even think about photographing? Locate a comfortable old photograph of yourself and recall what you did another way. Envision these schedules reviving. Or, on the other hand, picture acquiring direction from an older, more astute self later on in the wake of contacting her required weight.

- **Get rid of cravings.** Subliminal specialists utilize the intensity of emblematic symbolism on a standard premise, welcoming subjects to put sustenance desires on fleecy white mists or inflatables in sight-seeing and send them up, up, and away. On the off chance that you can direct off your eating routine from McDonald's brilliant curves, trance inducers comprehend that a counter-image can control you back. Welcome your psyche to flip through its picture Rolodex until you develop as an indication of yearnings throwing out. Push.

- **There are two preferred procedures over one.** A triumphant mix is entrancing and Cognitive Behavioral Treatment (CBT) with regards to getting more fit and holding it off, which patches up counterproductive thoughts and practices. Clients learning both lose twice as much weight without falling into the lose-a-few, recuperate-more trap of the health food nut. On the off chance that you've at any point kept up a sustenance journal, you've officially endeavored CBT. They monitor everything that experiences their lips for possibly 14 days before my clients learn mesmerizing. Each great trance inducer comprehends that raising cognizance is a principle move for the tyke towards suffering change.

- **Modify and then change.** The late pioneer of spellbinding, Milton Erickson, MD, focused on you. To change the lose-recuperation, the lose-recuperation example of one customer, Erickson recommended that she put on weight first before losing it—an intense sell today, except if you're Charlize Theron. Simpler to swallow: Modify your craving for high calories.

Shouldn't something be said about some solidified yogurt rather than 16 ounces of dessert?

- **Like it or not, it is the fittest for survival.** No proposal is sufficiently able to supersede the nature of survival. Similarly, as we like to believe, it's the fittest survival, despite everything we're modified for survival in case of starvation. A valid example: a private dietary mentor needed a proposal for her dependence on a sticky bear. The advisor attempted to clarify that her body felt that her life relied upon the chewy desserts and wouldn't surrender them until she got enough calories from progressively nutritious food. No, she demanded, all that she required was a proposition when she dropped out.
- **Practice makes perfect.** There are no washboard abs delivered by one Pilates class, and one spellbinding session can't shape your eating routine. Be that as it may, discreetly rehashing a useful suggestion 15 to 20 minutes daily can change your eating, especially when combined with moderate, regular breaths, the foundation of any program of social change.

CHAPTER 31:

The Virtual Gastric Band Program

The Virtual Gastric Band program is a Hypnosis strategy that reproduces the impacts, results, and advantages of a traditional gastric band or gastric bypass surgery. Initially created in Europe, the method requires no clinic remain or recovery period to acquire the ideal weight loss results. All change is designed, made, and actualized in the oblivious personality of the customer.

This healthy and regular choice of weight loss surgery has a 95% achievement rate. Analysts broadly perceive hypnosis as an extremely protected, consistent, and charming condition of profound physical and enthusiastic unwinding. The Virtual Band Hypnosis recommendations cause the oblivious personality to accept the stomach is a lot littler, the size of a golf ball, as though the gastric band was introduced precisely. It keeps the customer from over-eating and results in weight loss with a quantifiable decrease of muscle to fat and inches. However, there is no eating routine.

The motivation behind this hypnosis system is to assist individuals with eating littler bits and appreciate the solid changes they will naturally have the option to make, without hardship and consuming fewer calories. Most get-healthy plans include disposing of the nourishment's individuals cherish and can prompt disappointment because numerous individuals can't support an eating routine arrangement that makes them feel denied. At that point, they frequently eat more than they did before their "diet" disappointment and recover the weight. The focal point of the Virtual Gastric Band Hypnosis program isn't explicitly on what number of pounds are lost yet instead on dress size decrease, the capacity to eat limited quantities of nourishment, and perceiving when one has had enough to eat, feel fulfilled and quit eating. The typical result is that by eating limited nourishment quantities and halting when full, weight loss and littler apparel sizes will generally happen. Logically, it isn't easy to eat far less nourishment and not get thinner and apparel sizes.

Study Result

In mid-March and early April, two preliminaries started utilizing the Virtual Gastric Band program. One investigation bunch had five members, and the other had three members. The program comprised of 4 hypnosis sessions, one every week for one month. Every individual was given the necessary "Golden Rules of Success" to track with specific Hypnotic proposals to diminish partition sizes, drink a lot of water just as inspiration to practice all the more frequently. All were told to tune in to an extraordinary pre-recorded hypnosis CD in any event once day by day for 28 days to help the positive, enthusiastic, and physical changes wanted.

The goals of everything being equal and customers were to be and feel more beneficial, eat better, and decrease their garments' size. A few members had diabetes and, additionally, pre-diabetic. All members were female and extended in age from the mid-30s to the late-50s. Most ladies had small kids at home, yet all were working ladies with occupied lives. Their weight loss goals ran from at least 40 lbs. To more than 100 lbs.

Session 2 Results

Multi-week after the first Virtual Gastric Band Hypnosis "surgery" session, each member revealed numerous positive changes, including a few changes not identified with proper dieting or weight loss. All members detailed they were progressively loose, ate littler bits, drank more water, and saw their considerations, behavior, and feelings identified with nourishment and eating had changed significantly. The enthusiastic eating defined with every member or customer permanently halted by and large or was incredibly abridged. Most detailed, they perceived a "full inclination" and had the option to quit eating, usually. Some saw a deep-rooted propensity for eating immediately had changed. They ate all the more gradually and making the most of their nourishment more. One member acknowledged she never again wanted to eat ice-cream daily, which had been a propensity for a long time. Another took a large portion of her nourishment home from a café, which astonished her. Some detailed that they dozed better. One member, a pre-diabetic medical attendant with thyroid issues, never again wanted Chinese nourishment and turned out to be sick after eating a limited quantity of her preferred food, pasta. It was a reaction like many experiences after a traditional surgical gastric band procedure. She conventionally would have had a few bits; however, one part was a lot for her. Her coffee utilization was decreased from 5 cups to under 1 cup every day. She lost 6 lbs.

Furthermore, never again had overpowering desires for desserts or starches. Another member said she saw that "full signal" and now eats far less. Her garments fit her all the more serenely, and the fixation on nourishment is no more. Another saw that her preferred greasy, overwhelming nourishments didn't taste tantamount to they used to. She is presently happy with far less nourishment, drinks load of water, and sees positive changes in her reactions and musings toward food.

Session 3 Results

Now, members had been tuning in to their CD for about fourteen days. All members announced it was simpler to eat little parts, eat all the more restoratively, dispose of enthusiastic eating, drink more water, and feel progressively loose. One lady quit her 1+ pack of everyday smoking propensity and didn't encounter withdrawal or passionate eating. Another quit her half-year nicotine gum propensity. There had been no proposals for halting smoking or consummation nicotine reliance during the hypnosis procedures. One individual lost 8 lbs. Another lost 4 lbs. in 10 days, without consuming fewer calories. Another lost 2 lbs. in any case, her garments fit her so much better that she believes she may have lost one full dress size. Everybody felt more in charge and ready to quit eating when fulfilled.

All except one individual experienced weight loss or having their dress fit all the more approximately, yet she announced that she was looser and more joyful than she has been in quite a while.

Session 4 Results

One preliminary group had encountered their final hypnosis session of the Virtual Gastric Band Hypnosis program. Most members in that group had encountered their hypnosis session also. Around then, different members had encountered only 3 sessions and a few just 2 sessions. That implies members had been utilizing the program and altering their behavior for only 3 a month and a half.

Everybody saw enhancements in their dietary patterns and decisions. Most eat all the more gradually, eat littler bits, are increasingly loose, and have wiped out their enthusiastic eating. They feel definite and certain that the Virtual Gastric Band Hypnosis program has, at long last, permitted them to be in charge of their eating behavior.

The Virtual Gastric Band Hypnosis program helped every member and customer be in charge of their nourishment decisions and part size. Any individual who needs to eat more beneficial and shed pounds might be a contender for this new and specific Hypnosis program. When stoutness and the subsequent medical problems cost the American public and insurance companies millions, this might be a straightforward, unwinding, and fruitful approach to set aside money and lives without "going under the knife."

Virtual Gastric Band Hypnosis can be utilized by nearly any individual who wants to eat all the more restoratively to achieve weight loss goals in a characteristic and loosening way. It isn't essential to be a contender for the gastric band hypnosis program to use this entrancing methodology for change. The Virtual Band Hypnosis program is an amazing and regular approach to come back to a perfect load without surgery and deprivation.

CHAPTER 32:

Emotional vs. Physical Hunger

There is a significant contrast between emotional and physical hunger, which is by all accounts obscured by numerous individuals of us nowadays. Emotional hunger implies that you go to food to stay away from awkward feelings or to increase a pleasurable one. Regularly, it means that you eat how you feel and your body needs. Physical craving implies that you eat when your organization signs to you that you are eager. As a rule, when we are ravenous, we can quit eating when we are fulfilled, and before we are awkwardly full.

Usually, we can see instances of emotional hunger by understanding a portion of our sentiments.

- Is it true that you are eating for solace or out of dejection or trouble?
- Is it true that you are exhausted?
- Is it true that you are attempting to soothe restless or discouraged sentiments?
- Is it true that you are attempting to smother a hurting heart?

It might be challenging to decide whether we are eating because of our feelings. Notwithstanding, instances of physical yearning are substantially simpler to identify and depend on our sensations.

- Our stomach snarls, and we feel that empty sensation in our stomachs

- Your body feels powerless, or vitality appears to all of a sudden go down
- Glucose gets low, and you may start to feel precarious
- Sentiment of tipsiness

On the chance that you can figure out how to viably tune in to your body, you will everlastingly be liberated from being a captive to nourishment. Adaptable counting calories and knowing your signs for enthusiastic and physical yearning will make you feel more responsible for your eating and less subject to sustenance to support your temperaments or feelings. In the long run, you will most likely decide how eager or full you genuinely are. You can prepare yourself to quit eating before you are excessively full and to not go to sustenance when you are not ravenous. Check-in with yourself during your feast and acknowledge when you feel fulfilled, regardless of whether it implies not completing your dinner. Make sense of a part of the arrangement custom you can do to flag that you are done. Have a go at putting your napkin over your plate, pushing the plate away, or just state that you are done for all to hear.

A large number of us have battled with passionate eating and have learned how to break free from the cycle to make an upbeat and sound relationship around sustenance. Go through these tips to accompany your very own arrangement to enable you to distinguish the contrast among enthusiastic and physical yearning with the goal that you can get in shape, have more vitality, and create sound propensities around eating.

Bad Eating Habits

Everyone has unfortunate propensities, particularly with regards to eating. A few of us nibble relentlessly while we work. Others are inclined to swallowing a brew or three consistently, then smashing out on the sofa. Over a couple of us appreciate 12pm snacks generally scrumptious lousy nourishments like fallen angel's sustenance cake, cheddar, or salami cuts. Be that as it may, regardless of whether you're a by and significant stable person, odds are you unwittingly take part in propensities that are negative to your well-being and your build.

Bad eating patterns genuinely consume your well-being. They can make you fat, languid and by and large unfortunate. However, cutting them without any weaning period could be horrendous, in any event to your mind, so we'll investigate great options compared to probably the most well-known terrible dietary patterns. Pursue these proposals and change your negative behavior patterns into great ones.

Drinking natural product juice

When you were a child, your mother was continually guiding you to drink your juice. It's beneficial for you, isn't that so? Genuine, pure natural product juice has loads of nutrients, yet it also has a great deal of sugar, which is typically more sugar than the organic product it originated from. What's more, sugar vitality, when not utilized promptly in the body, is put away as fat. Drink a couple of natural product juice glasses, and you'll accumulate calories like a snowball gathers snow when it moves downslope.

Bad eating pattern solution: Eat the entire natural product

Eat the whole of organic products. A natural product is filling and has less sugar than organic product juice. Furthermore, it contains a more significant number of nutrients and supplements than pure syrup. It also contains fiber that will top you off and cause the sugar to gradually enter your circulatory system, which implies that your body will be less inclined to store it as fat. Whenever you need a glass of Tropicana, get an orange.

Enthusiastic snacking

You enthusiastically nibble on chips, wasabi rice wafers, and Cheetos while you work. The propensity may enable you to consume ventures, yet it likewise allows your body to store fat. Also, most tidbits are very salty and won't support your hypertension. Any way you see it, nibbling throughout the day is awful for you.

Wrong eating pattern solution: Manage your snacking

Try not to carry the entire pack to your work area. Instead, take a limited quantity of your bite and set the rest away. Or then again purchase single-sized packs, so you don't expend a major sack by eating thoughtlessly. Another tip is to monitor your nibbling. Each time you go after the sack, mark it down or make a solid, mental note. This will enable you to acknowledge precisely the amount you eat during the day. It tends to calm and may give the inspiration you have to decrease snacks radically. Likewise, it might break your three major dinners into five little ones, which will keep your digestion revved and enable you to feel full for the day and enable you to kick nibbling inside and out.

Break Free

Negative behavior patterns are difficult to break, mainly when they include sustenance. A couple of straightforward substitutions, be that as it may, can transform your unfortunate propensities into great ones. After some time, you're eating regimen will wind up lighter, more beneficial, and increasingly nutritious, and you'll feel and put your best self forward. So, kick those propensities; it'll be helpful for you.

Here are more, just in case:

Starving Yourself

Starvation often comes before and after binging. Skip breakfast, and your body has been "starving" for 12 to 18 hours, which makes you over-eat again and make your body store a significant part of the nourishment as fat, as it cannot consume it for vitality.

Binging

When nourishments are low in fiber and high in sugar or salt and somewhat hydrogenated Trans fats, the inclination is to over-devour. When eating five to six little suppers daily of high fibered crisp organic products, vegetables, entire grains, vegetables, seeds, and nuts, the outcome is consuming more calories and putting away less fat because your body's temperature is raised all the more now and again. Binging on refined prepared foods is most likely the best reason for obesity.

Sugar, White Flour, Caffeine, and straightforward starches

Sugar raises (glucose) levels, making your body produce insulin and change your metabolic rate. The individuals who eat a great deal of white flour and sugar items, stacked with empty calories, will store increasingly fat and have a harder time consuming it. Caffeine likewise raises the insulin levels, hindering the fat consuming procedure that begins toward the beginning of the day, and backs off for the day. Eating basic sugar starches late in the day advances fat stockpiling and glucose swings. Eating high fiber entire nourishments as a late-night bite can help keep up an enduring glucose level to give your body profound rest.

Not Drinking Enough Water

Water is critical for your synapses and each organ in your body (counting your skin) to work appropriately. For your body to consume fat, it needs eight glasses of unadulterated water day by day. Water not just fulfills your thirst; it diminishes craving and flushes out poisons. Fluids, for example, pop and espresso exhaust your waterway. Do drink your water. It makes your entire body feel better!

Absence of Exercise

Our bodies were made to move, so the less you crave for taking a walk, the better you will feel after taking a walk! Exercise expands our digestion to help consume the food we eat as vitality.

Not Knowing What You Eat

The vast majority don't consider the number of low fiber calories and how much awful fat they expand day by day, particularly on the chance that they frequently eat in eateries. Those overabundant calories get put away as fat.

Skipping Breakfast

You would argue to the ends of the earth that it's your stomach that reveals to you when you are full. By eating chewy foods in a casual way, you will be significantly less prone to indulge.

In case you are committing any of these Bad Eating Habits, tenderly and affectionately change to a more beneficial way of life. You will be happy you did.

CHAPTER 33:

The Disadvantages of Emotional Eating

Emotional eating mostly occurs when food becomes a person's go-to response to specific external or internal emotional cues. It tends to respond to stressful, difficult feelings by eating, even when you are not experiencing actual physical hunger. Rather than staying intact with their emotions and the discomfort that comes with these emotions, an emotional eater will run through a big bag of chips, several bars of chocolate, a large pizza, and a whole jar of ice cream to distract themselves from their emotional pain.

The foods that emotional eaters crave, often referred to as comfort foods, are characteristically high-calorie or high-carbohydrate foods with minimal nutritional value. Roughly 40% of people tend to have increased appetites when faced with stress, while about 40% eat less when they are stressed. 20% experience no change4at all in the amount of food they eat when exposed to stress; hence, you'll find that stress is associated with both weight loss and weight gain.

In situations of intense stress and emotions like sadness and boredom, emotional eaters usually believe with firm conviction. That food is the answer to all the problems they can face, and that it is a great way to relieve stress in that it gives them the energy that they need. This over-dependence on food gets typically to the point where it is not very healthy anymore.

Emotional eating is an issue that cuts through both genders. However, research studies have revealed that it is more common to women than men and that emotional eaters tend to incline more towards sweet, salty, fatty, and generally high-calorie content foods. Usually, these foods are not very healthy and should always be eaten in medium-sized portions and moderated. Emotional eaters especially over-indulge in these unhealthy foods and ten times out of ten it ends up affecting their health negatively.

Consequently, researchers have now accepted that positive emotions are part of emotional eating as negative emotions are. Eating in response to emotions can be very problematic and with plenty of shortcomings. Here are some of the more distressing immediate effects:

1. Intense Nausea

Since food binging, and more specifically, the feeling of the food in the stomach provides a short-term distraction to the emotions that they are trying to avoid, more often than not, emotional eaters eat up very quickly. As a direct result, they end up overeating. This causes them to experience stomach pains or nausea a little while later, and this can last for a day or two after the actual eating.

It is important to note that the initial problem causing them the stress is not solved; it's just misery piled up on more misery.

2. Feeling Guilty

Every once in a while, using food as a reward or as a pick-me-up, or as a means to celebrate is not necessarily a bad thing. After all, any psychologist or life coach will tell you that it is essential to celebrate the little wins in life; and if good food is your way of celebrating, then you can munch away because the Lord knows you deserve it.

However, when eating becomes your primary mechanism for coping with emotional stress, when your very first impulse whenever you are angry, stressed, upset, lonely, bored or exhausted is opening up the refrigerator, you will find yourself stuck in an unhealthy cycle where the real feeling and the root of the problem causing these feelings are never really addressed.

Furthermore, what's paradoxical with emotional eating is that after the emotional 'danger' has passed, and the emotional eater has stuffed their faces with all the comfort junk food they could find, they are usually filled with guilt and remorse for what they have done. In most cases, this guilt leads to lowering their self-esteem, and yet another emotional eating outburst.

3. Weight-Related Health Issues

I am sure you don't need me to tell you how the unchecked eating of foods with high calorie and carbohydrate content affects our bodies, but I will tell you all about it, just for good measure.

There is plenty of well-researched and well-documented evidence elaborating on the many negative health effects, both the short-term and long-term, of eating and overeating these unhealthy foods. Generally, the foods we crave during the emotional binging feats are high in salt, sugar, saturated fats, and everything else that is worthless to the body. Sure, there are some healthy fast foods, but even those still have pretty high sugar, salt, and trans-fat content.

High-carbohydrate foods increase the demand for insulin in the body, which, in turn, promotes even more hunger within a short period after eating. As a consequence, this causes one to eat more calories than necessary in their next meal, which FYI, is not cool: cause and effect.

Besides, consuming high levels of salt can have an immediate impact on the proper functioning of a person's blood vessels. And that's just in the short-term. In the long run, high salt consumption often increases blood pressure, making them more susceptible to strokes, kidney diseases, heart attacks, and other cardiovascular problems.

On the same severe and gloomy note, we got to talk a little about saturated or Trans fats. These are manufactured fats that are created during food processing, and they are commonly found in cookies, pastries, pizza dough, crackers, and fried pies. Do not be misinformed. There is NO amount of healthy saturated fat. Repetitive eating of foods that contain these fats decreases your HDL (good kind cholesterol) and increases your LDL (bad kind cholesterol) and to be frank, and you don't want to know what kind of peril this puts your heart into.

Diabetes, High Cholesterol, High Blood Pressure, Obesity, and Insulin resistance are but some of the irreversible health problems that can result from repetitive and unchecked emotional eating outbursts. I think we can all agree that it is not worth it to risk your health to hide your emotions.

CHAPTER 34:

Stopping Emotional Eating

Emotional eating occurs typically when your food becomes a tool that you use in responding to any internal or external emotional cues. It's normal for human beings to tend to react to any stressful situation and the difficult feelings that they have. Whenever you have stressful emotions, you tend to run after a bag of chips or bars of chocolate, a large pizza, or a jar of ice cream to distract yourself from that emotional pain. The foods that you crave at that moment are referred to as comfort food. Those foods contain a high calorie or high carbohydrate with no nutritional value.

Do you know that your appetite increases whenever you are stressed, and whenever you're stressed, you tend to make poor eating habits? Stress is associated with weight gain and weight loss. When you are under intense stress and intense emotions like boredom or sadness, you tend to cleave unto food. Now that's emotion napping, and it is the way that your body relieves itself of the stress and gets the energy that it needs to overcome its over-dependence on food. Usually, get you to the point whereby you don't eat healthy anymore.

Emotional eating is a chronic issue that affects every gender, both male and female, but research have shown that women are more prone to emotional eating than men. Emotional eaters tend to incline towards salty, sweet, fatty, and generally high-calorie foods. Usually, these foods are not healthy for the body, and even if you choose to eat them, you should only eat them with moderation. Emotional eating, especially indulging in unhealthy food, end up affecting your weight.

Emotional eating was defined as eating in response to intense emotional emotions. Many studies reveal that having a positive mood can reduce your food intake, so you need to start accepting that positive emotions are now part of emotional eating in the same way that negative emotions are part of emotional eating.

How to Stop Emotional Eating Using Meditation

You already know what to eat, and you already know what not to eat, and you already know what is right for your body and what is not suitable for your body. Even if you're not a nutritionist or a health coach or a fitness activist, you already know these things. But when you are alone, you tend to engage in emotional eating, and you successfully keep it to yourself and make sure that no one knows about it. It is just like you surrender your control for food to a food demon, and when that demon possesses you, you become angry, sad and stress at once and before you know what is happening, you have gone to your fridge, opened it and begin to consume whatever is there.

As strong as you, once this food demon has possessed you, it will convince you that food is the only way to get out of that emotional turmoil that you are facing. So, before you know what is happening, you are invading your refrigerator and consuming that jar of almond butter that you promised yourself not to consume. And just a few seconds that you open the jar of almond butter, you take the bottle, put it in your mouth, and close the door again. And you do it again and again and again, and before you know what is happening, you have leveled the jar up to halfway, and not a dent has been made on the initial in motion that you were eating over.

Now before you know it, if your consciousness catches up with you. You start to feel sad, guilt, and shame. The almond butter that you were eating didn't help you that much, not in the way that you wanted it to help you. So, if there is anything you need to realize, you now feel worse than you were one hour ago. And so, you make a promise that you won't repeat this again and that this is the last time that this will happen.

You promised yourself never to share an entrance with that almond butter again, but then you realize that this is what you have been doing to the gluten-free cookies, to that ice cream, and hot chocolate before now. If this is your behavior, then you'll be able to relate to this. Emotional eating is a healthy addition that you must stop. It is more of a habit and one not easy to control. So, there is hope for you if you are engaging in emotional eating today. You have to be able to have control by yourself and over your emotional eating. There are many strategies that you can use to combat that emotional eating, and one is meditation.

Now when it comes to emotional eating and weight management, it is essential to acknowledge the connection between our minds and our bodies. Today we live in a hectic and packed world that is weighing us down. However, mindful meditation can be a powerful tool to help you to be able to create a rational relationship with the food that you eat. One of the essential things about overcoming emotional eating is not to avoid the emotions, but rather to face them head-on and accept them the way they are and agree that they are a crucial part of your life.

If you want to stop emotional eating, then you need to be able to shift your beliefs and worthiness. You need to be able to create a means to cope with unhealthy situations. It is essential to note that meditation will not cure your emotional eating completely. Instead, it will help you to examine and rationalize all the underlining sensations that are leading to emotional eating in your life. For emotional eaters, the feeling of guilt, shame, and low self-esteem are widespread.

Frequently these negatives create judgment in their mind and triggers unhealthy eating patterns, and they end up feeling like an endless self-perpetuating loop. Meditation helps you to be able to develop a non-judgmental mindset about observing your reality. And that mindset will help with you and suppress your emotions negative feelings, without even trying to suppress them or comfort them with foods.

Develop the Mind and Body Connection

Meditation will help you to develop the mind and body connection. And once you're able to create that connection, you will be able to distinguish between emotional eating and physical hunger. Once you can differentiate between that, you'll recognize your cues for hunger and safety. You will instantly tell when your hunger is not related to physical hunger. Research indicates that medication will help to strengthen your prefrontal cortex, which is the part of the brain that helps you with will power. That part of the brain is the part of the brain that allows us to resist the urge is within us. Mindfulness will help the urges to eat even when they're not hungry.

By strengthening that prefrontal cortex, you'll be able to get comfortable at observing those impulses without acting on them. If you want to get rid of an unhealthy habit and start building new ones, you need to be able to work on your prefrontal cortex, and you can only do that with meditation. Once you start meditating, you will begin reaping the benefits. You will learn how to be able to live more in the present. You'll become more aware of your thinking patterns, and in no time, you will be able to become conscious of how you treat food. You'll be able to make the right choice when it comes to food.

CHAPTER 35:

Eliminate Cravings

Imagine a scenario in which you could disconnect from your desires, seclude them and send them away? Some weight reduction hypnotic systems assist you with doing this. For instance, you may be approached to imagine sending your yearnings state on a ship ceaselessly out to the ocean. Recommendations can likewise help you reframe your cravings, and figure out how to oversee them all the more adequately.

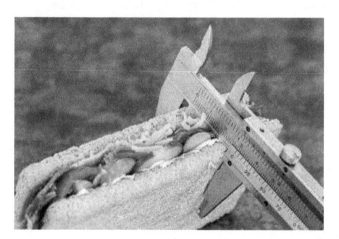

Weight Loss

The initial step of utilizing entrancing for weight reduction: Identifying why you aren't accomplishing your objectives. How does this work? Regularly, a subliminal specialist will ask you inquiries identified with your weight reduction, such as questions concerning your eating and exercise habits.

This information gathering recognizes what you may require help chipping away at. At that point, you'll be guided through acceptance, a procedure to loosen up the brain and body, and go into a condition of entrancing. While in entrancing, your psyche is exceptionally suggestible. You've shed your basic, conscious personality—and the subliminal specialist can talk straightforwardly to your unconscious thoughts.

In hypnosis, the hypnotherapist will furnish you with positive proposals, insistences and may request that you envision changes. You can attempt it right now with our many weight loss entrancing chronicles! Positive recommendations for weight loss entrancing may include:

- **Improving Confidence.** Positive proposals will engage your sentiments of certainty through empowering language.
- **You are picturing Success.** During hypnosis, you might be approached to imagine meeting your weight loss goals and envisioning how it causes you to feel.
- **You are reframing Your Inner Voice.** Entrancing can assist you with restraining an inward voice who "wouldn't like" to surrender unfortunate nourishments, and transform it into a partner in your weight reduction venture who's fast with positive recommendations and is progressively balanced.
- **You are tapping the Unconscious.** In the hypnotic state, you can start to distinguish the oblivious examples that lead to undesirable eating. You can turn out to be progressively mindful of why we are settling on undesirable nourishment decisions and bit control and build up increasingly careful procedures for settling on nourishment decisions.
- **They are fighting off Fear.** Hypnotic recommendations can assist you with subduing your dread of not making weight reduction progress. Fear is a No. 1 reason individuals may never begin in any case.

- **Distinguishing and Reframing Habit Patterns.** Once in hypnosis, you can inspect and investigate ways you use eating and "turn off" these automatic reactions. Through rehashed positive insistences, we can start to slow and eventually totally evacuate programmed, oblivious idea.
- **You are growing New Coping Mechanisms.** Through entrancing, you can build up increasingly stable approaches to adapt to pressure, feelings, and connections. For instance, you may be approached to picture an upsetting circumstance and afterward envision yourself reacting with a stable bite.
- **You are practicing Healthy Eating.** While entrancing, you might be approached to practice settling on the right dieting decisions, for example, approving taking nourishment home at a restaurant. It enables these sound decisions to turn out to be progressively programmed. The practice is additionally useful for controlling yearnings.
- **You are settling on Better Food Choices.** You may want and love undesirable nourishments. Hypnosis can assist you with beginning to build up a taste or inclination for more beneficial choices, just as impact the bit sizes you pick.
- **You are expanding Unconscious Indicators.** Through reiteration, you may have learned how to muffle the signs your body sends when you feel full. Hypnotherapy encourages you to become increasingly mindful of these pointers.

Changing Eating Habits

There are specific ways that we tend to consume our food. Some of these ways are not beneficial to us at all, and they create more harm to our bodies. Most times, we tend to ignore the time factor that eating requires. We barely look at the decisions that we make regarding food. All we do is to make decisions. Having an eating routine is essential. Nutritionists have advised us of the correct ways to consume our food.

One of them is that it is wrong to drink water immediately after a meal. First, you have to allow the food to settle, and after that, you should only drink water for some minutes. On the other hand, they advise that fruits should be consumed before meals for them to benefit your body rightfully. When you consume them together with your meals, they will not have the impact they would have if you had eaten them before your meal.

Most of these healthy facts are simple and easy to follow. It's just that we choose not to support them. Additionally, you tend to consume your foods in those moments that you should not be consuming it. For instance, you tend to eat a lot of food at night, and the only activity you will do is sleep. You will find out that much of the food that you eat is not well utilized in the body, and they tend to waste away. The result is that you end up gaining more weight due to the poor eating habits that you're making.

So, meditation will allow you to realize the impact of the decisions that you're making concerning food and help you to change how you make those decisions. You will recognize that you have some poor eating habits and you will decide to change them for the sake of your health and so that you will be in the right shape and weight.

What Are Good Eating Habits to Weight Loss

Do you struggle to eat well nourishment?

Do you attempt to imagine you appreciate eating soundly, however following two or three days, you truly miss your ordinary nourishments?

Do you think that it's hard to eat well nourishment reliably?

If you truly need to create smart dieting propensities, at that point, this straightforward standard hypnosis audio can support you.

Also, to our "stop comfort eating" title, this will change your whole demeanor towards nourishment. Dissimilar to the stop comfort eating collection where a ton of the attention is likewise on creating mental quality and self-discipline to oppose urges, this collection truly centers around this side of things more to assist you with developing good dieting propensities by re-wiring how you consider nourishment on a more profound subconscious level.

You will think about the negatives of eating an unfortunate eating routine. As opposed to seeing desserts, cheap food, or simply your preferred greasy nourishments as alluring, you will think about the negatives—the weight you will pick up, the negative well-being suggestions, and how low and self-basic you will feel after you have completed solace eating.

You will, likewise, usually think about the positives of proper dieting— how it will assist you with losing weight, improve your well-being, and how awesome and positive you will feel about yourself that you figured out how to defeat your solace eating inclinations! This straightforward change from negative to positive reasoning will profoundly affect your dietary patterns, and you will think that it's a lot simpler and considerably more characteristic to eat strongly.

You will turn out to be progressively predictable in your dietary patterns. You will stop "yo-yoing" between eating soundly, not all that strongly and pigging out. You will typically eat a significantly more adjusted, and sound eating routine, substantially more reliably.

Finally, smart dieting will quit being a struggle for you as you build up the sort of attitude shared by the individuals who eat steadily without contemplating it. This last change in mentality and convictions will transform you, decrease your waistline, and change how you consider nourishment until the end of time.

What to Expect

If you are new to hypnosis, at that point, you will locate this a wonderful encounter. You will turn out to be increasingly looser as you proceed to tune in. Relying upon your learning style, you could conceivably recollect all aspects of the experience; you will anyway consistently stir feeling revived and positive.

Short term

Over a short time, you will encounter genuine, substantial outcomes practically straight away. You will get yourself less powerless to enticements, and simply settling on better nourishment decisions usually. You will feel significantly more positive about yourself and your capacity to remain "on track" and create enduring, positive, smart dieting propensities.

Long Term

After some time, the hypnotic recommendations will construct and make perpetual, enduring changes to your examples of reasoning and conviction sets related to yourself, abstaining from excessive food intake, and nourishment. You will steadily get one of those individuals who eat strongly regularly. You won't fight or need to "be acceptable," you will generally eat a reasonable, sound eating regimen. In light of this, you will wind up shedding pounds, getting more advantageous and more advantageous, and capitalizing on life!

CHAPTER 36:

Enhance Your Motivation

Your journey is going to start with your motivation level. Many things are possible, but it feels like almost nothing is when you lack motivation. Getting out of bed morning after morning, trying to find the strength to make it through the day, can make it as hard as trying to climb a mountain on some days. Motivation can be found in many different things, but it will always come from our minds. What we're passionate about, the things that matter, motivates us to make it through the day.

The first thing you are going to want to do to motivate yourself is to change your attitude into a positive one. When we look at the world through a gray lens, we can easily see everything as terrible. When you hate one thing, that hate starts to grow and spread into other parts of your life. We can't look at life through rose-colored glasses either, because we don't want to make ourselves ignorant to reality. We have to look at the world, in our life, head-on, as it is objectively. When we can do this, it will be much easier to take on the new things that present to you every day.

Give yourself time to prepare to be motivated, too, not just to start the weight loss. First, you have to get in the right mindset. Then, you can prepare for your meal plan and exercise regimen before starting. If you try to force yourself into it, you might sometimes make it even harder to get started.

As humans, we like to be independent. Not everyone is interested in being told what to do, and we sometimes seek to be defiant in ways, even against ourselves. Sometimes in our heads, the things we're being told to do won't be our ideas and can instead simply be the pressures of society, our peers, and our parents. Their voices can still get so deep in our heads that we will mistake them for our own and easily get frustrated with what we're telling ourselves.

It can seem like an internal battle when you are trying to get motivated. There's the part of you that knows what you have to do, and then there's the voice that's telling you not to do it. To just sit around and wait for tomorrow. Motivation is all about silencing that voice and building one of encouragement.

Don't allow any regret into your life or the future. Regret can be such a wasted emotion. It is not. There is a psychological purpose for regret. It causes us to look back on our mistakes and question our motives for doing certain things. Regret can teach us how to be better in the future. However, too much regret can lead to a lot of time wasted. Some individuals will be so regretful over certain decisions that it consumes their entire life. If you want to move forward and be motivated, not just about weight loss but with everything in your life, you must learn how to let go of regret. Feeling it in the first place isn't wrong, but don't entertain it anymore. Think of it like someone that you pass at the grocery store, someone that you want to still is respectful towards even though you aren't very fond of him or her. Instead of talking to them and inviting them out to dinner, simply smile at them and keep walking. This is how we have to learn to process all feelings of regret, and emotions of guilt and shame as well. Simply let it passes, but do not allow it to stay past its welcome.

You are the person that you are right now because of the life that you've lived. It can be easy to think, "Oh, I should have done this," or "if only I had gone with the other option." However, if we hadn't made that one choice, then our lives would be incredibly different than what they are now. Each thing we've experienced, the decisions we've made, and the thoughts that we've had are all like ingredients that go into what makes us who we are. When you can learn to love yourself and the person that you've become, then it will be easier to build that motivation because you'll let that guilt and regret losing.

Look at what motivates you right now, at this very second. What's the first thing that comes to mind? Maybe it is wanting to make a loved one proud or providing for your child. Perhaps your motivation is getting your bills paid or merely making your next meal. Whatever it is, this can tell you a lot about what drives you in this life. When you become aware of all the motivating factors in your life, it will be a lot easier to use these images and ideas when you are struggling in certain situations. If nothing comes to mind at all, then it is time to do some soul searching. At the very least, wanting to make ourselves happy should be a motivator. Feeling good and looking better is all I need to motivate me on some days; however, others require a little more work.

Honestly, sometimes food was a motivator for me. I would tell myself that if I could avoid fast food all week and eat healthy Monday-Friday, that Saturday, I could go crazy. I told myself it didn't' matter if I wanted to drive myself through Taco Bell, Wendy's, and KFC all in one week. Whatever I decided for Saturday would be fine, as long as I stayed resilient against my Monday-Friday cravings. If I struggled on Wednesday and just wanted to skip the salad I brought to work and walk to the fast-food joint across the street, I would remind myself that I could get it on Saturday. When I would diet in the past, I would think that I had to cut all bad food out for the time being. It would drive me crazy! Eventually, I realized that I had to give myself looser restrictions and remind myself that it wouldn't be too long before I could have fast food again, which helped keep me motivated throughout the week, rather than always thinking about the food that I wanted.

What would end up happening was that I felt so good about myself for eating healthy all week that I wouldn't want to ruin my streak to keep up the diet. I would get to Saturday and think to myself that I had done so well all week, why ruin it now? I might still occasionally go out to dinner with my family on the weekends and get something that isn't great for me, but then this was a reward. I realized that motivation would breed more motivation. The easier it was for me to get started with the things I want and stay focused on my goals, the more this strengthened my willpower. There are always going to be hard days, but I remind myself that this is part of the process.

CHAPTER 37:

Great Techniques to Reach Your Ideal Weight

1. You jot down each move when you go through the techniques; it is essential. Get a pen and paper, and let's work through the techniques step by step.
2. Have you ever tried weight loss in the past? Did you succeed? That was the product of your preceding attempt to lose weight, now try to define what you've done. If you haven't been successful, be frank with yourself, and list the reasons that contributed to your failure.
3. Identify future weight loss plan's strengths, shortcomings, incentives, and risks. Twenty percent of your muscles will spur you on to your target weight, following the ideals of the 80/20 rules.
4. Set the expectations. Be sure how you plan to make your ideal weight come true. Your targets must be clear, observable, achievable, practical, and time-bound. Here's the contrast between what a good is and perhaps a wrong goal.
5. Write a plan of action for how you'll accomplish your goal—word of caution here. You need to get your action plan written down. You'll be failing without writing down your course of action.

Plan of action:

- Weigh myself and record weight in my diary before I launch my program for rapid weight loss.
- Weigh myself at 7 pm every Monday and record how much I weigh in the diary.
- Walk at least 1 mile in the neighborhood every evening between 5 pm and 6 pm.
- Drink 10 cups of water (100 MLS per glass) a day.
- Eat breakfast high in fiber content any day of the week.
- Listen to hypnotic audio message weight loss before I get off to bed.

6. Implement the Course of Action. Act and do the acts. You have to act, or you're never going to achieve your goal.
7. Read your written target and the action plan each morning when you wake, and then you go to bed in the evening. This will get you working on your plans. Create copies of the target and plan of action and put them all over the house to always remind you.
8. Take a look at your growth. Concentrate on your strengths, persevere, and remain consistent.
9. Visualize yourself to have weight loss.
10. Let's be optimistic. Never doubt your efforts to lose weight. Never seek to focus on your shortcomings.

Be bold in incorporating many weight-loss strategies in the action plan, like hypnosis and some others.

The Risk of Rapid Weight Loss

Most individuals who would like to lose weight wants to make it happen as soon as possible. After all, the same thing that helps us gain weight just does it due to eating pleasure. And weight loss is viewed as painful.

And the more quickly you can shed the extra weight, the better, right?

Incorrect. Quick weight loss is only one long-term failure recipe. If you have a strict low-calorie diet or have prolonged fasting, your body feels it is in danger. People led a life of festivity or famine in the earliest days of hunter-gatherers.

Typically, the body would go into a frustrating process in times of drought, holding on to fat until it could find another source of food.

An extreme diet will lead to weight loss since your body will begin to use fat reserves only after your food reserves are burned up. But that's going to slow this process fast.

The rapid weight loss is not only a fat loss. There is a lot of depletion of the gas. You get hydrated beneath, and your body changes even more. Dehydration generates significant health issues. Another major problem is the lack of muscle.

Muscle failure is challenging to recover from. Building only one kilo of muscle needs lots of exercises. But if you do a drastic weight-loss plan, you will lose it quickly.

When you start a deficient calorie diet, one example would be to lose 4 kilograms in a week. It may be two kilograms of fat, one kilogram of muscle, and one kilogram of air. You think this diet can't be managed, so you quit. You've put the four kilos back on within a few weeks.

But most likely it will be one kilo of oil and three kilograms of fat due to it's easy to put on fat ante tryout to put on muscle. You are now back at your old weight. And you've got more fat and less muscle. That means you'll have less capacity to burn fat.

You will lose some muscle with every subsequent weight-loss effort.

The secret to proper weight loss is to gradually and sustainably lose weight. Your body can comfortably cope with just half a kilo per week. Plus, you'll preserve your muscle mass if you do routine exercise. Also, make sure that you are adequately hydrated. This offers you the most excellent chance to achieve your perfect weight and hold it.

Over the years, due to stage hypnotists and media, hypnosis can help you lose weight Hypnosis has earned a bad reputation. It is time to change this as hypnosis is a compelling technique if you want to alter your personality. Knowing how to use hypnosis is the perfect way of preventing the use of it. If you've tried hypnosis of weight loss but refused to use this approach because of anxiety, don't let it deter you any longer. All that you heard about hypnosis is nothing but myths.

Most of these people would love to be smaller, but none would like to do some job. Typically, these are people who have tried many diets, and they can't lose weight or lose the weight they want for any reason.

Hypnosis is an advantageous method that helps people like you quickly and easily lose weight. Hypnosis is often associated with stigma due to confusion and misconceptions, but hypnosis is a hugely successful method of helping with weight loss.

Weight gain is mostly attributed to overeating and lack of physical activity. The issue is, the signs of the problem are these and not the cause. The cause is concealed underneath the surface, and virtually every diet only discusses the symptoms of the surface rather than the actual cause.

Emotional or behavioral problems typically caused unnecessary eating and lack of weight gain – causing activity. That may be an urge to hide from the world and not be heard, so you're gaining weight. It could be an urge in the past to punish yourself for any actual sin or imagine it. This might be almost anything, so it's going to be a source of emotional or emotion.

Although you can lose weight by dieting and through your exercise, it would be difficult to hold the weight off unless you also tackle the psychological issues that caused the weight loss initially.

The first misconception concerning hypnosis is that the methods are all alike. There could not be anything further from the facts. Authoritarian hypnosis, "You get sleepy," is what most people think about when they hear about this process. Very few people work with this kind. They are looking for a doctor who uses such approaches as clinical counseling and communication while you're attempting weight loss hypnosis. The oppressive hypnotist also scares away people by dictating what they will do. The behavioral hypnotizer, on the other hand, works for you. He is trying to understand better you're eating habits and how it affects your weight issue. The keys to this approach are motivation and positive reinforcement.

Hypnosis misconception number two centers around the subliminal messages. Subliminal messages are those you don't listen to. Among other stuff, they're potentially found in ads that you use. There has been a lot of discussion about this sort of post. In reality, at one point, people assumed that LP records contained subliminal messages, and they were afraid that many musicians would be listening to children. The subliminal messages do not work if you care and think about it. Only because you hear anything doesn't mean that you can act on it. Work is carrying this out. Subliminal messages aren't working.

The third myth relating to hypnosis is widespread. Many people think no tool will hypnotize them. This approach will support an incredibly large portion of the population. It is known that it is impossible to captivate even those with deficient intelligence or those with brain damage. Whether or not you can be hypnotized is more a hypnotist factor, not your hypnotizing capacity. To be successful, a hypnotist must be versatile.

Myth number four of hypnosis is that this is a weird practice that you encourage everyone to do to your brain and body. In reality, hypnosis is nothing more than using your normal dream state, the one often refers to as REM (rapid eye movement), intentionally. Sleep is a form of hypnosis you commit to every day. Hypnosis of weight loss works since it's normal.

The fifth myth relating to hypnosis is that you lose control of both the mind and body during the process. We've all seen television shows depicting a person clucking like a chicken while being hypnotized. Real hypnosis is nothing more than a calming condition where you are intensely concentrated. By trying to take your attention away from the specialist, you may stop the process. It could not be any simpler.

It is here that hypnosis comes into its own. Hypnosis helps to dig into the subconscious mind and address the problems that cause an increase of weight.

Hypnosis aid can be accessed in two ways.

Next, you should see a clinical hypnotist and also have one session on one. These are very successful but can be a little costly. You need to make sure that you locate a suitably trained and competent hypnotist. You won't usually need more than 5-8 sessions to lose weight permanently. If a hypnotist tells you to need more than that, then shop around a little bit more. The easiest way to find a successful clinical hypnotist is to give a personal recommendation.

The most rapid effect is provided by using both vocal and subliminal. The spoken form leads you through hypnosis sessions, which is best listened to when you will not be disturbed. The subliminal variant can usually be heard everywhere, as long as there are no binaural beats. When it has binaural beats, then relaxing ramps up and should not be heard when driving or running machinery.

All the rage among today's Hollywood stars is hypnosis for weight loss, and rightly so. Not only are they drop-dead magnificent and ideally physically fit to see spectacular and rapid results using this form, but by getting into the Hollywood secret on average every day, Joes like you and I lose pounds and inches quickly.

In a psychological research evaluation, it has been found that over 90% of participants who engaged in weight loss hypnosis trials lost significantly more weight than those who did not undergo any form of hypnotic therapy. The numbers speak for themselves, very quietly.

CHAPTER 38:

Weight Loss Exercise

There are two things you should do to drop weight, and among those, we've covered quite extensively at the moment, which is ideal for eating and filling your body with good, clean water. The other point you've got to do is make your body move.

You do not need to buy a subscription to a fitness center to get a workout. There are several things that you can regularly do that can help kick your body into losing weight, and you can do other routines to lose weight on your own.

Do not be discouraged when you start working out, whether in the house or at a gym, if you do not see results as soon as possible.

When you start exercising, if you push your body too hard, you can end up with injuries. There's no plan for your bones, joints, and tendons for the exertion you put on them. Don't assume that if you push yourself hard for a few exercises, you'll be shedding money; however, this method doesn't work for the body. Constant and slow wins the race when it comes to exercising.

Check your weight before you start exercising, just don't use it as a reference for understanding exactly how much weight you shed. Its weight varies all day long. You could end up being stopped only by scrutinizing your weight every day.

If you're slimming down, the best way to understand is by checking your garments' fitness. Another means to know if you're weight reduction is to start repositioning where you typically twist your belt.

When you inspect your weight and your clothing fit periodically, you're motivating yourself. Buy a some new running shoes or a brand-new pair of jeans on your own. This will certainly help to keep your motivation going as you pursue your goals of weight loss.

Take a day off from working out to allow your body to relax and repair. Your body needs a week-long day of rest.

Forfeit 30 minutes every day in the next days for the exercise because that will help you maintain your weight; however, you need a total of 4 days of 30-minute exercise to start losing weight, and five days a week is also much better.

Get the necessary work out details, and note the practices you can do from home. There is plenty of detailed research on a workout, so you can select what will most likely help you achieve your fat-burning goals. Choose or surf the website from your local bookstore or collect some publications about wellness and conditioning to find out more and burn the preferred variety of calories you try to shed every week.

Try to find a working-out friend. There would be someone who is just as committed to fitness and weight loss as you are. One of the advantages of having a dedicated partner is that you've got someone to give account to. You wouldn't want to disappoint your partner at the workout.

When your body is informing you, you've had enough, relax. If you've been working out for a considerable amount of time, you're sure to start getting signals from your body. It is particularly important when you are just getting started with your exercise routine.

Do so slowly if you want to increase the duration of your workouts. The same holds for your workout strength.

Pick an exercise regimen that suits your lifestyle. Everyone has different occupations and different lifestyles. There is no time to collect, which you need to find out or not. Decide which time suits you best. If you enjoy exercising late before going to bed, do it, or if you wish to apply early in the morning.

Stroll around, don't stand around. If you can walk around, then do it. Because they move regularly, people who are pacers do a lot of excellent themselves. Pacing helps you think as well.

Don't sit and stand if you can. When you can stand comfortably, you'll eat more calories in that way than if you'd sit. The TV and the couch are a loss to weight. If you are inclined to become a couch potato, do not lean upon it. Don't put such a comfortable chair in front of the TV so you won't be investing so much time in it. If you're a computer addict, the same applies to the computer.

If you work where most of the time you rest, stand up and stretch out every half hour or so. Most workers today are in front of a computer, so you need to relax instead of an elevator or escalator using the stairs. These are awesome conveniences, yet they are making us extremely careless. Taking the stairways may be faster than waiting on a lift to open up.

Smoking cigarettes doesn't add to your weight; however, it does lead to unpredictable consumption. Ten minutes of cardio a day is suitable for many people; you can accomplish this through different techniques other than running. If for physical reasons you can't run, then try a 15-minute fast walk to stay fit.

If you have time, you can walk around anywhere. Consider walking there or riding a bike if there is not much work or the grocery store away. It can take you longer, but at the same time, you're getting your exercise in.

Hide from the push-button control. Remotes are bad too when slimming down is involved. If you haven't had a remote, you might not turn on the TV, which suggests you might find much more energetic points to do.

If you take public transportation, get off a block, and walk the remaining distance before leaving. This is a great way to squeeze in a walk before and after work, or on the way to a different destination. Perform pelvic twists to match your stomach.

Indeed, you wouldn't do these with anyone else, but they're the right action to get your body ready for more big grinds from your tummy. It is also excellent on the muscle mass in the back and keeps your loosened rather than tight.

Suck in your tummy, walking. But do your utmost to preserve the tummy put in, walk correctly. You will soon begin to feel the tightening of those muscles.

Just how the diaphragm's breathing is performed correctly is amazing and can help relax the abdominal muscles. Most people use a shallow breath approach because it is, and oxygen is good for the brain.

Yoga-exercising trial. Yoga is a great way to reduce your weight and reduce your levels of stress and anxiety. Yoga exercise teaches you how to manage your muscle mass and get more muscle mass control.

Stamina training is burning more fat than the credit history people give it. When you work with muscle structure, they start shedding fat to sustain the development of muscle mass. Please realize that your choice will not be an exact tool in weight-loss determination when you gain muscle mass because muscle tissue is more than fat consideration—taking two of the staircases at once, instead of singly. This creates that you need to exert more on your own and increase your heart rate. Bring your beloved dog on a stroll because that might be a good workout for you both.

Undertake a dance lesson. This could be a ballroom dance where dances such as tango, fox, or salsa trot can be found. Such dances are fast-paced and will get you on the move. Even slow dance in the ballroom is a lot of workouts and will tone your legs. Or, you should take a lesson on aerobic dance. Do you recognize the number of Professional Dancers who are overweight?

Swim whenever possible. Swimming is a great way to get your cardio workout, and it's low to no effect on your joints, which is great for people who have bone weakening or joint problems.

Play tennis or basketball. Playing is a perfect way to get into shape. It's also extra fun working out in a competitive atmosphere with another person. Undoubtedly, you'll be more inspired to push yourself, and you'll lose more calories, but don't overdo it.

Always start your exercise with a 5-10-minute warm-up and end with a 5-10-minute cold. Your body needs to get to a certain amount of heart price before it reacts positively to the rest of the workout.

Don't lug your cell phone or wireless phone with you. If it calls, then go for it. There are numerous comforts in life, and we always have everything we need at our fingertips, yet for the midsection, this is certainly negative.

If your loaf, extend your legs a little by standing on your toes, and then gradually descend to your heals. Also, you should stretch your buttock muscle tissues, but maybe when no one else is looking.

Know what areas you need to work on and what areas are your perfect properties before going to bed, undress, and look at yourself before the mirror. Taking an inventory of yourself can keep you inspired in your workout ventures. Often, don't forget to follow up on any brand-new muscle tone you may have or on various other changes you've made.

Don't slouch around in your chair. Try to sit up straight and erect at any time. Slumping over is bad for the back and gives you a thin, limp body. Make it a point for both sitting and standing with an excellent pose.

Most people want to target their bellies and fully do away with that area. Unfortunately, we can't detect a decrease. A breathing exercise to help tighten those tummy muscles is one point that you can do.

Take the deep breath you can, and tuck your belly as far as you can at the same time. Hold it for a few secs, and weep slowly afterward. Don't let this out so fast that your stomach flops out.

This is not fantastic. Seek to take a similar breath every time you believe about it. It is ideal for some 50-60 times a day. This will allow you to lose a total of one inch within 20 days roughly.

Do not stop yourself from eating and working out properly by throwing on unfitting garments. Wearing the wrong clothes will make you turn up more meaningfully than you are. This often consists of fitness wear. When you put on clothes that fit, you can then go shopping for smaller clothing, and sell your little-used bigger clothes in a consignment store, or take them to Goodwill to be sold to a person who can use them.

CHAPTER 39:

Tips and Tricks

To achieve your weight-loss goals, you must be willing to let any fear and doubt you have about hypnotherapy. It is not something that you can second guess, particularly not its effectivity and results-driven orientation. It is a solution used for many different reasons, even other than weight loss. Hypnotherapy for weight loss can help you overcome a negative relationship with food, one that may have formed over a period or throughout your entire life. It is something that can present you with proper results and that you can always be sure of.

Although it is not a diet or weight loss supplement, it fulfills a similar supporting role and serves as the foundation for a more mindful lifestyle. Since the method thereof is focused on replacing old negative habits with new positive ones, it helps one to overcome challenges faced when trying to lose weight.

Whether you want to opt for a one-on-one weight loss for hypnotherapy session or listen to audiobooks online, both can serve you usefully.

Before you dive into the hypnotherapy world, you should know that there's a lot more to it than you may have initially thought. Much like Yoga and meditation, in general, it serves a higher purpose as it leads you on to a mindful path of physical, mental, and emotional wellness.

Tips for Hypnosis for Weight Loss

- **Find the right hypnotherapist for weight loss for you.** How would you go about doing this, you may ask? Instead of going the obvious route of searching for hypnotherapists online in your area, why not ask for recommendations instead? What's better than asking a friend, family member, or acquaintance to recommend you a good hypnotherapist for weight loss? If no one knows a hypnotherapist that is known for the outstanding jobs they perform, you may want to check with your doctor and ask for advice. They should be able to recommend a qualified and results-oriented hypnotherapist for weight loss. To ensure you have the right hypnotherapist once you've found one, be sure to check with yourself whether their consultation felt as though it was thorough, whether the hypnotherapy program was adjusted to meet your needs if there were any, and whether the practitioner was helpful and answered all of your questions. When hypnotherapists allow for space between sessions, it's also an indication that you're dealing with a good hypnotherapist.
- **Don't pay any attention to advertising.** We live in 2020, which means that everything we see online is taken seriously. However, it shouldn't be. People are oblivious and susceptible to accepting everything they read or hear, but not everything can be trusted when it comes to advertising. Advertising should, ever so often, be disregarded and not taken too seriously as it can be very misleading. It's always better to conduct your research before you accept that something is a sure way or not. In the case of hypnotherapy, since there are so many negative associations related to the practice, it's best to find out what's it all about yourself. As you can see from this useful set of information about hypnotherapy for weight loss, it is entirely safe and probably nothing negative that you expected it to be.

- **Get information about training, qualifications, and necessary experience.** Before you pick a hypnotherapist, you must be sure about their essential information first. Do they run their practice or operate independently? Are they certified and have a license? Ensuring that they also adhere to ethical standards, most preferably recommended by other medical physicians, you'll be assured that you are dealing with someone who knows what they are doing.
- **Before choosing one hypnotherapist, talk to several first.** Perhaps one of the best ways to determine whether a hypnotherapist is best suited for you is to speak with a few of them over a phone call first. This will take some effort, but it will be worth it in the end. You have to consider whether they can relate to you, care about your well-being, and listen to your concerns, whether they are personable, accommodating, and professional. If they tick all the boxes, then you're good to go.
- **Don't fall for any promises that may sound unrealistic.** If a hypnotist tells you that their therapy session will help you lose weight fast, don't even bother going to a single session. In reality, hypnosis for weight loss is a process that takes time. It can take anywhere between three weeks, up to three months to see your physical body change and lose weight. Since your body and mind should first adjust, you need to allow time to do so. Hypnosis for weight loss isn't a fad, nor is it a means of losing weight overnight. It's also essential to avoid hypnotherapists who suggest they will make you lose weight. Since they will only be talking during the session, what they're telling you is not true whatsoever. However, what you can expect from a professional and authentic hypnotherapist is a professional individual who takes responsibility for helping you get where you want to go. This person should help you access your subconscious mind with ease, and help you bring it on board with a proper weight loss plan and possibly an exercise routine.

- **Is your hypnotherapist of choice multi-skilled?** Although hypnosis is a terrific tool and can alter the mind's way of thinking about food, it goes hand-in-hand with nutrition. This is something you need to consider, mainly whether your hypnotist has a good understanding of what it takes to lose weight sustainably and healthily. Many people focused on starting a weight loss journey don't necessarily know what they should do or what they should eat. When looking for a hypnotherapist, look for a self-help coaching or some psychotherapy qualification, as well as a qualification/background in either nutrition or cognitive behavioral therapy.
- **Find out the time you should engage in a program.** This is quite important as hypnotherapy can become quite expensive if you're going to a professional for one-on-one sessions. If you prefer going to a professional rather than conducting the sessions at your home, you can choose to spread your sessions overtime to make it more affordable. Even though you may think that the sessions become less useful to achieve the overall effect, it works more effectively as your mind and body require time to adjust. Time is also needed as you change your old habits and replace them with new ones.
- **Ask your hypnotherapist if they can provide you with a program to maintain your progress at home.** A recording mainly helps to allow you to spread out sessions over time. Listening to your weight loss hypnosis recording will keep you in check and help you stay motivated and focused.
- **Ask your hypnotherapist, if he can tailor-make your hypnotherapy weight loss program for you.** If he agrees to it, you can expect a weight loss hypnotherapy program that is much more effective than individualized hypnosis. It offers treatments that may work better than ones that cater to everyone. Since every person tailor-make is different compared

to others, this makes a lot more sense. Sure, the general program will work, but a personalized one could offer you better results.

- **Ask whether your program includes an introduction session.** Starting with hypnotherapy for weight loss, you don't want to dive right into it. It's essential to take the necessary time, even if it's just an hour, to establish your needs and concerns regarding your current habits, lifestyle, and goals with your hypnotherapist. Ensuring that they care about your well-being and results instead of just taking you through the session is equally important. Taking the time to talk to your hypnotherapist and getting to know them better will help you feel more at ease and form a foundation of trust before starting with your hypnotherapy sessions.

- **Establish the costs involved before starting with your sessions.** Ensuring you know how much an initial consultation and each session costs will be another essential factor you must consider before choosing a hypnotherapist. Considering the cost, consider an overview of their program compared to other potential weight loss programs, review the cost solely based on the quality of service you'll receive, and take into account that you can spread your program over weeks instead of going to a few sessions a week.

- **Lastly, you should view hypnotherapy as an investment in yourself and well-being, rather than an unnecessary expense.** The context for this thought will realize once you engage in or complete your program.

CHAPTER 40:

The Final Weight Loss Puzzle

We can all be thin when we choose to, but most of us have been brain-washed with weight-loss companies and diets that we tend to ignore our bodies and instead follow medical establishments blindly. Our bodies are also wiser than the several varieties of diets in the market. However, with diverse information reporting to us how unhealthy foods will affect our weights, we have turned deaf ears on what the body is communicating.

The secret to becoming naturally thin is to follow four basic rules of life. The rules will guide you on when to eat, how to eat, what to eat, and how much you need to eat to avoid weight gain. These habits will not only enable you to eat whatever you crave but also ensure that you have the healthiest body.

1. Eat Only When You Are Hungry

When you choose to starve your body, you might begin to lose weight only for a short time. The body will react immediately by slowing down the metabolism process to ensure that enough fats are stored. This is usually aimed at allowing the body to survive for a longer period until it refeeds.

As soon as you begin eating, the boy will naturally store up all the food to prepare itself for the next starvation. This means that when you continuously eat after a starving period, all the food will be stored in the form of fats, thereby resulting in weight gain.

Also, some people may find themselves overeating once they move beyond a period of starvation. The body is usually hungry, and it is always difficult to control how much one eats, causing an influx in the number of calories that the body can contain. In such a case, you may find yourself gaining back all the weight you gained during starvation, but also end up gaining even more.

So, the bottom line is when you are hungry, you should EAT without hesitation.

2. Stop Eating When You Are Full

Another important step towards attaining a slim body is always to stop eating when you feel full.

One of the ways to know when you are full is to put your spoon or fork down between your bites. The automatic cycle of hand-to-mouth as people eat may cause overfeeding. Once you take a bite, give your spoon or fork rest to tune into your body's cues. You will be able to tell when you are full and satisfied.

An important tip to always stop eating when feeling full is turning off any distractions while eating. Studies have shown that people tend to eat 14 times more when they watch TV. This is associated with a lack of mindful eating that makes us unable to control our food intake.

3. Only Eat What You Crave

With the ongoing love-hate relationship we have with food, eating what you want, not what you think you should, sounds like an imaginary piece of cake. We often forget that eating is one of life's simplest pleasures. Deprivation of certain foods makes them all the more attractive to you. Eating what you want creates a balanced relationship with all foods. Most diabetics, when asked, what food they miss the most are those restricted by the doctors: salts, sugar (sweetened food), and white grubs. This is because their relationship with these foods created a tension that upset the balance. Listening to your body releases you from the guilt and anxiety that come from not following a strict dietary plan.

Enjoying food is essential because then you can listen to when you have had enough. Provided you are hungry, you are free to eat whatever you want and thoroughly enjoy it. Trust your gut because you are no longer what you eat but why you eat. The reasons you eat make a world of difference in informing your meal decisions, when to eat, what to eat, and when to stop. A few elements make food pleasurable: smell, taste, temperature, substance, presentation, and texture. When you crave for a cheesy, warm, savory meal, a crispy, cold salad will not do the trick. You will not receive the same satisfaction from it as much as you expected with the warm meal.

Denying yourself foods that you like often leads to over-eating when you get the chance to eat them and the foods you are currently "permitted" to eat. The reason for this is because you wind up looking for satisfaction elsewhere. The pleasure you expect to feel with certain foods is not easily substituted with different foods. Also, eating meals, you do not like would lead you to eat quickly to finish, which is not necessarily a responsible thing. Eating slowly helps you listen to when you become full.

When you enjoy your food, the following happens:

- You digest your food better. Your gastrointestinal system relaxes, releasing more digestive juices. When you eat something with guilt, your body is under stress, and that tension puts a strain on the digestive tract causing it to be that much slower and triggering gut issues like bloating.
- You will be satisfied with less.

- You absorb more nutrients. When you enjoy the food, absorption of nutrients takes effect mainly because the entire digestive tract is working at optimum capacity.

We are fully aware of our nutritional needs. Most people worry that if they always gave in to their cravings, they might never make healthy decisions. The contrary is true. Your body is always asking for different things at different times of the day and through the weeks. Any food that does not cause you pleasure should not form any part of your meal.

4. Eat Consciously and Enjoy Every Bite You Make

Eating consciously involves mindfulness with every food you buy, prepare, serve, and consume. Most people eat far too quickly to induce the feel-good hormone that is discharged with feelings of pleasure. Eating fast then makes you overlook the signs of satisfaction that your body is hinting at you, and you end up stretching out your stomach and putting on weight. The same pleasure you chased fleetingly disappears, and the guilt takes hold. To alleviate the guilt, you crave food, and the vicious cycle continues.

Mindfulness provides a balance between overeating and undereating while making you consciously aware of every bite and the sensations that accompany it. It is impossible to do something unless you know exactly what you are doing. That said, it is more important to feed your hunger than to feed your face. Unconsciously gulping down food like a barn animal brings about unwanted concerns of the physical, psychological, and emotional nature.

To reclaim your consciousness when eating:

- Start with your grocery shopping. Make sure you only purchase the foods you thoroughly enjoy.

- Exercise regular self-observation and be compassionate to yourself in case you catch yourself slipping.
- Allocate time to meals. Take about thirty minutes to an hour out of your day to sit down and enjoy your food.
- Avoid multitasking and distractions during meal times. Avoid eating in front of the fridge or the TV. Sit down with your food as the only thing in front of you and engage your senses.
- Always serve your meal on a plate or a bowl. Avoid eating from the packaging.
- Take small bites and chew thoroughly while engaged in every mouthful.

The focus would be to shift your mind from just thinking about food to taking yourself on an Epicurious journey. Eating consciously leads to emotional health, along with:

- Reducing stress on the body and the mind.
- Eating deliberately according to researchers, helps you reach your optimal weight by cutting the excessive eating.
- Healthy blood sugar levels.
- Improved relationship with food.

Exercising mindfulness in food as well as life generally leads you to do the right things properly.

Food is food. There is no "good" nor "bad" (unless it is inedible), and at this point, it fails to qualify as food. When we remove the stigma associated with food cravings, we become liberated and begin to fully enjoy our experience with food. Mindful eating might be new to Western culture, but it is a tried and tested technique in the Asian culture over a long period.

When our limiting inner dialogue on food no longer guides us, we can cultivate new thoughts based on our conscious eating- freed from the shackles of deprivation of certain types of food. Our approach to food and eating experiences becomes something to which we can look forward. Awareness with food gives a pause allowing us to consider our impulses and reactions from time-to-time. To unlock mindfulness eating, ask yourself how you relate to food and be frank with yourself. It is also noteworthy to note that not all people have the same dynamic relationship with food.

CHAPTER 41:

Hypnotherapy Techniques

Hypnotherapy is the use of hypnosis in patients who have discomfort or difficulties within their minds. Those using hypnotherapy claim patients experiencing a trance are much more likely to listen to the advice given to them. Some disorders hypnotherapy treats include pain, stress, obesity, fatigue, and amnesia. While many of these disorders are mental-related, certain physical illnesses may also be managed. Hypnotherapy is a procedure the Ancient Egyptians and Indians used to do. The activity in these cultures would also have a religious feel, and the activity included both music and dance.

Some claim the patient-therapist relationship can trigger problems. The patient may want to please the therapist, or they may think they don't like them. Many of these arguments, however, are contradictory since hypnotherapy usually happens in a medical facility. Several rising techniques are used in this procedure. Age regression is a key technique. The hypnotist will attempt to restore the patient to a previous state emotionally, and this is always done to help the patient recover what they've lost.

The second method used in hypnotherapy is called revivification. In this approach, the hypnotist can help patients recall their previous experiences. For example, the hypnotist will ask a patient if they've ever been fishing, and if they've been, they'll start remembering the time they've been fishing, and the hypnotist won't need to build a new state. Another common hypnotherapy approach is called directed imagery.

This approach can lead the patient through a pleasant experience. The hypnotist also repeats such ideas or principles to get the patient to embrace them, and this is called repetition.

Overall, people are more comfortable in a dream state. Research has shown that when a person can imagine what they want, they're far more likely to get it. In this case, the hypnotist aims to help the patient achieve the desired objective. Hypnotherapy is based on the word "Hypnos," and this was the Greek god of sleep. This method was mainly used to support people psychologically and was not widely known until the 19th century.

Hypnotherapy for Weight Loss

The subconscious mind has immense control over the actions of our bodies. And over our subconscious mind, we have great control. But are we sure of how to use it? Will we understand our minds enough to handle it correctly and take advantage of this advantage for us? We may ask someone to use it for us if we do not.

The conscious mind can drive an idea by repetitive thoughts into the subconscious mind. In a certain amount of time, the idea is set such that the subconscious mind pushes the body to act on the plan.

This is the basic concept on which this theory is based. A hypnosis specialist will also aid us if we cannot do this ourselves (fix an idea into the subconscious). Of course, it's much easier to say than to do.

Firstly, since weight loss hypnotherapy can sound like a good idea, but it can make the difference between success and failure to find the right therapist. Seek to get positive advice from close friends or experts in the area.

Secondly, because old habits die pretty hard, and you can only hope that you are close to the desired results after several weeks or even months of intensive treatment. Thirdly, that at the beginning of your new body, you will feel very nervous, and you will wake up to ideas "plants" inside your mind that get stronger and stronger. This could take some time to get used to.

In all of this, we can conclude that although weight-loss hypnotherapy can seem a pretty easy process before you go into the theory, there are a few things to consider. For one, I don't want anyone to worry about my subconscious mind.

Reasons Why Hypnotherapy for Weight Loss Works

For too many people, weight loss is the ultimate (and unattainable) target. Dozens of products are available on the fitness market-supplements, dietary plans, workout programs, and even "miracle" solutions. Most of these goods will not achieve the desired outcome since weight loss is a complex operation.

Hypnosis of weight loss is one viable alternative. In comparison to other eating plans and drugs, it provides a comprehensive solution. Hypnotherapy discusses the physiological causes of overweight persistence and thus produces positive outcomes.

Good Encouragement

All the limitations are traditional weight loss. You'll learn what foods to avoid, what bad habits to give up, and how to regularly track your progress. In these cases, constructive energy would be absent.

Hypnosis in weight loss focuses on the positive. It shifts underlying patterns of thought. Instead of thinking that burgers will make you fat, you will discover that carrots will improve your health and provide essential vitamins to your body.

Positive hypnotic advice teaches you how to love your body and enjoy good health. It is much easier to maintain the system if you are happy and positive about it.

Coping with Stress

Will you want to eat more any time you are tired, nervous, lonely, or depressed? If so, you're unhealthy with food and relying on the wrong mechanism of coping.

Hypnosis allows you to uncover the triggers for stress, anxiety, and even self-pity. These emotional factors overtake you and form your relationship with food. Auto-consciousness allows you to escape circumstances that make you feel bad. Furthermore, you learn how to cope without turning to food. A healthier coping strategy is always enough to lose weight and lead to a healthy lifestyle.

Benefits of Hypnotherapy for Weight Loss

The food industry is a billion-dollar industry and shows no sign of a slowdown. How many diets have you just tried to boom to the biscuit tin?? Who doesn't realize that less and more is the secret to weight loss? Certainly, we do not lack 'details.' So, why the battle? I will let you in the secret because when it comes to making permanent changes, your conscious mind (which is your willpower) is tight, your unconscious mind is here the real powerhouse. When you remember all of the above, and it has not changed yet, it's doubtful you'll change it either, so it might be time to try weight loss hypnotherapy.

- Emotional eating.
- Eat when you're not hungry.
- Compulsive eating (wondering why you are doing this but can't stop).
- The cycle of compulsion-guilt-punishment.

Your unconscious biases (which you don't know about, but are revealed during hypnotherapy for weight loss) motivate your food relationship. As youngsters, we may have been told "to finish everything on our plates," and these old messages can still be played. Or maybe we grew up with a mother who troubled her weight, or perhaps we saw food as "love," We comforted ourselves and "love" today when we felt weak, depressed, anxious, or lonely.

It's not about diets, it's about feelings, and how you 'use' food to change them, this is why weight loss hypnotherapy works so well for feelings and thought patterns. For women, food is also their choice of medicines.

It might well be time to dive and try hypnotherapy to lose weight for true independence and an improved, safe link to food and exercise for life.

Is Hypnotherapy the Answer for Weight Loss

For all the demands modern lives impose on individuals, weight loss can be challenging to achieve. It is no wonder that men, women, and even children are feeding on the road more and more. The standard Western diet known as S.A.D. is high in sugar, fat and simple carbohydrates, and chemical additives. This diet makes people obese and triggers a diabetes epidemic and other associated diseases. People are traveling less. The average citizen is busy and exhausted, but not enough physically.

Stress is a significant factor in poor lifestyle choices and can lead to bad habits. Individuals who have gained weight are mindful of what they are doing, but it is difficult to find encouragement if the burden keeps piling. We just want someone else to stay in their bodies (with a healthy diet and workout habits) for a little while to help push things in the right direction. Hypnosis will help here. The new person who resides inside his body may be them!

Hypnosis operates at a subconscious level by giving the subconscious mind clear suggestions. Good ideas to encourage weight loss, research at an unconscious level to build new attitudes, principles, and traditional thought so that consumers can make healthy decisions. Hypnosis helps a positive lifestyle transition leading to the reduction of body weight. It's so good, therefore. Diets have shown long-term ineffectiveness while modifying the diet and maintaining habits leads to positive results in weight loss.

Hypnosis strategies for weight loss typically include reinforcement of motivation and confidence building phrases as well as clear instructions for a healthy lifestyle. Hypnosis exercises often use visualization techniques to help the client "see" his target weight and "feel" what it looks like. This makes them successful. If a person can think he can lose weight, he can. Sadly, many people have attempted many diets and failed, losing their self-confidence and desire to take away their importance. Weight loss hypnosis focuses on how people feel when they lose weight, their willingness to do so, and adopting a new, healthier lifestyle.

Hypnosis deals with multiple individuals differently. Some people respond to suggestions very easily and adjust them consistently for a long time, resulting in faster weight loss. However, some take longer and longer sessions to retrain the subconscious mind and alter their perceptions about themselves, what they are willing to do, and what they want to do. To change their lifestyle successfully, people want to do it. Persons with hypnosis to lose weight will find that it offers several potential health benefits that are not specifically linked to weight loss. Hypnosis soothes the mind, nerves, and the entire body. It relieves anxiety and reduces tension. The recommendations include confidence and self-esteem that help every aspect of customer's lives. People who use hypnosis for a particular purpose also consider several unintended advantages. The gentleness of the approach also offers a healthy, supportive, and simple way to support a child or teenager with excessive weight.

Conclusion

Most people claim that weight loss hypnosis is a simple way to solve weight issues. People are also attracted by hypnosis because they feel they don't have to do any workouts, can eat whatever they want, and all they have to do is close their eyes and lose weight in minutes. That's just not true.

No magic pills are available to lose weight, be it by hypnosis or some other form of weight loss. It is not possible to lose weight immediately after only one hypnosis session. A well-trained and professional hypnotist takes many sessions to achieve the best possible outcomes.

Several websites on the Internet say that weight-loss hypnosis will produce dramatic results after just one session. Most people are likely to be insulted by this argument because everybody knows it is not possible to lose the weight overnight—no matter how successful the hypnotist is.

Practicing weight loss hypnosis was another method for those who want to shape their bodies as they wish. There are also men who don't like their own body image. This leads to loss of self-esteem and confidence. Some people prefer to use workouts and other lifestyle strategies to achieve their ideal body shape. Unfortunately, few tests are churning out. That is why people who understood the technique of mental strength resort to hypnosis to lose their body mass. You will find an absolute guide on how to use that method to attain the correct body shape on the internet. It is up to you to use your brain's strength to understand how useful it can be for you.

Hypnotizing is generally known to remove the inner self concentration. It generally happens in the same way as in a trance. Slimming hypnosis is an operation performed with the aid of the hypnotherapist. In this case, the person who wants to slightly repeat the messages given to him in the form of sentences, phrases, or even pictures may do so verbally. Mental images often play a major role in achieving the same result.

One thing you must remember is that your mind needs to concentrate more as you go through the hypnotizing process. In certain states, the mind and the subconscious state are very sensitive. You are well-positioned to react suggestively to the circumstances which lead you to your ideal body so that the best results can be obtained in a very short period of time. It is an activity that many people can do effectively with much less effort.

The research centers and interested stakeholders have performed many studies. Research has shown that people typically achieve fair outcomes using this form of hypnosis. This method can also lose up to an average of 2.7 kilograms.

Hypnosis, however, does not always function well on its own. You will take into account other behaviors that can effectively improve your weight loss. Take the best diet plan with your nutritionist's support. Not just this, you should do the workouts that will reduce your excess weight. In addition, you will try to follow a balanced lifestyle, which would help you in the end. Regulate your sleep hours, for example, and avoid any bad habits.

If you use this routine and use all the tricks, you get the best performance. Ultimately, you learn to regulate your mind to lose weight. You train your subconscious mind to decrease your body mass, and if you practice this cycle, it will happen.

CPSIA information can be obtained
at www.ICGtesting.com
Printed in the USA
LVHW052029210221
679514LV00001B/31